Focused Intensive Care Ultrasound

OXFORD CLINICAL IMAGING GUIDES

Published and forthcoming

Acute and Critical Care Echocardiography
Edited by Claire Colebourn and Jim Newton

Focused Intensive Care Ultrasound
Edited by Marcus Peck and Peter Macnaughton

Practical Perioperative Transoesophageal Echocardiography, Third edition
Edited by David Sidebotham, Alan Merry, Malcolm Legget, and Gavin Wright

Point of Care Ultrasound for Emergency Medicine and Resuscitation
Edited by Paul Atkinson, Bob Jarman, Tim Harris, Justin Bowra, and David Lewis

Focused Intensive Care Ultrasound

Edited by

Marcus Peck

Consultant in Anaesthesia and Intensive Care Medicine,
Frimley Park Hospital, Surrey, UK

Peter Macnaughton

Consultant in Intensive Care Medicine, Derriford Hospital, Plymouth UK

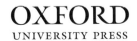

OXFORD
UNIVERSITY PRESS

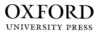

Great Clarendon Street, Oxford, OX2 6DP,
United Kingdom

Oxford University Press is a department of the University of Oxford.
It furthers the University's objective of excellence in research, scholarship,
and education by publishing worldwide. Oxford is a registered trade mark of
Oxford University Press in the UK and in certain other countries

Published in the United States of America by Oxford University Press
198 Madison Avenue, New York, NY 10016, United States of America

British Library Cataloguing in Publication Data

Data available

Library of Congress Control Number: 2018961647

ISBN 978–0–19–874908–0

Printed in Great Britain by
Bell & Bain Ltd., Glasgow

Foreword

The continuing expansion of the use of ultrasound in the care of critically ill patients, enhanced by the development of machines combining sophisticated technology with diminishing size, has brought with it the need for physician guidance in where and how to use it. In this book, editors Marcus Peck and Peter Macnaughton have brought together a cast of experienced and talented clinicians known for their expertise in ultrasound teaching in the realm of Intensive Care medicine to deliver such guidance. Importantly, their approach extends beyond teaching basic FoCUS to a broader perspective, extending into a problem-based approach covering advanced techniques, a role in performing selected procedures, and aspects of governance that are so important in attaining quality studies. The subject matter is covered in a comprehensive and readily readable format, accessible to both the novice and the seasoned user. Access to online motion clips, aligning with the text, is a great advantage.

This book is an excellent resource for any and every physician undertaking ultrasonography in the critically ill patient. It should be kept readily accessible at all times.

Anthony McLean
Professor and Head Intensive Care Medicine
Nepean Hospital, University of Sydney
Australia

Preface

Ultrasound has exploded into mainstream clinical practice worldwide, yet few existing texts deliver exactly what intensive care clinicians need to get started with it. Some are oversimplified, many lack any physiological background, and most are either too advanced, assuming too much basic knowledge, or focus too much on applications that are unrelated to intensive care practice.

As more and more clinicians take up this important skill from scratch, the need for a holistic text is clear. So we set about designing one.

We created this book in the knowledge that any new clinical skill must be learnt in the busy 'real world' of intensive care medicine, so we made sure that each chapter stays focused on exactly what readers need to know.

We aimed to cover all relevant aspects of focused ultrasound, cardiac and lung in particular, from their foundations right up to more advanced-level scanning, while making this threshold absolutely clear, where necessary, so that readers know when they are in borderline territory. This distinction sets this text apart from others and is designed to enable readers to progress as safely as possible.

We commissioned authors with a strong track record in ultrasound teaching and clinical care, and asked them to share their insights on both, which keeps the text rich and relevant throughout. The language used is simple and easy to read.

Knowing how to acquire and interpret ultrasound images correctly is important; understanding how to integrate this information into the clinical situation is paramount. To help readers recognize key pathologies and know when to intervene, every clinical chapter includes discussion of normal and abnormal physiology.

We have covered key anatomical areas of the body. However, we understand that patients do not present with discrete anatomical abnormalities, and so we have also included a section on how to use ultrasound to assess a patient with common problem-based scenarios, such as cardiac arrest, acute respiratory distress syndrome, and failure to wean from mechanical ventilation, to name just a few.

We also recognize that in intensive care medicine, the use of ultrasound goes beyond its diagnostic capability, and so we have included a section on procedural ultrasound with 'how to' guides for all common ultrasound-guided interventions.

We hope that we have produced a resource that you will find useful, either as someone new to ultrasound or someone with more experience who wants to progress your ultrasound skillset.

Contents

Abbreviations   xi

Contributors   xv

Practising beyond focused cardiac ultrasound   xvii

Digital media accompanying the book   xix

SECTION 1 ULTRASOUND-BASED

1. Focused ultrasound   3
2. Physics of ultrasound   9
3. Image optimization   17
4. Artefacts   25

SECTION 2 STRUCTURE-BASED

5. Transthoracic echocardiography, sonoanatomy, and standard views   35
6. Transoesophageal echocardiography, sonoanatomy, and standard views   47
7. Left ventricular assessment   55
8. Right ventricular assessment   69
9. Atrial assessment   81
10. Pericardial assessment   89
11. Aortic valve assessment   97
12. Mitral valve assessment   107
13. Intravascular volume and cardiac output assessment   117
14. Lung ultrasound, sonoanatomy, and standard views   125
15. Pleural assessment   133
16. Lung assessment   141
17. Aortic assessment   151
18. Vascular assessment   161
19. Abdominal assessment   169

Contents

SECTION 3 **PROBLEM-BASED**

20. Haemodynamic instability — 179
21. Cardiac arrest — 185
22. Dyspnoea and hypoxaemia — 193
23. Failure to wean from mechanical ventilation — 199
24. Trauma — 205
25. Advanced echocardiography: sepsis — 211
26. Acute kidney injury — 217
27. Acute respiratory distress syndrome — 225

SECTION 4 **PROCEDURE-BASED**

28. Vascular access — 237
29. Percutaneous tracheostomy — 245
30. Pleural drainage — 251
31. Pericardial drainage — 257
32. Paracentesis — 261
33. Lumbar puncture — 267

SECTION 5 **GOVERNANCE-BASED**

34. Governance in point-of-care ultrasound — 273

Index — 279

Abbreviations

A2C	apical two-chamber (view)
A3C	apical three-chamber (view)
A4C	apical four-chamber (view)
A5C	apical five-chamber (view)
ACP	acute cor pulmonale
ACS	acute coronary syndrome
AF	atrial fibrillation
AKI	acute kidney injury
ALS	advanced life support
AMVL	anterior mitral valve leaflet
AR	aortic regurgitation
ARDS	acute respiratory distress syndrome
AS	aortic stenosis
Asc Ao	ascending aorta
ASD	atrial septal defect
ASE	American Society of Echocardiography
ATP	adenosine triphosphate
AUROC	area under the curve of the receiver operating characteristic
AV	aortic valve
BLUE	Bedside Lung Ultrasound in Emergency (protocol)
BSA	body surface area
BTS	British Thoracic Society
CBD	common bile duct
CC	cricoid cartilage
CCA	common carotid artery
CFA	common femoral artery
CICV	can't intubate, can't ventilate
CKD	chronic kidney disease
cm	centimetre
cmH2O	centimetre of water
CPIS	Clinical Pulmonary Infection Score
CPO	cardiogenic pulmonary oedema
CPR	cardiopulmonary resuscitation
CSF	cerebrospinal fluid
CT	computed tomography
CTM	cricothyroid membrane
CUSIC	Core Ultrasound in Intensive Care
CVC	central venous catheter
CVP	central venous pressure
CW	continuous wave
Cx	circumflex artery
1D	one-dimensional
2D	two-dimensional
3D	three-dimensional

dB	decibel
DC	direct current
DD	diastolic dysfunction
DI	dimensionless index
DIVC	distensibility index of the inferior vena cava
dL	decilitre
DPL	diagnostic peritoneal lavage
DVT	deep venous thrombosis
ECG	electrocardiogram
ECMO	extracorporeal membrane oxygenation
EDA	end-diastolic area
EDV	end-diastolic volume
EF	ejection fraction
EM	emergency medicine
EMG	electromyography
EPSS	E-point to septal separation
ESA	end-systolic area
ESV	end-systolic volume
FAC	fractional area change
FAST	Focused Assessment with Sonography for Trauma
FICE	Focused Intensive Care Echo
FoCUS	focused cardiac ultrasound
FS	fractional shortening
g	gram
G	gauge
HCM	hypertrophic cardiomyopathy
HFpEF	heart failure with preserved ejection fraction
HFrEF	heart failure with reduced ejection fraction
Hz	hertz
IAS	inter-atrial septum
ICS	Intensive Care Society
ICU	intensive care unit
IHD	ischaemic heart disease
IJV	internal jugular vein
iNO	inhaled nitric oxide
INR	international normalized ratio
IPPV	intermittent positive-pressure ventilation
IU	international unit
IVC	inferior vena cava
IVCDI	inferior vena cava distensibility index
IVS	interventricular septum
IVSd	interventricular septum dimension
J	joule

kg	kilogram
kHz	kilohertz
LA	left atrium
LAA	left atrial appendage
LAP	left atrial pressure
LBBB	left bundle branch block
LDH	lactate dehydrogenase
LFT	liver function test
LP	lumbar puncture
LSV	long saphenous vein
LUS	lung ultrasound
LV	left ventricle
LVEDA	left ventricular end-diastolic area
LVEDD	left ventricular end-diastolic diameter
LVEDP	left ventricular end-diastolic pressure
LVEF	left ventricular ejection fraction
LVESA	left ventricular end-systolic area
LVH	left ventricular hypertrophy
LVIDd	left ventricular internal dimension in diastole
LVIDs	left ventricular internal dimension in systole
LVOT	left ventricular outflow tract
LVPWd	left ventricular posterior wall dimension
LVSD	left ventricular systolic dysfunction
m	metre
MAPSE	mitral annular plane systolic excursion
MHz	megahertz
M-mode	motion-mode
mmol	millimole
MR	mitral regurgitation
MRI	magnetic resonance imaging
ms	millisecond
MS	mitral stenosis
MV	mitral valve
MVO	mitral valve obstruction
MVR	mitral valve replacement
NAP4	fourth National Audit Project of the Royal College of Anaesthetists
NCEPOD	National Confidential Enquiry into Patient Outcome and Death
NICE	National Institute for Health and Care Excellence
PAA	proximal ascending aorta
PAOP	pulmonary arterial opening pressure; pulmonary artery occlusion pressure
PAP	pulmonary arterial pressure
PASP	pulmonary arterial systolic pressure
PAT	pulmonary acceleration time
PCI	percutaneous coronary intervention
PCR	polymerase chain reaction
PD	pulse duration
PDA	posterior descending artery
PDT	percutaneous dilatational tracheostomy
PE	pulmonary embolus
PEA	pulseless electrical activity
PEEP	positive end-expiratory pressure
PFO	patent foramen ovale
PHT	pulmonary hypertension
PICC	peripherally inserted central catheter
PISA	proximal isovelocity surface area
PLAPS	postero-lateral alveolar/pleural syndrome
PLAX	parasternal long-axis
PLR	passive leg raising
PM	papillary muscle
PMVL	posterior mitral valve leaflet
POCUS	point-of-care ultrasound
PPV	positive pressure ventilation
PRF	pulse repetition frequency
PSAX	parasternal short-axis
PW	pulsed wave
RAP	right atrial pressure
RCA	right coronary artery
RI	resistive index
RV	right ventricle
RVEDA	right ventricular end-diastolic area
RVEF	right ventricular ejection fraction
RVH	right ventricular hypertrophy
RVI	right ventricular inflow (view)
RVO	right ventricular outflow (view)
RVOT	right ventricular outflow tract
RVSP	right ventricular systolic pressure
RWMA	regional wall motion abnormality
s	second
S4C	subcostal four-chamber (view)
SAAG	serum-ascites albumin gradient
SAM	systolic anterior motion
SAX	short-axis (view)
SBT	spontaneous breathing trial
SCV	subclavian vein
SEC	spontaneous echo contrast
SFA	superficial femoral artery
SIRS	systemic inflammatory response syndrome
SIVC	subcostal inferior vena caval (view)
SPL	spatial pulse length
SPT	suprasternal
SS	suprasternal (view)
SSAX	subcostal short-axis (view)
STj	sinotubular junction
SV	stroke volume
SVC	superior vena cava

SVI	stroke volume index	TT	tracheostomy tube
SVV	stroke volume variation	TTE	transthoracic echocardiography
TAPSE	tricuspid annular plane systolic excursion	TV	tricuspid valve
TC	thyroid cartilage	UK	United Kingdom
tdi	thickness of diaphragm	US	ultrasound
TDI	tissue Doppler imaging	USGVA	ultrasound-guided vascular access
TGC	time gain compensation	VAP	ventilator-associated pneumonia
THI	tissue harmonic imaging	VATS	video-assisted thoracoscopic surgery
TOE	transoesophageal echocardiography	VC	vena contracta
TPN	total parenteral nutrition	VF	ventricular fibrillation
TR	tricuspid regurgitation	VSD	ventricular septal defect
TRV	peak velocity of tricuspid regurgitation jet	VTI	volume–time integral; velocity–time integral

Contributors

Shirjel Alam, Registrar in Cardiology, Royal Infirmary of Edinburgh, Edinburgh, UK

David Ashton-Cleary, Consultant in Intensive Care and Anaesthesia, Royal Cornwall Hospital, Truro, UK

Russell Barber, Consultant in Anaesthesia and Intensive Care, Lincoln County Hospital, Lincoln, UK

Colin Bigham, Consultant in Intensive Care and Anaesthesia, Derriford Hospital, Plymouth, UK

Andrew R Bodenham, Consultant in Anaesthesia and Intensive Care, Leeds General Infirmary, Leeds, UK

Stefanie Bruemmer-Smith, Consultant in Occupational Health and Health Management, BAD GmbH, Zentrum Potsdam, Berlin, Germany (previously Consultant in Intensive Care Medicine, Brighton and Sussex University Hospital Trust, UK)

Thomas Clark, Consultant in Anaesthesia and Intensive Care, Torbay Hospital, Torquay, UK

Andrew Constantine, Registrar in Cardiology, North West Thames Deanery, London, UK

Carlos Corredor, Consultant in Cardiothoracic Anaesthesia and Intensive Care, Barts Heart Centre, London, UK

Paul Diprose, Consultant in Cardiac Anaesthesia and Intensive Care, University Hospital Southampton, Southampton, UK

James Doyle, Consultant in Intensive Care, Royal Surrey County Hospital, Guildford, UK

Nick Fletcher, Consultant in Cardiac Anaesthesia and Intensive Care, St George's Hospital, London, UK

Michael Gillies, Consultant in Intensive Care, Royal Infirmary of Edinburgh, Edinburgh, UK

Lewis Gray, Consultant in Intensive Care and Anaesthesia, Royal Victoria Infirmary, Newcastle, UK

Tim Harris, Professor of Emergency Medicine, QMUL and Barts Health NHS Trust, London, UK

Alex Harrison, Consultant in Intensive Care and Nephrology, Royal Sussex County Hospital, Brighton, UK

David Hendron, Consultant in Anaesthesia and Intensive Care, Ulster Hospital, Belfast, UK

Nicholas Ioannou, Consultant in Intensive care, Anaesthesia, and ECMO, Guy's and St Thomas' NHS Foundation Trust, London, UK

Gajen Sunthar Kanaganayagam, Consultant Cardiologist, Imperial College Healthcare NHS Trust and Chelsea and Westminster NHS Trust, London, UK

Justin Kirk-Bayley, Consultant in Intensive Care and Anaesthesia, Royal Surrey County Hospital, Guildford, UK

Ahmed Labib, Consultant in ECMO, Intensive Care and Anaesthesia, Hamad General Hospital, Doha, Qatar

Peter Macnaughton, Consultant in Intensive Care, Derriford Hospital, Plymouth, UK

Paul Margetts, Consultant in Intensive Care and Anaesthesia, Derriford Hospital, Pymouth, UK

Ashley Miller, Consultant in Intensive Care and Anaesthesia, Royal Shrewsbury Hospital, Shrewsbury, UK

Craig Morris, Consultant in Anaesthesia and Intensive Care, Royal Derby Hospital, Derby, UK

Prashant Parulekar, Consultant in intensive care, acute and general medicine, William Harvey Hospital, Ashford, UK

Marcus Peck, Consultant in Anaesthesia and Intensive Care, Frimley Park Hospital, Frimley, UK

Susanna Price, Consultant in Intensive Care and Cardiology, Royal Brompton Hospital, London, UK

Benjamin Reddi, Consultant in Intensive Care, Royal Adelaide Hospital, Adelaide, Australia

Conn Russell, Consultant in Anaesthesia and Intensive Care, Ulster Hospital, Belfast, UK

Michaela Scheuermann-Freestone, Consultant Cardiologist, Hampshire Hospitals NHS Foundation Trust, Basingstoke, UK

Jennie Stephens, Consultant in Acute and Intensive Care Medicine, Royal Cornwall Hospital, Truro, UK

Guido Tavazzi, Consultant in Anaesthesia, Intensive Care, and Pain Medicine, Fondazione IRCCS Policlinico San Matteo, University of Pavia, Pavia, Italy

Kelly Victor, Senior Cardiac Physiologist, Guy's and St Thomas' NHS Foundation Trust, London, UK

Andrew Walden, Consultant in Intensive Care and Respiratory Medicine, Royal Berkshire Hospital, Reading, UK

Practising beyond focused cardiac ultrasound

Echocardiography has a shallower learning curve than other applications of ultrasound. It takes time to become competent in focused cardiac ultrasound (FoCUS), and considerably longer to master advanced echocardiographic applications. Consequently, the knowledge and skill gaps between FoCUS and comprehensive echocardiography are is large. So how should these be overcome?

Firstly, consider your goals. A comprehensive examination will usually be the investigation of choice, so whenever possible leave the experts to be experts and refer for a definitive opinion. When a more limited study is appropriate, know the limits of ultrasound and your ability to use it.

Stay within your competence. Focusing on identifying acute, severe pathology, and resisting the urge to grade less severe pathology, will minimize your risk of over- and under-reporting and the potential for causing harm. And whenever you see significant pathology or something that you are not sure about, refer for comprehensive echocardiography.

Stay involved. Learning a new skill is one thing; keeping it is another. Disuse atrophy is a real problem in ultrasound, at all levels, and the best way to avoid this is to keep scanning actively. Another is teaching.

Stay supervised. This is the key to safe practice, and the more contact you have with comprehensive echo providers, the better. Keep a logbook, share your interesting cases, and, if possible, attend your institution's echo meetings. While we may practise as self-regulating practitioners, being part of a community makes us better at what we do. The support you receive from experts will enable you to progress safely.

Stay learning. Continuing your professional development is an expected part of modern healthcare provision. Deepening or broadening your interest in ultrasound will bring you, and your patients, great rewards. We embrace this ideal in this book.

What defines expertise and the threshold between basic and advanced echocardiography remains open to debate and may vary geographically. However, it is widely understood that spectral Doppler represents a technical boundary, certainly for the purposes of this book.

To help guide you beyond FoCUS, this book introduces 'next step' concepts, in an advanced section at the end of every echocardiography chapter, while highlighting the potential pitfalls involved. If you are interested in practicing these clinically, please make sure that you have good local supervision and the governance infrastructure around you, to do so as safely as possible.

Digital media accompanying the book

Individual purchasers of this book are entitled to **free** personal access to accompanying digital media in the online edition. Please refer to the access token card for instructions on token redemption and access.

The corresponding media can be found on *Oxford Medicine Online* at: www.oxfordmedicine.com/focusedicu

Videos

There are over 70 videos of transthoracic echocardiography and ultrasound (see example below). These show assessment of aspects of organ structure and function, common problems, and procedures, with specific reference to critical care patients. Cases demonstrate the views you can expect to see and how to interpret these to inform management, interventions. and hopefully outcome.

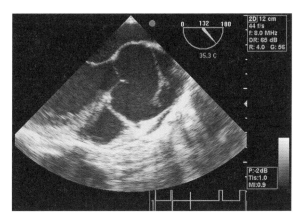

Throughout the book, videos are noted with this symbol, so you can easily find the corresponding material online: 📹 Video

Multiple choice questions

Sixty self-assessment questions, arranged into an interactive online test, help you retain what you have read and revise for exams. This symbol is noted at the end of each chapter to remind you to test your knowledge online: ✅ Test

Share this resource

If you are interested in access to the complete online edition, please consult with your librarian.

SECTION 1

Ultrasound-based

Focused ultrasound

Marcus Peck and Peter MacNaughton

Introduction

The development of focused ultrasound (US) has been rapid due to the combination of push by the proliferation of affordable technology and pull from interested frontline clinicians, keen to use it in their own setting. Despite initial concerns from traditional users about its validity and safety, focused US has been widely recognized by relevant professional organizations in Europe, North America, and Australasia. What was once regarded with scepticism is now becoming embedded into everyday clinical practice, limited only by each health system's capacity to deliver training and governance.

This chapter will define focused US, outline its scope, and explain why it is so important in contemporary intensive care practice.

Development

'Real-time' US technology was first developed in the mid 1960s, with the advent of fast B-mode technology, produced by the German company Siemens. Japanese technology companies led its commercial promulgation in the 1970s, and by the early 1980s, there were over 45 manufacturing centres worldwide. Improving image quality and portability encouraged widespread uptake of US into mainstream clinical practice, and machines began to decentralize from radiology departments into clinics run by other specialties such as cardiology and obstetrics. In the 1990s, rapid development of the telecommunication and personal electronics markets enabled US technology to take huge leaps forward,

with increasing miniaturization and affordability, to produce the kind of point-of-care machines that we are familiar with today.

Emergency medicine (EM) was the first specialty outside the aforementioned to utilize focused US at the bedside. During the early 1990s, numerous position statements from EM's professional organizations called for clinical uptake and research in the area, and scanning for abdominal free fluid in trauma (now known worldwide as FAST) became widespread.

In the 2000s, multiple EM guidelines were developed, endorsing best practice in US training and delivery. Other specialties (including anaesthesia, surgery, and respiratory medicine) recognized the potential of US to improve patient safety, and US became a standard of care for procedures, such as central venous access and pleural drainage, that had been previously performed using surface landmark techniques.

Since 2010, focused US has exploded into mainstream clinical practice. EM and intensive care medicine have developed training programmes specific to their fields, and many useful protocols have been created to evaluate various anatomical areas (heart, lung, abdomen) and clinical settings (undifferentiated shock, trauma, cardiac arrest).

Since pioneering work in the 1980s, lung US (LUS) has emerged as an extremely useful imaging tool in the critically ill that, in experienced hands, can approach the accuracy of computed tomography (CT) scanning. LUS is becoming an increasingly used tool for the routine assessment of the patient with acute respiratory failure, with many professional bodies calling for it to become a standard of care and incorporated into the training programmes of those working in the intensive care unit (ICU). LUS has considerably more clinical utility and accuracy than the stethoscope, and it can be viewed as the twenty-first century replacement to this 200-year-old device.

Definition

This refers to the use of basic US techniques by non-experts as an extension of their clinical examination to dichotomously answer ('yes/no' or 'present/absent') questions designed to detect major, time-critical diagnoses that are relevant to their scope of practice and impact on immediate clinical management. In the critical care setting, such diagnoses are usually life-threatening and responsive to remedial interventions.

The goals of focused US are to gain better physiological understanding and reduce diagnostic uncertainty as early as possible.

Importantly, focused US can be performed rapidly in any clinical environment, without transferring the patient or relying on specialist input, which may not always be immediately available. Repeated study by the same observer enables them to monitor deterioration or evaluate clinical response to interventions, all in real time.

Focused US uses mainly two-dimensional (2D) imaging to 'eyeball' structures and detect the presence (or absence) of clinically relevant pathophysiology in a qualitative or semi-quantitative manner in patients with symptoms or abnormal signs.

Focused US contains very little measurement, which has the potential to introduce error, and no spectral Doppler, which requires considerable training for accurate use. Borderline areas, depending on perspective, include the use of M-mode and colour flow Doppler. This book will consider M-mode measurement to be within focused US, and all Doppler assessment (including colour flow) to be an advanced US technique.

A noteworthy distinction between focused US and traditional, comprehensive US is the degree to which the operator assimilates the patient's acute physiology and organ support into the diagnostic process.

Operators who understand critical illness are well placed to interpret US findings in clinical context, and this integrative approach is why focused US is potentially so effective.

It is fundamentally important that the operator refers to a specialist for comprehensive assessment if they detect pathology outside the scope of focused echo.

Terminology

Given that focused echo has such multi-specialty and international roots, it is no surprise that it is described in so many different ways. Literature abounds with references to 'bedside', 'handheld', and 'point-of-care' US, to name a few. As international practice has become increasingly joined up, two terms have prevailed.

'Point-of-care ultrasound' (POCUS) describes the use of focused US at the patient's bedside for diagnostic or therapeutic purposes, and it may encompass the heart, lungs, pleura, abdomen, or major vessels. POCUS describes a 'goal-directed' US examination that can be performed quickly at the bedside, using portable US equipment, to identify easily recognizable pathology. POCUS examinations should be seen as an extension of the clinical examination, as their results interpreted in conjunction with information from the history and rest of the clinical examination. This is in contrast to traditional comprehensive US examination that is usually undertaken by an imaging expert without such detailed information.

'Focused cardiac ultrasound' (FoCUS) is the term used to describe focused echocardiography, regardless of the operator, machine, or location. This term distinguishes it from 'comprehensive' echocardiography, which is a complete, systematic, quantitative examination performed by fully trained individuals, usually within the cardiology domain, with the knowledge and expertise to use all advanced echo modalities. It also distinguishes it from 'limited' echocardiography, which describes a study limited in its number of images (not scope), performed by experts with advanced echo techniques to answer specific questions that are beyond the scope of focused echo.

Training, competence, and accreditation

There is a diverse range of training programmes world-wide, each designed to meet local needs. Common threads include blended learning with online material, a hands-on course, mentored practice, a logbook of between 20 and 50 cases, depending on the field (e.g. abdominal, lung, cardiac, etc.), and some form of final triggered assessment.

In response to the increasing use of US examination by non-radiologists/ultrasonographers, the United Kingdom (UK) Royal College of Radiologists developed recommendations for training in 2005 and updated them in 2012. Of note, they accepted the potential benefit, and supported the role, of focused US examination to assess specific clinical questions undertaken by clinicians with limited training, compared to a specialist sonographer. They proposed three levels of US training that have since been incorporated into the guidance issued by many other professional bodies and organizations.

Level 1 represents the most basic level of training and should ensure that the practitioner can:

- Perform the examination safely and accurately
- Recognize and differentiate normal anatomy and pathology
- Diagnose common abnormalities
- Recognize when a second opinion (from a level 2- or level 3-trained practitioner) is required.

Level 2 training and practice equates to a much more experienced practitioner who should be able to recognize and diagnose almost all conditions within the relevant organ system (e.g. lung, abdomen). Level 2 practitioners would be involved with training and supporting level 1 practitioners.

Level 3 is advanced US practice, representing a clinician with a specialist interest who takes tertiary referrals from level 2 practitioners and has other evidence of advanced practice such as undertaking specialist US examinations and being active in US research.

Validated tools to determine competence are currently lacking. The American College of Emergency Medicine stated in 2009 that 'methods of determining competency include traditional testing, testing using simulator models, videotape review, observation of bedside skills, over-reading of images by experienced sonologists (expert physicians who perform and interpret US examinations), and monitoring of error rates through a quality assurance process'.

In the UK, there has been considerable investment in EM 'finishing schools' as a means of testing competence to a national standard, and there is interest in simulation both for echo training and assessment, particularly for transoesophageal echocardiography (TOE).

Indications

Indications for POCUS depend on the patient's symptoms, signs, and clinical setting (Table 1.1), as well as their suspected pathophysiology (Table 1.2).

Internal validity

US performed by operators with limited training and minimal experience has been consistently shown to be superior to clinical examination for detecting left ventricular systolic dysfunction, valvular disease, and pericardial effusions. Other cardiac conditions listed in Table 1.2 are less well validated but are considered by experts as legitimate targets for POCUS, because evidence suggests that novices can detect them and they have important implications in a critically ill patient.

POCUS has greatest validity in haemodynamically unstable patients. In the setting of undifferentiated shock or hypotension, it demonstrably improves

Table 1.1 Common indications for POCUS

Symptoms	Signs	Clinical setting
Chest pain	Hypotension	Cardiac arrest
Shortness of breath	Shock	Penetrating cardiac injury
Abdominal pain	Dyspnoea	Blunt abdominal trauma
Oligo-anuria	Hypoxaemia	Stable penetrating abdominal trauma
Collapse	Ascites	Pre-hospital/resource-limited areas

Table 1.2 Pathophysiology readily detected by POCUS

LV enlargement	Consolidation
Left ventricular systolic dysfunction	Atelectasis
Right ventricular enlargement	Cardiogenic pulmonary oedema
Right ventricular systolic dysfunction	Non-cardiogenic pulmonary oedema (ARDS)
Pericardial effusion/tamponade	Pulmonary fibrosis
Volume status	Pleural effusion
Gross valvular abnormalities	Pneumothorax
Large intra-cardiac masses	Abdominal aortic aneurysm
Significant LVH	Peritoneal free fluid
Significant RVH	Hydronephrosis
Significant atrial dilatation	Cholecystitis

ARDS, acute respiratory distress syndrome; LV, left ventricular; RV, right ventricular.

diagnostic accuracy, shortens time to diagnosis, and leads to a change in clinical management in approximately 50% of cases.

Acute respiratory failure remains one of the most common reasons for admission to ICU. Traditionally, imaging the lungs in order to confirm the diagnosis and assess progress meant a choice between chest radiography and CT scanning. The former, although relatively easy to perform, has limited sensitivity and specificity, and the latter is impractical, costly, and not without risk in the critically ill patient.

LUS is more accurate than chest X-ray at ruling in or out a pneumothorax, identifying the interstitial syndrome (pulmonary oedema), and confirming the presence of consolidation (in mechanically ventilated patients). In experienced hands, the sensitivity and specificity of LUS approach those of CT scanning. A standardized focused lung examination (the 'BLUE Protocol') has been shown to be a highly accurate tool for the initial assessment and diagnosis of patients with acute respiratory failure. Pulmonary oedema results in specific US signs that change much more rapidly with its evolution and resolution and are more sensitive than the signs seen on chest X-ray.

US will readily identify free fluid and is the gold standard for assessment and treatment of pleural, pericardial, and intra-peritoneal fluid.

Risks and limitations

Exposure time and energy transfer in focused US are extremely low, and so the risk of tissue injury, thermal or otherwise, is insignificant.

The main concern is that misinterpretation can potentially result in harm to patients. Over-interpretation may cause introduction of unnecessary therapy, and under-interpretation may cause omission of appropriate therapy, definitive investigations, or specialist input. Importantly, utilization beyond the scope of POCUS [e.g. quantification of aortic stenosis (AS)], without the necessary training and supervision to perform this, may well lead to inaccurate conclusions and harm. Safeguards for each of these problems include the provision of adequate training, competency assessment, and robust local governance to ensure that practice stays within appropriate boundaries (Chapter 34).

POCUS is not designed to answer every clinical question, and to practise safely as an operator, one must recognize the limitations of POCUS and one's own expertise. Referral to a fully qualified expert is essential for anything beyond its scope. However, if one keeps within these boundaries, practising POCUS is safe and cost-effective and produces unparalleled insight into the physiological status of critically ill patients.

✔ Multiple choice questions

Interactive multiple choice questions to test your knowledge can be found in the Online appendix at www.oxfordmedicine.com/focusedicu. Please refer to your access card for further details.

Further reading

Frankel HL, Kirkpatrick AW, Elbarbary M, *et al*. Guidelines for the appropriate use of bedside general and cardiac ultrasonography in the evaluation of critically ill patients—part I: general ultrasonography. *Critical Care Medicine* 2015;**43**:2479–502.

Levitov A, Frankel HL, Blaivas M, *et al*. Guidelines for the appropriate use of bedside general and cardiac ultrasonography in the evaluation of critically ill patients—part II: cardiac ultrasonography. *Critical Care Medicine* 2016;**44**:1206–27.

Via G, Hussain A, Wells M, *et al*. International evidence-based recommendations for focused cardiac ultrasound. *Journal of the American Society of Echocardiography* 2014;**27**:683. e1–33.

2

Physics of ultrasound

Benjamin Reddi and Nick Fletcher

Introduction

To be able to use US effectively, one must be able to understand the physics on which it is based. These fundamental principles dictate the choice of probe and how to use it, which buttons to press and how to set them, and whether or not the images obtained are interpretable.

This chapter will describe the US wave, how it is produced, and what effect body tissues have on it as it passes through the body. It will describe the key principles that underpin image resolution and discuss the importance of the US pulse. The advanced section will introduce how Doppler US and aliasing are produced.

The ultrasound wave

To generate a US image, a transducer probe emits high-frequency sound waves, then detects the echoes of the waves as they are reflected from tissue interfaces throughout the viewing field. Sound waves are generated as the local displacement of particles forms a repeated sequence of pressure peaks (compressions) and troughs (rarefactions).

Waves are defined by the following physical properties (Figure 2.1):

- Frequency (f)—the number of waves passing a fixed point per second, measured in hertz (Hz). The dynamic range of audible sound spans 20–20,000 Hz, compared to 2–10 MHz for commonly used medical US. The reciprocal of the frequency is the time taken for a wave to pass a specified point—the period (T)—measured in seconds.

- Wavelength (λ)—the distance between equivalent points (e.g. troughs or peaks) of two adjacent waves, usually in the order of tenths of a millimetre.

- Propagation speed (c)—the product of frequency and wavelength, inversely related to the density and elasticity of the propagation medium. Elasticity tends to vary more than density in human tissues and is hence the dominant influence (Table 2.1). When interpreted by the US receiver, a reflected wave is assumed to have travelled at 1540 m/s, the average propagation speed in soft tissues. When a wave passes between media of different density/elasticity, the frequency remains the same, but λ changes according to the equation $c = f \times \lambda$.

- Amplitude—the excursion of pressure peaks and troughs from the average, measured in units of pressure. The power of the sound wave (measured in watts) is proportional to the square of the amplitude and determines the biologic effect of a sound wave. The amplitude of a reflected wave dictates the brightness of the corresponding dot on the US image.

The ultrasound transducer

The transducer receives electrical energy and emits acoustic energy. When acoustic waves are reflected from a tissue interface, the transducer converts acoustic energy back into electrical energy to be interpreted by the image processor. Transduction depends on the piezoelectric effect—electrical energy

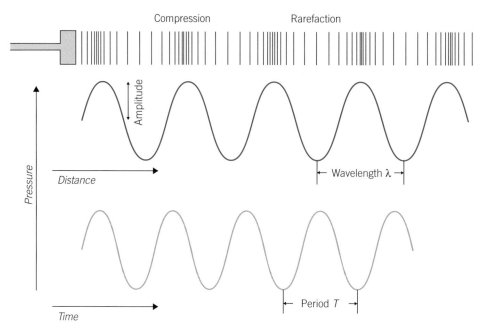

Figure 2.1 A schematic demonstrating the nature and properties of sound waves. Note the alternating compression and rarefaction of the transmission medium. Wavelength, frequency, and amplitude are the fundamental properties of each ultrasound wave.

Adapted from Mr G Leech with permission.

pulsed across an ultrasonic crystal causes the crystal to deform slightly, producing the vibration underlying the US wave. The crystal vibrates at its natural resonant frequency, specified by modifying the mechanical properties of the crystal. In turn, returning sound waves cause the crystal to oscillate, generating the electrical signal required to construct a US image. The time taken for a reflected pulse to return to the probe depends upon the depth of the tissue interface from which it has been reflected and determines, in turn, the position of the associated dot on the US image.

A group of active US-producing piezoelectric crystal elements within the transducer, termed an array, is cyclically activated and inactivated in phase, each activation cycle producing an arc of US lines. A spatial sequence of juxtaposed lines allows a 2D image or 'frame' to be compiled. A temporal sequence of frames generates a real-time sequence of images. The lateral resolution of the image is determined by the line density (typically 100+ across the sector), and temporal resolution by the frame refresh rate (typically up to 100 Hz), discussed further in The ultrasound pulse and limits of resolution.

Linear probes have a rectangular face that emits and receives parallel beams generating a rectangular image of high resolution. Curvilinear probes have beams that fan out across the imaged sector to broaden the field of view; however, this diminishes line density and degrades image resolution at increasing depth. Echocardiography probes require a small footprint to fit between the ribs but must be able to image

Table 2.1 Velocity of sound in various transmission media

Tissue	Velocity (m/s)
Air	330
Fat	1450
Water	1520
Blood	1570
Muscle	1585
Bone	4080

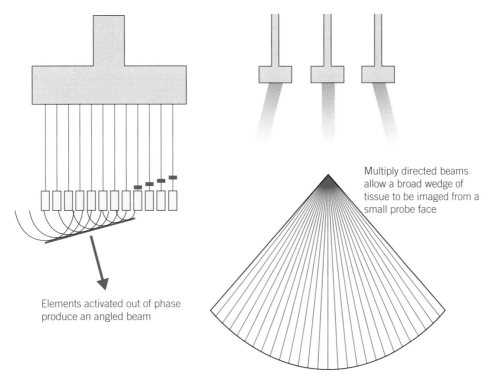

Figure 2.2 A schematic demonstrating how the phased array ultrasound transducer works. An electrically mediated delay in transmission of each transducer element allows an ultrasound beam to be swept across the field multiple times per second. In particular, this will help to accurately track fast-moving sections of cardiac tissue.
Adapted from Mr G Leech with permission.

the breadth of the heart. This is achieved using 'phased array' technology. The probe contains a linear array of sound wave-producing elements that pulse slightly out of phase; the resulting wavefront ripples from the probe at an angle (determined by the phase difference between adjacent wavelets). Repeating the process with different phase differences allows multiply directed beams to be generated from the same elements, imaging a broad wedge of tissue (Figure 2.2) with the electronically steered beam.

The interaction between sound waves and tissue

As sound passes through a medium, the intensity of the wave diminishes as it is absorbed, reflected, diffracted, and refracted (Figure 2.3). Signal attenuation is measured in decibels (dB), the logarithm of the ratio between the intensities of the initial and attenuated signals. Signal intensity is proportional to wave amplitude ($I = kA^2$; units J/s/cm^2). Any medium has a characteristic attenuation coefficient. Since signals are progressively attenuated as they penetrate the tissue, and attenuation is also proportional to the signal frequency, the attenuation coefficient is expressed as dB/cm at 1 MHz. On average, soft tissue has an attenuation coefficient of 1 dB/cm at 1 MHz, equating to losing around 20% of signal intensity per centimetre penetration for a 1-MHz signal.

Absorption: sound energy is dispersed as heat when vibrating molecules jostle against one another, generating friction. Absorption is more pronounced at higher frequencies and in more viscous tissue.

Signal reflection is the basis of US imaging. A sound wave is reflected when it encounters an interface between media of differing acoustic impedance Z (Table 2.2). The difference between acoustic impedance of adjacent media (acoustic mismatch) determines the proportion of the signal that is reflected. Acoustic impedance is a function of the density and the speed of sound through a medium.

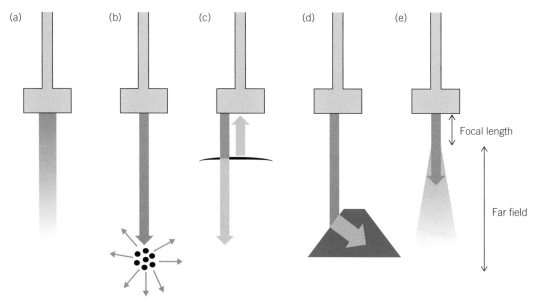

Figure 2.3 A schematic demonstrating how an ultrasound wave travels into body tissue. The signal is attenuated by a number of differing mechanisms: (a) absorption, (b) scattering, (c) reflection, (d) refraction, and (e) diffraction.
Adapted from Mr G Leech with permission.

Air-filled structures and bone tend to reflect almost all sound waves, effectively obscuring deeper structures. Furthermore, the acoustic mismatch between soft tissue and air mandates the use of a coupling medium between the probe and the skin, e.g. an US gel.

Specular reflectors have a smooth surface and are broad, relative to the wavelength of the US beam. Examples include the kidney, spleen, pericardium, and cardiac valves, which generate clear US images when the incident angle is 90°. Objects with irregularities, presenting a surface less than a wavelength in size, tend to scatter US beams in many directions,

e.g. lung and myocardial tissue—this can be helpful in imaging structures not perpendicular to the US beam. Indeed, backscatter and diffuse reflection produce most clinical images. Red cells are smaller than US wavelength, scattering the beam in all directions and reflecting very little back to the transducer. That becomes important, however, in Doppler interrogation of blood flow (Chapter 2).

A US beam is refracted or deflected from its path when it meets an interface between two media that propagate the wave at different speeds at anything other than a 90° angle of incidence. The ratio of incident and transmission angles equals the ratio of propagation speeds. Refraction gives rise to important imaging artefacts (Chapter 3).

As the US beam propagates from a discoid transducer, it remains essentially cylindrical up to a certain distance, the near field length. Beyond this point—the far field, the wavefront spreads out (diffracts) in a conical pattern and the intensity diminishes as the power is dispersed over a greater area. The near field length is further and the extent of divergence in the far field smaller for high frequency beams transmitted from a large transducer face. The beam can be focused by means of a lens within the transducer, constricting the beam at the focal length at the cost of exaggerating

Table 2.2 Acoustic impedance of various transmission media

Medium	Acoustic impedance $(kg/m^2/s \times 10^{-6})$
Air	0.0004
Blood	1.61
Muscle	1.7
Soft tissue (average)	1.63
Bone	7.8

diffraction in the far field. Focusing thus improves lateral resolution at the focal point, reducing the spatial separation required for a pair of point reflectors to generate two distinguishable signals. Diffraction also occurs after reflection from a convex surface or transmission through a small aperture.

The ultrasound pulse and limits of resolution

The US image is constructed when waves are reflected back to the probe from a tissue interface. If waves were emitted continuously, it would not be possible to correlate the emitted with the received wave and hence identify the depth at which the reflection/tissue interface took place, the crucial step in generating the image. Instead, waves are pulsed briefly, each pulse containing only a few cycles (Figure 2.4). A relatively long period of silence follows each pulse, during which echoes are listened for. The time taken for pulse reflections to return to the transducer indicates the depths at which reflecting surfaces are encountered—the 2D image is constructed according to the arrival time of reflected pulses. The pulsed signal is described by the pulse duration (PD), the pulse repetition frequency (PRF), and the spatial pulse length (SPL). At higher

frequencies, the PD and SPL are shorter since both wavelength and period are reduced.

PRF is the number of pulses emitted per second (not to be confused with the transducer frequency). Its reciprocal is the pulse period. The depth of the US-viewing window dictates the maximum PRF; to unambiguously localize all the echoes in a field requires that a single pulse has time to traverse that field and back before the next pulse is emitted. For example, to distinguish all objects within a 10-cm viewing window, a single pulse must have time to travel 20 cm before the next pulse is emitted. Taking the average speed as 1540 m/s, the time taken to travel 20 cm is 0.2 m/1540 m = 0.13 ms and the maximum PRF required to generate an unambiguous image is 1 pulse/0.13 ms = 7.7 kHz. In turn, the PRF determines the temporal resolution of the moving 2D image. Remember each image is constructed from a sequence of juxtaposed scan lines, forming a frame. Temporal resolution improves, the faster the image is refreshed (higher frame rate); clearly, it takes longer to refresh each line when the pulse frequency is lower and the pulse period longer. Temporal resolution can be improved by reducing the imaging depth, narrowing the sector width, or reducing the density of scan lines.

SPL is the physical distance from beginning to end of the pulse, i.e. λ × number of cycles per pulse. At higher frequencies, the wavelength, and thereby SPL, is reduced. SPL is important because it determines the axial resolution of the US image, i.e. the ability to distinguish point reflectors at different depths. In order for two points at different depths to be distinguished, they must be separated by at least half the SPL, so that the two pulse reflections arrive at the transducer independently (Figure 2.5). Since the number of cycles per pulse is usually determined by the manufacturer, the sonographer can only improve the axial resolution by using a probe of higher frequency (and therefore shorter λ and SPL). The trade-off, as discussed in The interaction between sound waves and tissue, is the increased attenuation associated with higher-frequency signals. Hence, high-frequency probes are ideal for gaining detailed imaging of superficial structures, e.g. for guiding vascular access.

The ability to resolve two reflectors lying side-by-side—lateral resolution—is generally poorer than axial resolution. Resolving neighbouring objects requires

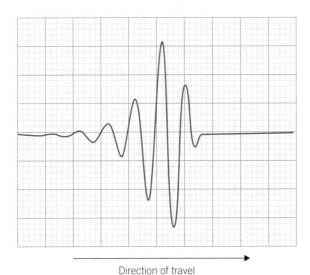

Direction of travel

Figure 2.4 A schematic of an ultrasound pulse that only contains a few waves of ultrasound.

Adapted from Mr G Leech with permission.

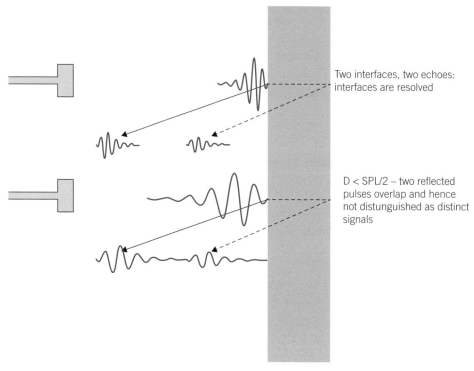

Two interfaces, two echoes: interfaces are resolved

D < SPL/2 – two reflected pulses overlap and hence not distunguished as distinct signals

Figure 2.5 A schematic demonstrating axial or range resolution. This is the ability of the ultrasound device to detect and display two separate points at different distances from the transducer. The pulse repetition frequency is an important determinant of this resolution.

Adapted from Mr G Leech with permission.

that they generate echoes from distinct US beams (Figure 2.6), i.e. lateral resolution is limited by the beamwidth. The beamwidth is reduced at lower frequencies (or longer λ) and narrowed by focusing and greater transducer aperture, such that:

Lateral resolution
= beamwidth at focus
= 2.4 (focal depth × λ)/aperture diameter

Linear probes used for vascular access typically have a shallow focal depth and high frequency (low λ). Curvilinear probes use lower-frequency US and a wide sector, allowing deep penetration and a broad field of view, albeit at the expense of axial, lateral, and temporal resolution.

Image pre-processing

Scan data can be manipulated during acquisition to optimize the image before storage:

- The dynamic range is the ratio of the maximum-to-minimum signal level expressed in decibels; increasing the dynamic range allows weaker signals

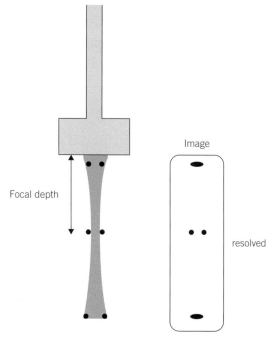

Image

Focal depth

resolved

Figure 2.6 A schematic demonstrating lateral resolution. Lateral point resolution is dependent on beamwidth. Beamwidth can be influenced by the setting of focal depth, which should be located just below the region of interest.

Adapted from Mr G Leech with permission.

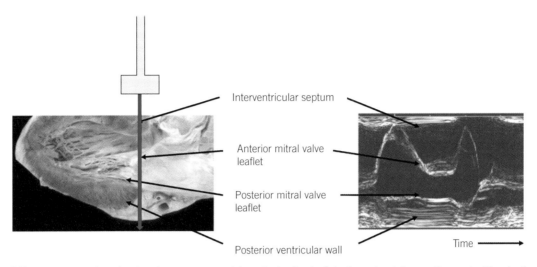

Interventricular septum

Anterior mitral valve
leaflet

Posterior mitral valve
leaflet

Posterior ventricular wall

Time

Figure 2.7 M-mode imaging showing the movement of the mitral valve leaflets throughout the cardiac cycle. The depth setting is on the *y*-axis, and time on the *x*-axis. Rapid anatomical movement can be better detected by the use of M-mode. Adapted from Mr G Leech with permission.

to be displayed, which, in a high-quality image, can promote distinction between areas of subtly differing echogenicity. However, in a poor image, narrowing the dynamic range eliminates weaker signals, enhancing the clarity of strong signals to produce a higher-contrast image. Contrast can also be augmented using edge enhancement, a filtering technique that accentuates the differences in signal strength between adjacent regions.

- Time gain compensation (TGC) allows adjustment of the intensity of signals returning from different depths to counter the effect of attenuation that would otherwise render deeper structures progressively fainter. TGC is typically adjusted, so that similar structures generate similar intensity images throughout the image, e.g. the myocardium at the front and back of the heart appears similarly bright.

Motion-mode imaging

In M-mode, a representation of depth and motion is generated from a limited number of crystals, producing a narrow US beam. The resulting one-dimensional (1D) frame is refreshed at thousands of Hz, giving excellent temporal resolution of structures transected by the beam. Graphically, the uni-dimensional image is represented on the *y*-axis followed in time on the *x*-axis (Figure 2.7). It is most useful in assessing pleural or cardiac valve motion, or modulation of chamber or vessel size over time, for instance changes in inferior vena cava (IVC) diameter during respiration. Disadvantages include difficulty seeing the image in spatial context and making accurate measurements in 1D while the beam/structure relationship shifts in 3D.

Advanced echocardiography

Principles of Doppler imaging

Doppler imaging allows visual representation of the direction, velocity, and character of fluid flow, yielding important haemodynamic information during echocardiography and vascular access. It is based on the concept that the frequency of a wave is modulated in proportion to the direction and velocity of a moving structure from which it is reflected. For instance, when waves echo from blood travelling away from the US probe, the distance and time between the reflected wave peaks is stretched out as each successive wave peak is reflected from red cells at a point slightly further away from the probe. Since the wave velocity remains constant and the wavelength has increased, the frequency is reduced in proportion to the velocity of the flow of blood, and this is known as the 'Doppler shift'. This shift is highly dependent on the angle of incidence between the flow and US beam, a major source of error when using this mode. Since flow velocity is proportional to pressure gradient, Doppler analysis allows the severity of valve stenoses to be estimated, while directional information allows identification of valvular incompetence.

Pulsed wave (PW) Doppler allows blood flow to be analysed at a discrete location, e.g. mitral inflow, but is limited in terms of velocity resolution. Continuous wave (CW) Doppler offers no spatial localization, but a far greater range of distinguishable velocities, and is used routinely to estimate gradients across stenotic valves. Colour flow Doppler enhances the 2D US image by portraying flow using colour, usually blue and red, for opposing directions and diminishing saturation with progressive velocity.

As well as gathering faint echoes from fast-moving red cells, pulsed wave Doppler can be used with a low-pass filter to pick up the relatively intense signal from slow-moving myocardium to depict the velocity of ventricular contraction and relaxation (Chapter 7). This is known as tissue Doppler imaging (TDI).

In PW and colour flow Doppler, there is a limit to the blood velocity that can be accurately detected and displayed by an echo machine. This is known as the Nyquist limit, which happens to be half the PRF. At velocities beyond this limit, aliasing is encountered.

When aliasing occurs in PW Doppler, the spectral display 'wraps around' the display, giving the appearance of flow in the opposite direction. When aliasing occurs in colour flow Doppler, it wraps around the colour spectrum, switching to the opposite colour or a speckled mosaic of either red and blue, and white or green, depending on the settings. Machine controls can be adjusted to eliminate aliasing, but at standard settings, it usually indicates fast or turbulent blood flow.

✅ Multiple choice questions

Interactive multiple choice questions to test your knowledge can be found in the Online appendix at www.oxfordmedicine.com/focusedicu. Please refer to your access card for further details.

Acknowledgement

We would like to acknowledge the significant educational contribution of past British Society of Echocardiography President Graham Leech (deceased), who provided some of the illustrations for this chapter.

Further reading

Armstrong WF, Ryan T, Feigenbaum H. *Feigenbaum's Echocardiography*, 7th ed. Philadelphia, PA: Wolters Kluwer Health/Lippincott Williams & Wilkins; 2010.

Hoskins PR, Martin K, Thrush A. *Diagnostic Ultrasound: Physics and Equipment*, 2nd ed. Cambridge (UK), New York, NY (USA): Cambridge University Press; 2010.

Otto CM. *Textbook of Clinical Echocardiography*, 5th ed. Philadelphia, PA: Elsevier/Saunders; 2013.

3

Image optimization

Carlos Corredor and Nick Fletcher

Introduction

Whether the target is the heart, lung, or abdomen, critical care patients can be difficult subjects to scan. US platforms are increasingly designed for auto-optimization of images, according to the clinical context. However, it is essential that anyone who wants to master US understands how to improve images using the main controls provided, a process known affectionately as 'knobology'.

Good decisions should be based on good images, and this chapter will describe how you can optimize the environment, probe selection, depth, gain, compression, focus, sector width, and zoom to obtain the best images possible.

The advanced section will introduce practical aspects of colour, pulsed wave, continuous wave, and TDI and present some of their many limitations, which explain why considerable supervision is required to develop skills in these modalities.

Pre-examination preparation

Performing echocardiography in the ICU poses challenges that are inherent to the critical care environment and the seriously ill patient. Time and effort spent beforehand minimizing the effect of these factors results in better image quality and yields better diagnostic information.

Space around the bed is often limited by the presence of other monitoring and vital equipment; the sonographer should adopt a comfortable position and reduce ambient light as much as possible to enable reduction of US gain. Other challenges to access include mechanical ventilation (causing large lung volumes),

surgical dressings, and drains, which can preclude some windows.

Minimal changes in patient position can usually improve sonographic windows and image quality. Repositioning the patient as close as possible to the left lateral decubitus position decreases the distance from the heart to the anterior chest wall. Raising the patient's left hand above their head increases separation between the ribs, improving the size of acoustic windows. In comprehensive echo, it is essential to have a working electrocardiogram signal, to accurately relate phases of the cardiac cycle to the electrical activity of the heart. This is not the case for focused echo. However, an ECG trace is still a useful guide.

Once ergonomics are optimized, it is crucial to adjust controls on the echocardiography machine to produce the best possible images.

The analogue US signal received by the transducer is modified before digitalization and display in the pre-processing phase. Further changes to the digital image can be performed in the post-processing phase; these modifications can alter the appearance of the stored image. The ability to perform post-processing image adjustments is limited by the machine, its settings, and the image quality obtained during pre-processing.

Pre-processing image controls encountered in most modern echocardiography machines include frequency, power output, gain, depth, TGC, compression, focus, sector width, and zoom (Figure 3.1). Frame rate is affected directly by the settings chosen in sector width and depth. Post-processing controls, including brightness, contrast, and grey scale, can be manipulated to improve the contrast resolution of the display.

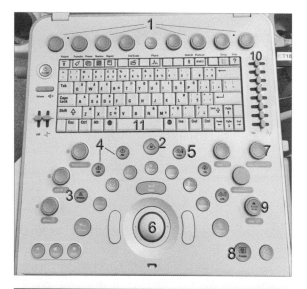

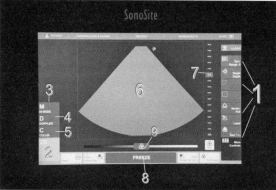

Figure 3.1 Control panels of two portable ultrasound machines—solid keys (above); touchpad (below).
(1) Navigation keys; (2) 2D selector; (3) M-mode selector; (4) spectral Doppler selector; (5) colour Doppler selector; (6) trackball; (7) depth; (8) freeze; (9) gain; (10) time gain compensation; (11) keyboard.

Reproduced with kind permission from Phillips and Fujifilm Sonosite.

Frequency

Transthoracic echocardiography (TTE) probes have relatively low frequencies of around 3.5 Hz; transoesophageal probes use higher frequencies of 3.5–7 Hz, as they are placed very close to cardiac structures. Curvilinear probes for abdominal and pleural scanning utilize 2–5 MHz, and linear array probes for vascular US use 8–10 MHz. The quality of image resolution is directly proportional to transducer frequency, with better resolution at higher transducer frequencies. The opposite is true for tissue penetration, which is higher at lower transducer frequencies.

Modern US machines automatically utilize tissue harmonic imaging (THI) to improve image quality. Harmonics are multiples of the original fundamental (or transmitted) frequency and are the result of the non-linear propagation of US waves through the tissues. The strength of the harmonic signals increases with depth, to a point of maximum intensity, and it is then attenuated by further increases in depth. The usual depth of cardiac structures coincides with the maximal harmonic frequencies, making this US property ideal for exploitation in echocardiography. Lateral resolution and endocardial definition are improved with the use of THI, which also reduces near field and side lobe artefacts and improves image quality in patients with suboptimal US penetration. Transmitted frequency and harmonic frequency can be altered on the echo machine, by switching between 'resolution', 'general', and 'penetration' settings, to account for different situations, such as the obese patient.

Depth

This control allows the user to set the maximum field depth of the image displayed. Reducing the depth setting will increase the frame rate and PRF. Therefore, adjusting the depth and width settings to visualize the entire structure of interest (but no more) will achieve optimal lateral and temporal resolution.

Gain

Gain is not dissimilar to the volume control encountered in audio equipment, in the way that it regulates the amplitude of the signal received. The returned echo signals can be amplified by adjusting the gain control. However, manipulating the gain control cannot compensate for poor reflected amplitude resulting from low power output or attenuation.

Excessive gain produces a very bright image, impairing the definition of adjacent structures. On the other hand, a gain setting that is too low may preclude visualization of poorly echo-reflective structures. The ideal gain setting will render an image where solid structures appear with a uniform intensity, and cavities full of blood appear as dark echo free space.

Time gain compensation

The interaction of US and tissue leads to loss of signal strength, known as attenuation. TGC aims to compensate for the effects of attenuation by allowing differential adjustment of gain at different depths of the US signal. The adjustment is performed by multiple sliding controls that are each responsible for a specific band of depth. Signals reflected by objects located far from the transducer are weak, and thus far-field gain is set higher than object located in the mid field. The signal from objects close to the transducer is stronger and requires setting of an even lower near-field gain. Optimal image acquisition requires frequent adjustment of the TGC control, depending on the area of interest for the observer (Figure 3.2).

Compression

The US display cannot process the same amplitude range of reflected signals that the receiver can. Therefore, the dynamic range of the incoming signal must be reduced. Dynamic range refers to the difference between the highest and lowest signal amplitudes, and variations of the standard grey scale are used to represent each value of amplitude. In this way, if the reflected signal is too weak and falls below the threshold of the system, it is eliminated. Similarly, very strong reflected signals are also eliminated, as they impair the ability to accurately discern all tissues in the image; in other words, they reach saturation.

The cardiac valves are dense structures that produce strong reflected signals. By contrast, the myocardium is a soft tissue that produces weaker signals. These weak signals require amplification, in order for them to have greater representation in the dynamic range. Some machines have auto-optimization functions, which utilize dynamic range. In others, the operator can modify the dynamic range to aid appreciation of subtle variations in weaker signals. Amplification of weaker signals, however, can lead to an increase in noise and degrade image quality.

Focus

The focal zone of the US beam can be adjusted electronically to converge at a desired point in relation to

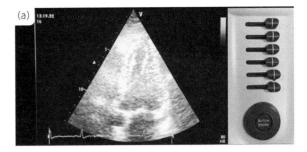

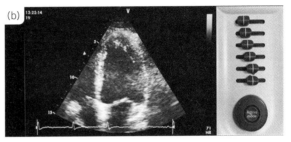

Figure 3.2 A4C images and TGC sliders demonstrating (a) inadequate and (b) optimal contrast adjustment.

the region of interest (Figure 3.3). Locating the focus point slightly deep to this will place the observed structures within the focal zone, which is the area of greatest US beam intensity and best lateral resolution (Figure 3.4).

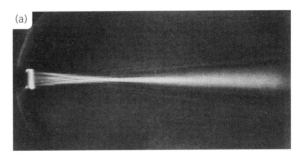

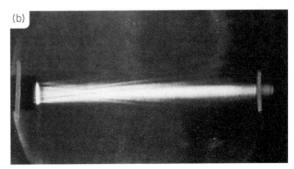

Figure 3.3 Schleiren photography visualization of ultrasound beams. (a) Short focal distances. (b) Long focal distances.
Images courtesy of G Leech.

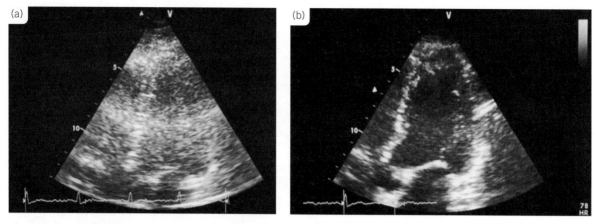

Figure 3.4 An A5C image centred on the left ventricle demonstrating: (a) inadequate focus position for visualization of the left ventricular apex; (b) optimal focus position for the above.

Sector width

Echocardiography machines usually display a standard 60°-wide image. This setting ensures that structures located on the lateral aspects of the image are seen. Narrowing the beamwidth improves frame rate and scan line density, resulting in better image resolution of central structures. The same is true for curvilinear probes. Some US machines allow for movement of the image sector without physically moving the

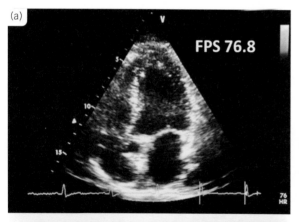

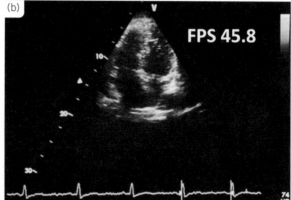

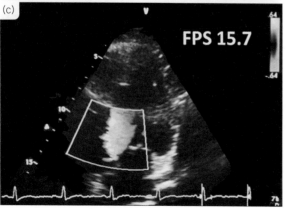

Figure 3.5 An A5C image illustrating reduction in frame rate. (a) A normal 2D image = FPS 76.8. (b) Excessive depth setting = FPS 45.8. (c) Use of colour flow Doppler = FPS 15.7. FPS, frames per second.

probe; these are known as phased array probes. This lateral steer control enables movement of the reduced image sector to the right or the left.

should be applied before freezing an image to ensure that write zoom is applied. Once the image is frozen, read zoom can be used to magnify it.

Zoom

Image magnification can be achieved in both the pre-processing (write zoom) and post-processing (read zoom) phases. Write zoom enhances the image by using a higher pixel density when digitizing the picture. By contrast, read zoom only magnifies the picture, without actually adding any additional data, and is the equivalent of using a magnifying glass. Zoom

Frame rate

Frame rate is often equated to temporal resolution for the purpose of echocardiography. Temporal resolution allows differentiation of an object that has moved over time. Frame rate can be increased by reducing the depth of the image or by reducing scan sector width. Simultaneous use of image modalities, such as colour Doppler and 2D, can significantly reduce the frame rate (Figure 3.5).

Advanced echocardiography

Colour flow Doppler

By convention, flow towards the transducer is displayed in red, and flow away from the transducer in blue. A well-known mnemonic is 'BART' ('blue away, red towards'). The sonographer can adjust different parameters, in order to optimize the information provided by the colour flow map; adjustments include:

- Box size and position—these can be adjusted to focus on a single structure or multiple flow streams simultaneously. A smaller colour box sector (less width and depth) has a higher frame rate, and thus better resolution.
- Baseline—different physiological or pathological flow patterns have specific velocity ranges that allow optimal display, and adjusting the zero baseline may be necessary when blood flow velocities lean more towards one direction.
- Scale—compression or expansion of the velocity scale within the Nyquist limits can improve visualization of the velocity range of interest.
- Gain—increasing gain can improve the definition of small jets but potentially create artefacts as a trade-off (Figure 3.6). Turning the colour Doppler gain dial upwards until aliasing is seen as speckles across the

whole sector, and then turning it down until this just disappears, obtains the ideal gain.

Pitfalls with colour Doppler

- Misinterpreting red and blue—when imaging vascular structures, red does not always mean 'arterial', and vice versa. Care must also be taken to avoid inadvertent selection of the colour invert option while scanning.
- Lowering the scale (or Nyquist limit)—this results in overestimation of the colour map area, and vice versa.
- Coanda effect—eccentric regurgitant jets that hug chamber walls will appear smaller than they should, leading to underestimation of regurgitant flow.
- Loading conditions—altering the pressure difference between cardiac chambers will alter the flow disturbance but this is independant of the degree of structural valve disease. An example of this is the apparent reduction in mitral regurgitation (MR) seen with colour Doppler after induction of anaesthesia, simply due to vasodilatation.

Spectral Doppler

CW and PW Doppler US display blood velocity as a parabolic curve. Blood flow towards the transducer

(a)
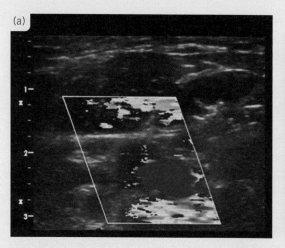

(b)
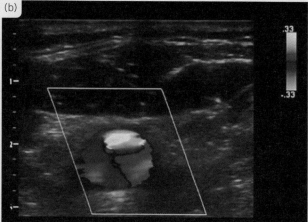

Figure 3.6 A PW Doppler image, taken from the left ventricular outflow tract in an A5C image, demonstrating: (a) aliasing; (b) aliasing resolved by setting the correct baseline. For a colour version of this figure, please see colour plate section.

is conventionally displayed above the baseline, and flow away from the transducer appears below the baseline. The operator can optimize these images by adjusting:

- Angle of interrogation—the incident angle of the US beam must be as parallel as possible to the direction of blood flow at the site being sampled. At 20°, the underestimate will be 6%, and anything above this is unacceptable.

- Baseline—the zero line can be shifted towards either the top or bottom of the display to enable the entire trace to be seen, as large as possible, for the purposes of tracing its volume–time integral (VTI). In PW Doppler, adjusting the baseline also helps to avoid aliasing by maintaining velocities within the limit of the scale (Figure 3.7).

- Scale—this can be modified, in conjunction with the baseline, to optimize waveform size (and prevent aliasing in PW Doppler).

- Gain—adjusting the degree of amplification of returned signals enables optimal display of the wave, with minimal background noise.

- Sweep speed—decreasing this produces multiple narrower traces on one screen, which enables variation in peak velocity to be observed.

Increasing this enables one large trace to be visualized, increasing its area and accuracy of VTI measurement.

- Tracing VTI curves—this is best done with a high sweep speed, using the baseline and scale to obtain the largest single trace possible. Care must be taken with the trackball (or touchpad) to trace accurately around the entire outer envelope of the spectral Doppler trace. Once this is done, the machine automatically estimates the peak and mean gradients.

Pitfalls with spectral Doppler

It has important technical limitations, in terms of image acquisition and interpretation, which must be fully understood before this information is used in a clinical context. These include (but are not limited to):

- Doppler alignment. In some valve lesions, blood flow can be eccentric, requiring non-standard views for accurate assessment. Any angle of interrogation will underestimate blood velocity.

- Truncated traces. When parabolic spectral Doppler traces are displayed with their tips blunted, or cut off completely, it suggests that the angle of interrogation is imperfect,

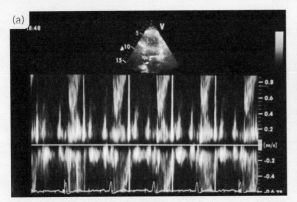
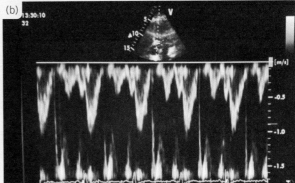

Figure 3.7 An image of the internal carotid artery with colour Doppler, demonstrating: (a) excessive gain causing speckling outside the blood vessel; (b) adequate gain setting with the colour signal limited to the contours of the artery. For a colour version of this figure, please see colour plate section.

and any estimations based on it will be underestimated.

- Range ambiguity. CW Doppler measures all velocities along the line (not at a certain point, as in PW Doppler). CW Doppler cannot confirm at which anatomical point the peak velocity was produced. In this way, medially directed MR can be easily misdiagnosed as AS.

- Effect of cardiac output on transvalvular gradient. Increased blood flow [sepsis, aortic regurgitation (AR)] will increase pressure gradients, based on the simplified Bernoulli equation, and overestimate the severity of AS. Reduced left ventricular contractility and ejection will underestimate AS for the same reason.

- Arrhythmias. In sinus rhythm, stroke volume can be considered the same from beat to beat. This is not the case in atrial fibrillation (AF), for instance, and this produces highly variable information, depending on which beat is evaluated.

Solutions exist to each of these problems, but they require considerable experience, and we refer the interested reader to an advanced echocardiography textbook, two of which are listed in Further reading.

Tissue Doppler

TDI is used in the assessment of ventricular long-axis function, both systolic and diastolic. Starting from an optimized A4C, clicking on TDI colours the image red and blue, depending on whether tissue velocity is towards or away from the probe. Clicking on PW overlays a sampling volume, which can be positioned at the annuli of either the mitral or tricuspid valves, depending on which ventricle is being assessed. Once this is activated, PW TDI produces a trace of tissue motion, in accordance with conventions described for spectral Doppler. Baseline, scale, gain, and sweep speed are all similar considerations.

Pitfalls with tissue Doppler

- Angle of interrogation—this is as important as it is in spectral Doppler. The TDI sampling line should be aligned with the longitudinal aspect of the ventricular wall of interest.

- Sampling volume—for accuracy, this has to be located at the valve annulus, not anywhere else.

- Regional wall motion abnormalities (RWMAs)—basal RWMAs at the sampling point will cause underestimation of global function.

✔ Multiple choice questions

Interactive multiple choice questions to test your knowledge can be found in the Online appendix at www.oxfordmedicine.com/focusedicu. Please refer to your access card for further details.

Acknowledgement

We would like to acknowledge the significant educational contribution of past British Society of Echocardiography President Graham Leech (deceased), who provided some of the illustrations for this chapter.

Further reading

Armstrong WF, Ryan T, Feigenbaum H. *Feigenbaum's Echocardiography*, 7th ed. Philadelphia, PA: Wolters Kluwer Health/Lippincott Williams & Wilkins; 2010.

Hoskins PR, Martin K, Thrush A. *Diagnostic Ultrasound: Physics and Equipment*, 2nd ed. Cambridge (UK), New York, NY (USA): Cambridge University Press; 2010.

Otto CM. *Textbook of Clinical Echocardiography*, 5th ed. Philadelphia, PA: Elsevier/Saunders; 2013.

4

Artefacts

Russell Barber and Nick Fletcher

Introduction

Image artefacts are an inevitable part of using US and are encountered almost every time a US device is used. Some are avoidable, being generated by poor scanning technique, while others arise as part of the intrinsic physical limitation of the modality. Either way, artefacts are that part of the image that are not anatomically real. Without appreciation of their existence and frequency, they can be deceptive and lead the physician down an erroneous, and potentially harmful, therapeutic pathway.

The ability to recognize and remedy potentially correctable artefacts is the most important safeguard against them. With knowledge and experience, physicians can even exploit artefacts and use them to their advantage in making a diagnosis.

This chapter will describe the technical assumptions that produce artefacts and explain acoustic shadowing, enhancement, and reverberation, including the origin of A-and B-lines. It will also describe near-field, side lobe, and mirror image artefacts and how to avoid them. Finally, it will introduce the concept of foreshortening and how off-axis imaging can produce false images.

Technical assumptions in ultrasound

Artefacts may be images of the wrong size, shape, brightness, or position. Anatomical structures that are not seen by the US machine are yet another form of artefact.

Artefacts are caused largely by the technical assumptions made by the machine when processing information from the US beam; some are listed below:

- The interrogating beam is thin and narrow, and all reflections that are detected by the transducer have originated only from this main central beam.

- US travels along a straight path, and there is only one direct path to and from the transducer.

- Within the human body, US travels at a uniform speed of 1540 m/s, and the depth of the reflector is accurately determined by the time elapsed between sent and received US, regardless of its transmission through fat, muscle, or blood.

- All reflections are received from each pulse of US before the next pulse is sent out.

Deficient images

Poor resolution

Resolution is the ability of the US processor to distinguish two objects; it may be axial, lateral, or temporal. In clinical practice, the most commonly encountered problem is that of lateral resolution, which is the ability to distinguish two objects that are side by side, perpendicular to the beam (Figure 4.1). In the presence of poor lateral resolution, two objects will appear erroneously merged as a single image. Reduction in image quality is a common encounter when viewing structures at depth. As well as significant attenuation and reflection of the signal, the US beam diverges at greater depths, so that images of deeper structures

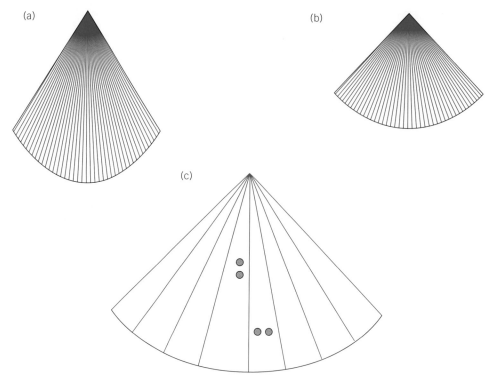

Figure 4.1 A schematic demonstrating the importance of scan line density. (a) and (b) demonstrate the effect of changing the sector depth setting on scan planes— increasing the line density improves resolution. (c) demonstrates how two neighbouring reflectors will be shown as one. In axial resolution, the reflectors lie one in front of the other, along the beam direction. In lateral resolution, the reflectors lie side by side, perpendicular to the beam direction.

Image courtesy of G Leech.

typically suffer from poor lateral resolution. To remedy this, the following are suggested:

- Use the highest frequency probe and settings, but this will be at the expense of penetration
- Use the focus, so the narrowest part of the beam images the area of interest.

Narrow the sector width and depth, to increase the scan line density and thus increase the frame rate.

- Use optimal gain settings, including the time gain control.

Acoustic shadowing

Even those new to sonography will be familiar with the loss of picture from acoustic shadowing. It occurs behind highly reflective structures or heavy absorbers of US such as ribs or mechanical prosthetic valves or even air. US cannot penetrate any further, creating a silhouette of echo dropout. Nothing can be seen from this US-void region, and a shadow is cast. Avoiding such blind spots is confined to finding a different acoustic window onto the area of interest or using a different scanning modality [e.g. TOE, CT, magnetic resonance imaging (MRI)] (Figure 4.2).

Edge shadowing

Acoustic and edge shadowing share the same consequences of impaired deeper tissue visualization. In edge shadowing, the shadow is a thin, hypoechoic line, extending out from the lateral edges of a fluid cavity or vessel wall (Figure 4.3). Although the precise mechanism of edge shadowing is unclear, it probably occurs from a combination of beam attenuation, refraction, and reflection.

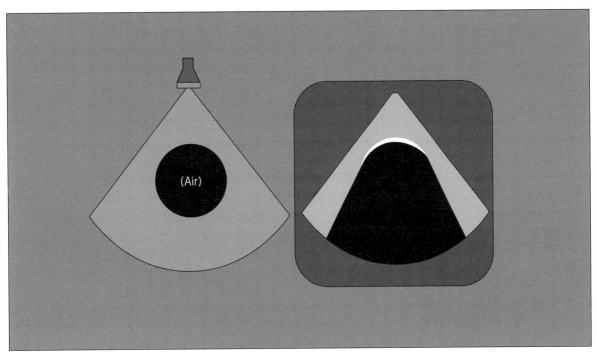

Figure 4.2 A schematic demonstrating acoustic shadowing. This diagram demonstrates the lack of ultrasound penetration when a poor transmitter or a strong reflector is in the beam.

Image courtesy of G Leech.

Degraded images

Reverberations

At each tissue layer, a US beam may be reflected, refracted, absorbed, or transmitted, and it must be

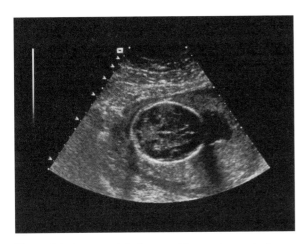

Figure 4.3 An antenatal ultrasound image demonstrating edge shadowing—attenuated signal behind the fetal skull.

Image courtesy of Infomed Research and Training Ltd.

appreciated that this occurs to both the interrogating beam and those US waves returning to the transducer. A returning US beam may be reflected from the under-surface of a tissue interface it passed through only a moment ago.

Reverberations are a phenomenon where returning US is reflected between two strong reflectors. Reflectors may be calcified tissue such as a stenotic mitral valve (MV) or a metallic mechanical valve (Figure 4.4). The US wave becomes temporarily trapped, as it bounces back and forth, before finally being transmitted through the upper tissue layer to be detected by the transducer. Meanwhile, the US machine does not account for this extended journey. Instead, it assumes the pathway has been direct and calculates the depth accordingly, giving rise to ghost signals. These typically take the form of one or more echoes directly behind the strong reflector. The distance between each ghost signal is the same, resembling rungs on a ladder, because they represent multiples of the true distance. It is not always possible to avoid reverberations, and using a different viewing

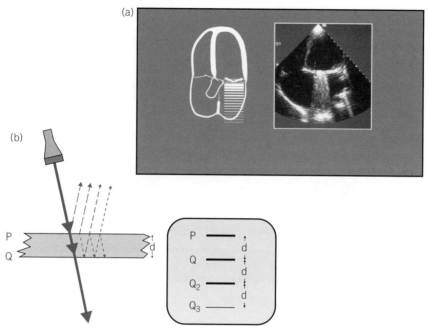

Figure 4.4 Schematics demonstrating reverberation artefacts. (a) An apical 5-chamber view showing multiple reverberations, caused by a mechanical mitral valve, producing artefacts within the left atrium. (b) A schematic of reverberation between two reflective planes (P and Q), causing successive artefactual lines (Q2 and Q3) at multiples of the distance (d) between them. Image courtesy of G Leech.

angle may be the only remedy. Turning down the gain attenuates the artefact, but also image acquisition.

A- and B-lines in lung ultrasound

Many of the features utilized as diagnostic indicators in LUS are, in fact, artefacts. A-lines are reverberations between the pleural surface and the surface of the transducer itself. Their depth is a multiple of the distance between the skin and the pleural line (Chapter 16).

It is hypothesized that B-lines in LUS are a form of reverberation (Figure 4.5a). Here the two highly reflective

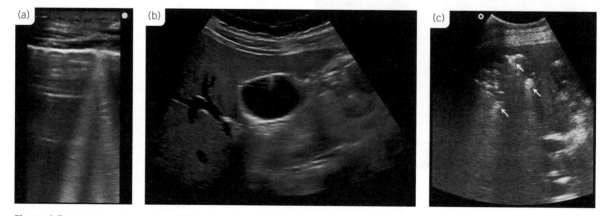

Figure 4.5 Images demonstrating different reverberation artefacts. (a) B-lines. (b) Comet tails. (c) Ring-down artefact. Images courtesy of R Barber and Christy Bembridge.

surfaces are the pleura and the interlobular septa. In non-oedematous and fibrotic states, the interlobular septa are not reflective. However, they become highly reflective in alveolar–interstitial syndromes. They may be also called lung comets, but this terminology is to be avoided, as it does not reflect their property of expanding to the bottom of the screen. B-lines are:

- Well defined and arise from the pleural line
- Move synchronously with pleural sliding
- Extend to the bottom of the screen without fading.

Comet tails

Comet tails are a closely related form of reverberation artefact (Figure 4.5b). Comet tails are commonly seen with metallic objects and calcified stone such as metallic clips and gall bladder calculi. Sequential echoes are so close together that individual signals are hard to see and they almost look to be continuous. They have a triangular, tapered tail, as attenuation diminishes their amplitude. They are much shorter-lived and so have relatively short tails. They fade in a manner similar to the tail of a comet.

Ring-down

Ring-down is used synonymously with comet tails, because they have a similar appearance on US (Figure 4.5c). However, strictly speaking, their formation is a product of a completely different physical basis. Liquid trapped between pockets of air bubbles vibrate after being bombarded with US. The liquid resonates or 'rings', creating a continuous sound wave that is transmitted back to the transducer. They hold diagnostic importance, as identification of this phenomenon suggests the presence of gas in some serious conditions such as aerobilia, Fournier's gangrene, or emphysematous pyelonephritis.

Acoustic enhancement

This is the reciprocal of acoustic shadowing and can be helpful in studying the more elusive deep body tissues. Fluid-filled structures permit unimpeded transit of US without dissipation by reflection or absorption, allowing an optimal window through which to study deeper structures. These deeper regions appear brighter than normal. Keeping a patient's bladder purposefully full is a commonly used technique to improve the imaging of

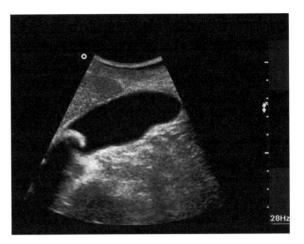

Figure 4.6 An image demonstrating acoustic enhancement. The time gain control may be needed to reduce the 'glare' visualized in deeper structures.
Image courtesy of Infomed Research and Training Ltd.

uterine structures (Figure 4.6). This is also why TOE gives such a good image of the mitral valve through the left atrium (LA). Be sure to adjust the time gain compensation on the console. Otherwise, these structures can look too intense; detail can appear washed out, or boundaries appear thickened.

False objects

Near-field clutter

This is due to acoustic noise near the transducer, resulting from high-amplitude oscillations of the piezoelectric elements, and it can make distinguishing structures within 1 cm of the transducer very difficult. It causes a fuzz-like appearance, and when this is seen in the left ventricular apex, it can be misinterpreted as an apical thrombus.

Side lobe artefact

Side lobes are unwanted offshoots of the central US beam. Side lobes are relatively close to the central beam, but of lower energy, and so require a strong reflector if their echoes are to be detected by the transducer. Since the US machine denies the existence of side lobes, it assumes that all returning signals originate from the central beam. As the interrogating beam scans from left to right, the strong reflector is smudged out as a curved line (Figure 4.7).

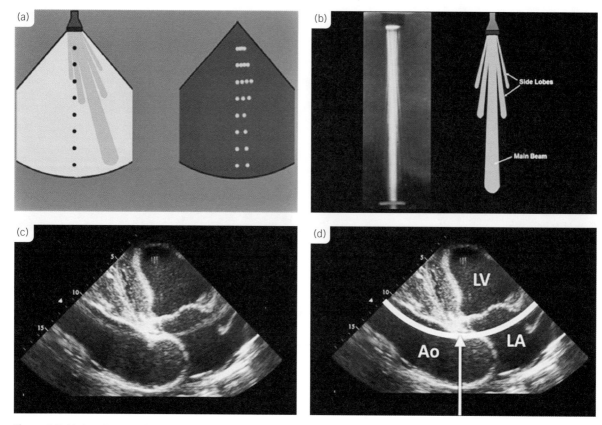

Figure 4.7 Various images demonstrating side lobe artefacts. (a) A diagram of how side lobes produce arcs, with their curvature always equidistant from the transducer. (b) Schleiren photography of side lobes. (c) An apical 2-chamber view with a side lobe artefact that could be misinterpreted as an aortic dissection. (d) The same image annotated (white band, artefact; arrow, strong reflector; Ao, aorta; LV, left ventricle; LA, left atrium). Note: the way that it appears to pass through anatomical planes reveals its artefactual nature.

Image courtesy of G Leech.

The nomenclature for artefacts is invariably defined and poorly structured. In practice, the term 'linear' artefact is often used to describe such ghost lines, without alluding to the underlying mechanism of production. Reverberations and side lobes can produce these lines, and mirror images of the LA can mimic an aortic dissection flap. When suspecting an artefact mimicking a dissection flap, consider the following:

- The 'flap' extends through the aortic wall and across normal anatomical boundaries.
- Colour flow does not show interruption of blood flow.

Mirror image artefacts

Mirror or multipath artefacts are created in a similar way to reverberations. Whereas reverberations are reflections back and forth within the path of the interrogating US beam, in mirror images, the beam is deflected away from the axis of the central beam.

The machine makes the same false assumption that the prolonged reflection time the US took to return to the transducer is due to depth, rather than it taking a 'scenic', indirect route. Consequently, a phantom mirror image is created on the other side, deep to the reflective surface (Figure 4.8). Real echoes are usually stronger and overwhelm the mirror effect.

Refraction artefacts

These are produced when the beam direction is refracted or bent, so that the object is displayed in the wrong place on the screen.

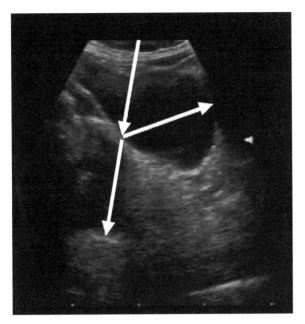

Figure 4.8 An image demonstrating mirror image artefact. A bladder wall producing a mirror image artefact behind it, the same shape and distance away as the opposite wall.
Image courtesy of Infomed Research and Training Ltd.

Measurement errors

Foreshortening

Foreshortening of the left ventricle (LV) is a commonly witnessed feature of echocardiography using the apical 4-chamber view. Failure to align the US beam exactly along the long axis of the LV creates a false apex. What appears to be the cardiac apex is, in fact, part of the distal ventricular wall, and the true apex often lies a rib space or two below this. Mistaking the apex leads to the incorrect calculation of the left ventricular cavity size and derived figures such as stroke volume and ejection fraction. Furthermore, the right ventricle (RV) will appear to be 'apicalized', adjoining the interventricular septum (IVS) close to the apex, creating the impression that it is enlarged. The clue to a false apex is its rounded shape, in comparison to the pointed true apex. The longitudinal length of the ventricle is shortened, in comparison to what it should be, and both atria look unopened and squashed. Although it is a useful landmark, palpating for the apex beat on the chest wall may not always direct you to the true apex. If the RV looks unexpectedly elongated down the IVS, in comparison to other views, then it probably is foreshortened. Rotating the patient fully onto their side or to a more supine position may remedy this. If the true apex cannot be found, the results should be interpreted with caution.

Oblique measurements of dimension

Vessels such as the IVC and aorta are considered to be circular in cross-section. Particular interest in the IVC diameter comes from its predictive value for fluid responsiveness, and this can greatly influence clinical decisions. Transmitting the US beam off the actual centre leads to the measurement of a chord, rather than the diameter, and so underestimates the true diameter. This is made even harder when the orientation of the probe and position of the IVC can vary with respiration. Furthermore, using M-mode for measurement is vulnerable to miscalculation when the vessel is not truly perpendicular. The same errors can apply to measurements of the left ventricular diameter.

✅ Multiple choice questions

Interactive multiple choice questions to test your knowledge can be found in the Online appendix at www.oxfordmedicine.com/focusedicu. Please refer to your access card for further details.

Acknowledgement

We would like to acknowledge the significant educational contribution of past British Society of Echocardiography President Graham Leech (deceased), who provided some of the illustrations for this chapter.

SECTION 2

Structure-based

Transthoracic echocardiography, sonoanatomy, and standard views

Conn Russell

Introduction

The heart is a complex structure, with only a finite number of windows through which it can be seen using US. Understanding cardiac sonoanatomy is essential for the provision of effective FoCUS. This chapter will describe from them the standard FoCUS views, including the anatomical structures one should expect to see and, importantly, how to obtain and optimize these images to extract the best diagnostic information. It will discuss cardiac axis, probe handling, and pitfalls in image acquisition. The advanced section will introduce additional views, used in comprehensive echocardiography, because these are readily obtained inadvertently during FoCUS scanning and can guide the operator back to standard views.

Ultrasound imaging of the heart

The position of the heart, surrounded by aerated lungs and the bony thoracic cage, makes obtaining diagnostic images with US challenging. Given these potential barriers, it is remarkable that the heart can be imaged at all, let alone with the level of detail possible from a full echocardiography study. Fortunately, several areas on the chest wall provide windows between the ribs, through which views of the heart can be obtained, with minimal interference by the lungs.

The left parasternal window takes advantage of the gap between the sternum and the pleural reflection of the left lung, while the apical window visualizes the heart where lung coverage is minimal. The suprasternal and subcostal windows image the heart from above and below the lungs, respectively. The cardiac phased array probe, with its small footprint, compared to traditional curved abdominal US probes, is designed to image between the ribs.

Orientation of the heart within the chest

It is important to appreciate that the long axis of the heart and the long axis of the body are different. The heart usually lies in a plane running between the right shoulder and the left hip, as opposed to the cranial–caudal long axis of the body. When describing long and short axes in echocardiography, these are in relation to the cardiac axis. The RV lies most anteriorly, while both atria lie superiorly, towards the right shoulder.

There is significant inter-patient variability in the position of the heart within the chest. Hyperinflation, caused by chronic lung disease or positive pressure ventilation, can displace the heart towards the feet. More extreme variations in cardiac axis can occur with conditions such as large pleural effusions, lobar collapse/resection, and dextrocardia, which may necessitate non-standard acoustic windows.

Probe orientation

Cardiology and radiology developed imaging conventions independently of each other, so they describe

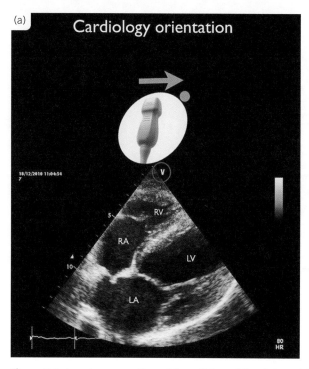
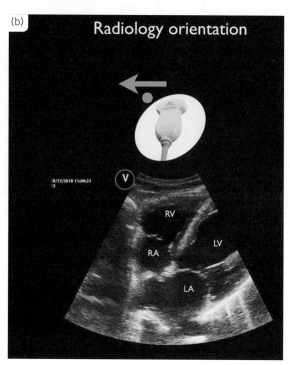

Figure 5.1 Imaging conventions: (a) cardiology; (b) radiology. LA, left atrium; LV, left ventricle; RA, right atrium; RV, right ventricle.

probe orientation differently, which is a common source of confusion when learning cardiac and non-cardiac US simultaneously.

By convention, in echocardiography, the field marker relates to the right side of the screen (as viewed by the operator), and the probe marker is pointed anywhere between the patient's shoulders and their left flank (Figure 5.1). In radiology, the field marker relates to the left side of the screen, and the probe marker is pointed either towards the patient's head or their right flank.

Once the type of probe is selected, the US machine will usually automatically select appropriate defaults, including marker orientation. Orientating the image to complex cardiac anatomy is difficult, particularly for novice echocardiographers, and using 'pattern recognition', from previous images and diagrams, is usually a more effective strategy for obtaining optimal views.

Probe kinematics

The echo probe can be manipulated in several ways to gain different angles through the heart and alter the

image obtained. A useful mnemonic for this is 'PART' (pressure, alignment, rotation, tilt). This textbook will use the following terms to describe probe kinematics:

- 'Footprint'—the point of contact between the probe and the skin
- 'Pressure'—the downward force applied by the probe to the patient. The 'ALARA' principle can be applied here, i.e. as low as reasonably achievable
- 'Alignment' (or 'sliding')—movement of the probe from one surface point to another, without changing any other aspect of its orientation
- 'Rotation'—twisting of the probe, clockwise or anticlockwise, from a fixed footprint
- 'Tilting'—non-rotational movement along the long edge of the probe from a fixed footprint, causing the object of interest to move 'out-of-plane'
- 'Rocking'—non-rotational movement along the short edge of the probe from a fixed footprint, causing the object of interest to move 'in-plane'.

Patience and deliberate movement of the probe, one manoeuvre at a time, pay dividends, particularly when scanning a patient on mechanical ventilation whose lungs intermittently veil the heart.

Improving image quality

Patient, operator, machine, and environmental factors all lead to difficulties with obtaining good-quality images. Suboptimal images are common in critical care due to poor patient positioning, background lighting, and the effects of mechanical ventilation.

A few general tips to aid in basic image acquisition:

- Firstly, decide whether to scan from the patient's left or right, and set the environment accordingly; each has obvious advantages and disadvantages.

- Get comfortable. Ergonomics are important for both your and the patient's comfort.

- The probe is usually best held like a pen using the heel of your hand as an anchor on the patient's chest to minimize unwanted movement.

- US gel improves contact with the skin. An excessive amount can lead to unwanted slipping of the probe across the chest wall.

- Usually, only small movements and gentle pressure are required to optimize the image.

- Imaging the patient in full expiration will usually improve parasternal and apical windows. Imaging in full inspiration may help subcostal views.

- Whenever possible, enter patient details and connect ECG leads to allow clip acquisition, storage, and optimal review. If an ECG is not available, or there are time constraints, the machine can be set to acquire a fixed recording time. However, expect these images to appear jerky on playback, due to clipping during an incomplete cardiac cycle.

Standard views

Comprehensive, departmental echocardiography is usually performed in a quiet, darkened room on a cooperative patient, and it can take an expert over 40 minutes to complete. All views are obtained systematically, according to a minimum dataset, and detailed quantitative interrogation of chambers and valves is routine. Such exacting standards are rarely necessary in the majority of acutely ill patients, in whom acuity of the clinical scenario often precludes a comprehensive study. However, it is possible to achieve sufficient images to answer specific focused questions in the majority of cases.

The focused echo exam is a simplified version of the comprehensive adult TTE dataset. It was designed to answer only the clinical questions relevant to diagnosis and immediate management. Standard focused views are:

- Parasternal long-axis (PLAX) view
- Parasternal short-axis (PSAX) view
- Apical four-chamber (A4C) view
- Subcostal four-chamber (S4C) view
- Subcostal inferior vena caval (SIVC) view.

Parasternal long-axis (PLAX) view

Useful for:

- Assessing gross left ventricular function
- Determining left ventricular chamber size
- Detecting anterior and posterior pericardial fluid
- Differentiating pericardial from pleural fluid.

Sonoanatomy

A portion of the right ventricular outflow tract (RVOT) is seen in the near field. The left ventricular cavity is contained anteriorly by the septal wall, posteriorly by the posterior free wall of the LV, and laterally by the MV, LA, and aortic valve (AV), all of which are seen on the right of the screen (Figure 5.2a and Video 1.1.1a ⊙).

In a true PLAX view, the apex of the heart should not be seen, and visualization of an apparent apex represents foreshortening of the LV. In the far field of a true PLAX view, it is not uncommon to see the anterolateral papillary muscle.

The anterior (AMVLs) and posterior mitral valve leaflets (PMVLs) are visualized, with the anterior leaflet closest to the AV. Only two AV leaflets are seen at any one time—the anterior one is always the right coronary cusp and, depending on probe position, the other is either the left or non-coronary cusp.

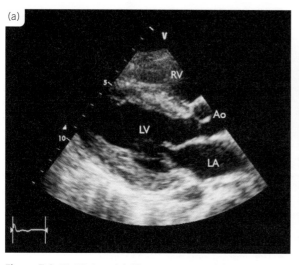
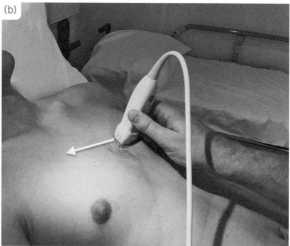

Figure 5.2 PLAX view: (a) 2D sonoanatomy; (b) probe position. Ao, aorta; LA, left atrium; LV, left ventricle; RV, right ventricle.

The descending aorta is seen in its short axis in the far field. It is important to include this in your image, because pericardial effusions will be seen above (anterior to) it and pleural effusions will be seen below and to its left.

Probe position and orientation

The PLAX window usually lies at the left sternal edge, anywhere between the second and fifth intercostal space. The scan plane is usually in a line running between the right shoulder and left hip, with the marker pointing towards the patient's right shoulder (Figure 5.2b). The probe should be held almost perpendicularly to the patient's chest wall.

Image optimization

The PLAX image is optimized by positioning the patient on their left side, with their left arm above the head and their breath held in expiration. These manoeuvres widen the rib spaces, bringing cardiac structures closer to the chest wall, but are seldom feasible in the acute setting. However, scanning a ventilated patient after they have been 'turned' to the left by the nursing staff can make a huge difference.

A foreshortened PLAX view cuts obliquely through the left ventricular wall and appears to show its apex on the left of the screen, which it should not. This can be improved by a combination of subtle tilting (to get both the MV and AV in view), rocking (to maximize the width of the ventricle), and rotation (to open up the ventricle, so that it goes off the left of the screen).

In a textbook PLAX view, the heart lies almost horizontally across the screen. In practice, it is often angled more obliquely. Trying another rib space can sometimes improve the image, but when this fails, the heart can be described as 'off-axis'.

Parasternal short-axis (PSAX) view

Useful for:

- Eyeballing left ventricular function
- Identifying gross RWMAs
- Comparing the size of both ventricles
- Identifying abnormal septal position and motion.

Sonoanatomy

Mid-papillary level

The best overall assessment of left and right ventricular function is obtained at this level. Here we see the uniformly thick walls of the LV and all its coronary artery territories (Figure 5.3a and Video 1.1.1b ⬤). The thin-walled, crescent-shaped RV is also usually seen, although dropout of the right ventricular free wall is common due its parallel alignment with the US beam.

At this level, the anterolateral and posteromedial papillary muscles are seen within the left ventricular chamber, in continuity with its endocardium. As

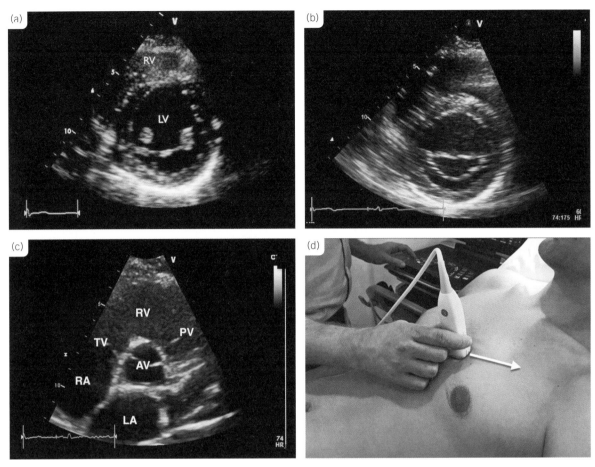

Figure 5.3 PSAX views: 2D sonanatomy at the (a) mid-papillary level, (b) mitral valve level, and (c) aortic valve level; (d) probe position. AV, aortic valve; LA, left atrium; LV, left ventricle; PV, pulmonary valve; RA, right atrium; RV, right ventricle; TV, tricuspid valve.

the beam is tilted further downwards, the papillary muscles disappear to produce the apical PSAX view.

Apical level

This view has little utility in FoCUS, but it can be readily found. You may notice increased twisting motion, when compared to the mid-papillary level.

> **Pitfall**
>
> The apex has increased radial contractility, compared to any other level, which is why global left ventricular ejection fraction should be assessed at the mid-papillary view.

Mitral valve level

Tilting the beam upwards from the mid-papillary level brings in a view sometimes referred to as the 'fish-mouth' view, so-called because the AMVL and PMVL open in resemblance to this (Figure 5.3b and Video 1.1.2c ⬤).

Aortic valve level

Tilting further upwards towards the chin reveals the AV in short axis, with the inflow and outflow of the right heart wrapped around it (Figure 5.3c and Video 1.1.2d ⬤). This view demonstrates both atria, the inter-atrial septum (IAS), the RV, and the main pulmonary artery, as well as the aortic, tricuspid, and pulmonary valves. This is an important view in advanced echocardiography, but it adds little value in FoCUS.

Probe position and orientation

The contact point on the chest wall is the same as in PLAX, but the probe is rotated 90° clockwise from it

(Figure 5.3d). Before rotation, placing the cursor (or an imaginary line) through the centre of the PLAX image sector will highlight the structures one should expect to see in cross-section after the probe is rotated. Once in PSAX, the probe marker usually points towards the patient's left shoulder, and tilting the beam up and down sweeps the image through the heart, generating the imaging planes described above.

Image optimization

A poor PLAX view usually means a poor PSAX view, so time taken optimizing the PLAX image before rotation is always well spent. Watching the screen while rotating the probe does not usually help optimize the image, and can distract the operator while the probe tilts, rocks, and slides off its window, causing the image to deteriorate. Somewhat counterintuitively, watching the probe (not the screen) can help to prevent this.

Subjects with poor windows in the upper chest (PLAX, PSAX) tend to have better lower windows (A4C, S4C), and vice versa.

Apical four-chamber (A4C) view

Useful for:

- Comparing the size of all four chambers
- Assessing longitudinal and radial function of both ventricles
- Atrial septal position and motion.

Sonoanatomy

All four chambers can be visualized simultaneously— the left heart on the right side of the screen, and vice versa. The normal LV is characteristically bullet-shaped, with a cylindrical base and a paraboloid apex. The normal RV is characteristically triangular-shaped, and its apex inserts into the interventricular septum (IVS) at approximately two-thirds of the length of the left ventricular cavity (Figure 5.4a and Video 1.1.2a 🎥).

In a true A4C, the IVS lies vertically and the atrioventricular valves lie horizontally. The apex is the thinnest part of the left ventricular wall and does not move during the cardiac cycle; instead, the rest of the heart moves up and down towards it. If the left ventricular apex is mobile and appears to be the thickest part of the LV, it is likely to be foreshortened.

Probe position and orientation

The probe should be positioned initially close to the 'apex beat' of the heart, with its marker directed to the patient's left, in line with the rib space, and the beam tilted up towards the right scapula (Figure 5.4b). However, the true apex is often found at least one rib space below this. More depth is usually required at this stage.

Image optimization

This view is often the most challenging to achieve in the supine position. Very small adjustments can transform an unidentifiable image into a useful one; unfortunately, these can also make a good image unidentifiable.

The ventricles can initially appear slanted. Lefttward slant can be corrected by a combination of medial re-alignment (along the rib space) and lateral rocking of the probe. Rightward slant can be corrected by lateral realignment and medial rocking of the beam. In an A4C view, the lateral wall of the RV is not always well seen, due to its parallel alignment with the US plane. This can be improved by realigning the beam laterally and rocking medially to form an 'RV focused view'.

If the atria are poorly visualized or if the coronary sinus appears in its long axis, running horizontally in the atrioventricular groove, then the beam must be too low. Tilting it upwards will bring the true A4C into view (Figure 5.4c). Further upward tilt opens up the aortic root, as it leaves the LV, to form the apical five-chamber view (A5C). If the A5C view is seen initially, then tilting slightly downwards should bring the A4C image into view (Figure 5.4d and Video 1.1.2b 🎥).

> **Pitfall**
>
> Foreshortening the ventricles gives a false impression of size and function. Sliding the probe to a lower rib space, and/or tilting the beam upwards, can correct foreshortened ventricles.

Subcostal four-chamber (S4C) view

Useful for:

- Rapid global assessment of cardiac movement or pericardial fluid in periarrest situations
- Evaluation of right ventricular wall thickness
- Situations when upper chest views are not possible (e.g. hyperinflation of the lungs).

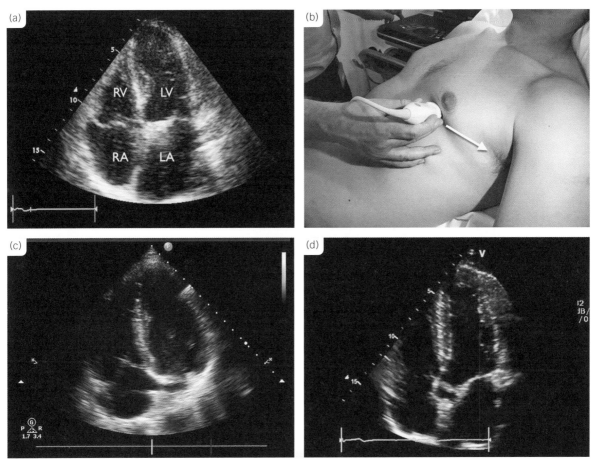

Figure 5.4 Apical views: (a) A4C view; (b) probe position for A4C; (c) with coronary sinus seen in the long axis (the beam is just posterior to A4C); (d) A5C view (the beam is just anterior to A4C). LA, left atrium; LV, left ventricle; RA, right atrium; RV, right ventricle.

Sonoanatomy

This resembles the A4C view leaning towards the right, and it contains the same anatomical structures, with the addition of the liver in the near field that acts as its acoustic window (Figure 5.5a and Video 1.1.3a).

Probe position and orientation

The probe is held almost flat against the stomach, to the right of the patient's xiphisternum, and pointed towards the left scapula, with the marker directed towards the patient's left flank (Figure 5.5b).

Image optimization

The patient should be supine, or slightly head-up, with their knees slightly bent to relax their abdominal musculature. Firm pressure is usually required, and this can cause some discomfort, especially in patients with abdominal pathology. Deep inspiration (or a mechanical inspiratory hold) may improve the subcostal view by displacing the heart caudally.

This is often the quickest view to obtain in an acute setting. However, recent abdominal surgery, dressings, drains, and abdominal pain can all make obtaining a subcostal view difficult, and sometimes impossible.

Subcostal inferior vena caval (SIVC) view

Useful for:

• Observing the size and collapsibility of the IVC to guide fluid therapy.

Sonoanatomy

The SIVC view visualizes the RA, IVC, and hepatic veins in their long axis (Figure 5.6a and Video 1.1.3b).

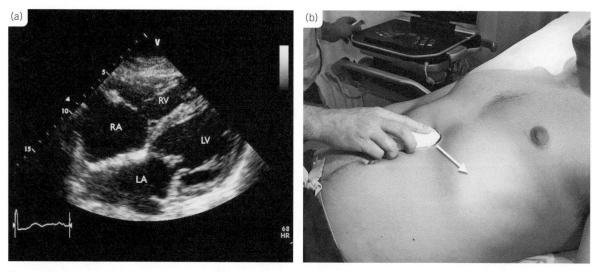

Figure 5.5 S4C view: (a) 2D sonoanatomy; (b) probe position. LA, left atrium; LV, left ventricle; RA, right atrium; RV, right ventricle.

Probe position and orientation

Obtain an S4C view with the RA in the centre of the screen, and slowly rotate the beam anticlockwise until the IVC is visualized in long axis as it passes through the liver (Figure 5.6b). Depending on the position of the heart, this rotation angle can be remarkably small—often well under 90° and occasionally as little as 30°. The IVC diameter and variability should be assessed visually or measured within 2 cm of the RA, immediately proximal to the hepatic vein.

Image optimization

Ensure that the true maximal luminal diameter is seen throughout the respiratory cycle. A clue to this is visualizing both endothelial margins of the IVC as sharp white lines, due to the bright specular reflection caused when the US beam is perpendicular to its walls.

> **Pitfall**
>
> The aorta can be mistaken for the IVC, as they run parallel to each other. The IVC must be seen to enter the RA (Videos 1.1.3b and 1.1.3d ⏺).

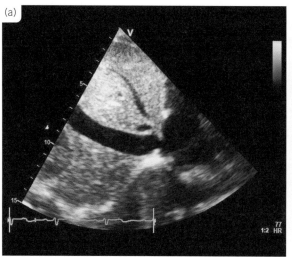
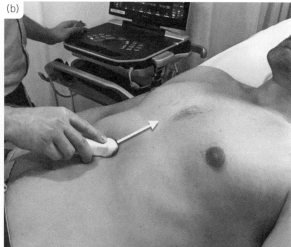

Figure 5.6 SIVC view: (a) 2D sonoanatomy; (b) probe position.

Advanced echocardiography

Once the practitioner has the grasp of basic echocardiographic views, it may be useful to gain experience by obtaining additional images, under supervision. These are:

- Right ventricular inflow (RVI) view
- Right ventricular outflow (RVO) view
- Apical two-chamber (A2C) view
- Apical three-chamber (A3C) view
- Subcostal short-axis (SSAX) view
- Suprasternal (SS) view.

Right ventricular inflow and outflow views

Both views can be found unintentionally when attempting to find PLAX, because they are so closely related to it. Once recognized, these views can act as useful landmarks to guide you back to PLAX.

The RVI view is achieved by tilting the beam downwards, towards the right hip, from the PLAX position. The RVI view visualizes the RA and tricuspid valve (TV) in the near field, and the anterior and inferior walls of the RV on the right and left sides of the screen, respectively (Figure 5.7a and Video 1.1.4b). It is useful for detecting tricuspid regurgitation (TR) jets and measuring their peak velocity, because they are often well aligned for Doppler assessment.

The RVO view is achieved by tilting the beam upwards, towards the left shoulder, from the PLAX position. The RVO view images the anterior wall of the RV, RVOT, pulmonary valve, and main pulmonary artery (Figure 5.7b and Video 1.1.4c).

Apical two- and three-chamber views

The A4C view visualizes the anterolateral and inferoseptal walls on the right and left sides of the screen, respectively.

Rotating the probe approximately 50° anticlockwise from A4C reveals the A2C view, which visualizes the anterior and inferior left ventricular walls on the right and left sides of the screen, respectively (Figure 5.8a and Video 1.1.2c).

Rotating the probe approximately 130° clockwise from A4C opens up the A3C view (also known as the apical long-axis view), which is similar in shape to PLAX and visualizes the anteroseptal and inferolateral ('posterior') walls on the right and left sides of the screen, respectively (Figure 5.8b and Video 1.1.2d).

In this way, the three apical views combined enable long-axis evaluation of all six left ventricular segments, providing the basis for comprehensive assessment of RWMAs and left ventricular ejection fraction (LVEF). The A3C view also has good alignment with the left ventricular outflow tract (LVOT), enabling measurement of

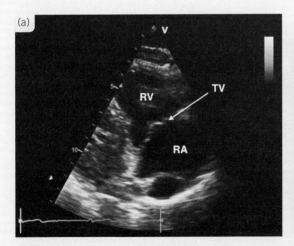
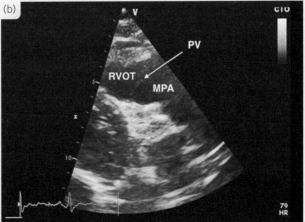

Figure 5.7 Variants on PLAX: (a) RVI view, 2D sonoanatomy; (b) RVO view, 2D sonoanatomy. MPA, main pulmonary artery; PV, pulmonary valve; RA, right atrium; RV, right ventricle; RVOT, right ventricular outflow tract; TV, tricuspid valve.

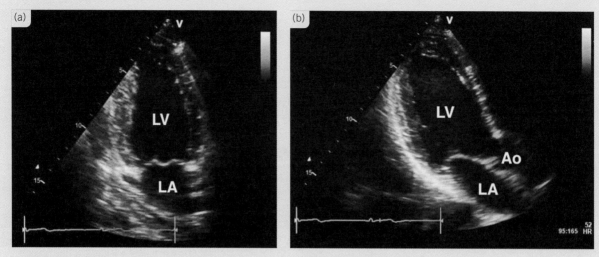

Figure 5.8 Variants on A4C: (a) A2C, 2D sonoanatomy; (b) A3C, 2D sonoanatomy. Ao, aorta; LA, left atrium; LV, left ventricle.

trans-aortic velocities, pressure gradients, and stroke volume.

Subcostal short-axis view

Anticlockwise rotation of 90° from the S4C view obtains a view similar in shape to PSAX, with all the same cuts, including the mid-papillary, MV, and AV levels, which can be found by tilting the beam up and down in exactly the same way (Video 1.1.3c 📹). The subcostal window is sometimes the only one available, and it can be an invaluable way to eyeball the ventricular size, shape, and systolic function in difficult situations. However, measurements are inadvisable in SSAX view, as it lacks the stability/reliability of other views.

Suprasternal view

The SS view can be obtained with the patient's neck extended and the probe placed in the suprasternal notch, rotated to the 1 o'clock position, and angled downwards towards the pelvis. It visualizes the arch of the aorta and its first three branches—the brachiocephalic, left common carotid, and left subclavian arteries (Figure 5.9). In intubated patients, obtaining a good image can be challenging, due to the presence of the endotracheal tube. However, the SS view is well aligned with the descending aorta, and so it can be a useful way to evaluate central blood flow using spectral Doppler in patients who are otherwise difficult to access with echo (e.g. pregnant patients or those in the operating theatre).

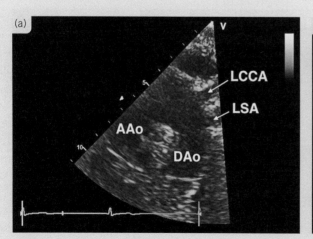
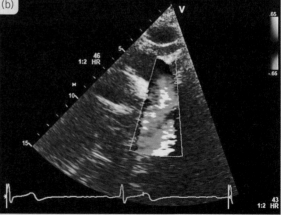

Figure 5.9 Suprasternal view: (a) 2D sonoanatomy; (b) with colour flow Doppler. AAo, ascending aorta; DAo, descending aorta; LCCA, left common carotid artery; LSA, left subclavian artery. For a colour version of this figure, please see colour plate section.

✓ Multiple choice questions

Interactive multiple choice questions to test your knowledge can be found in the Online appendix at www.oxfordmedicine.com/focusedicu. Please refer to your access card for further details.

Further reading

American Institute of Ultrasound in Medicine. Transducer manipulation for echocardiography. *Journal of Ultrasound in Medicine* 2005;**24**:733.

Anderson B. *Echocardiography: The Normal Examination and Echocardiographic Measurements*, 2nd ed. Brisbane: MGA Graphics; 2017.

Intensive Care Society. *Focused Intensive Care Echo (FICE)*. Available from: http://www.ics.ac.uk/ICS/fice.aspx [accessed 28 August 2018].

Jensen MB, Sloth E, Larsen KM, Schmidt MB. Transthoracic echocardiography for cardiopulmonary monitoring in intensive care. *European Journal of Anaesthesiology* 2004;**21**:700–7.

Wharton G, Steeds R, Allen J, *et al*. A minimum dataset for a standard adult transthoracic echocardiogram: a guideline protocol from the British Society of Echocardiography. *Echo Research and Practice* 2015;**2**:G9–24.

6

Transoesophageal echocardiography, sonoanatomy, and standard views

Nick Fletcher

Introduction

Transoesophageal echocardiography (TOE) was developed in the 1980s with the progression of endoscope and piezo-electric transducer technology. The oesophagus is an attractive site to place a US transducer, due to its proximity to the heart and great vessels. Unlike the surface windows, there is no intervening subcutaneous tissue, muscle, bone, or lung that produces the technical difficulty experienced when attempting TTE in critical care patients. There is not the same requirement to position patients, as TOE is normally performed in the supine position. In general, resolution of cardiac structures is enhanced and artefact is reduced with TOE, as compared with TTE. TOE may seem complex to those who are trying to master basic TTE. However, a simple understanding of how transducer rotation interacts with the position of the heart within the thorax will allow the learner to easily develop the basic concepts of TOE.

This chapter will describe the omniplane probe (with its scan planes) and indications, contraindications, and complications of TOE, before defining a scheme for focused TOE assessment in a critically ill patient. It will highlight the cardiac structures that are best imaged using either TTE or TOE, and outline specific clinical applications (including suspected aortic dissection, left atrial appendage (LAA) thrombus, mitral disease, and right ventricular failure) that lend themselves to TOE assessment.

TOE probe technology and use

A TOE probe is essentially a US transducer mounted inside the tip of a sealed endoscope without the optic fibres. Probes were initially monoplane, and then biplane, with limited movement of the transducer. All TOE probes are now omniplane, with continuous rotation of the transducer possible between 0° and 180°. There are two wheels mounted on the endoscope handle that enable anteflexion and retroflexion of the probe tip, in addition to lateral flexion in both directions (Figure 6.1). Three-dimensional (3D) TOE probes are now available, although their utility in critical care patients is not yet established. Compared to a fibreoptic endoscope, the TOE probe tip is slightly expanded, and care is needed when inserting it into the oesophagus. Jaw thrust or jaw lift is necessary to insert the probe, although many would recommend the use of a laryngoscope, as for endotracheal intubation. Whereas, in the outpatient setting, the procedure may be performed in the awake patient using topical anaesthesia, in the intensive care setting, sedation is essential and paralysis may be desirable. Additional care is required to ensure that the patient does not cause bite damage to the delicate probe casing. Regular visual checks of the probe and electrical testing are recommended. A system of probe decontamination and storage is necessary between episodes of use; this is normally arranged in line with the hospital infection control guidelines.

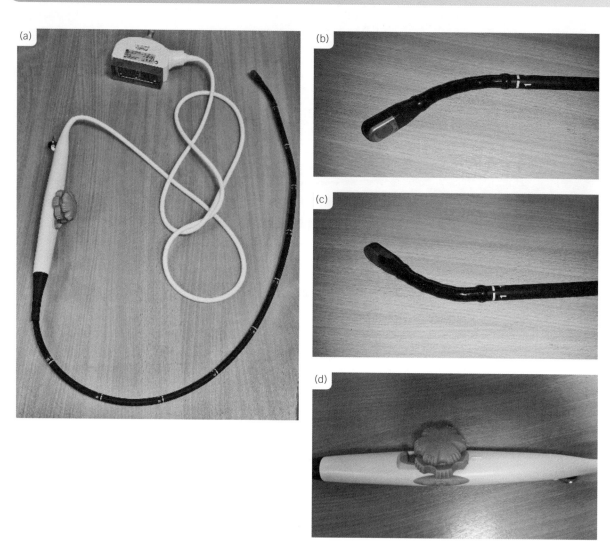

Figure 6.1 Various photographs of a TOE probe. (a) The whole probe. (b) The probe tip in anteflexion. (c) The probe tip in retroflexion. (d) The handle with control wheels and buttons for transducer rotation.

Reproduced with kind permission from GE Heathcare.

Contraindications and complications

The absolute contraindication to insertion of a TOE probe is obstruction of the oesophagus from adhesions or carcinoma. Effort should be made to exclude symptoms of dysphagia prior to initiating a scan. If resistance is felt on insertion of the probe, the probe should not be introduced any further. Relative contraindications include recent gastrointestinal bleeding, recent gastric surgery (including for weight loss), oesophageal varices, and pharyngeal pouch. Caution is required in the anticoagulated patient, although many such patients have undergone TOE examination without harm. If a patient is not already intubated and ventilated, then this should be considered

as the safest method of maintaining the airway during the procedure. Prior to this, the nasogastric tube should be suctioned to empty the stomach, and it may even be necessary to temporarily withdraw and reinsert it, to ensure it does not obstruct the US window.

Information on complications has been obtained mostly from cardiology or cardiac anaesthesia, and major adverse events—trauma to the oesophagus or significant bleeding—range in frequency from 1:1000 to 1:10,000. It is possible that this rate may be higher in frail critically ill patients, particularly if the operator is not experienced in probe insertion. It is essential that force is never applied; the probe should pass easily. Other complications that may occur include dental damage, sore throat, and minor bleeding. If there is concern that blood was seen on the probe, then haemoglobin levels should be monitored regularly.

TOE scan planes

The TOE US plane is displayed on the screen with a similar convention to TTE, with the apex of the field situated at the top. Right-sided cardiac structures are shown on the left side of the sector display, and a display of the transducer rotation angle is featured on the top left of the screen. The key difference with TTE is the posterior origin of the US sector. There are four main defined positions of the probe within the oesophagus at which images are obtained: the upper oesophagus, mid oesophagus, transgastric, and deep transgastric. At each position, the probe is first rotated, then the transducer plane is rotated to the desired position, and finally a little anteflexion or retroflexion may be applied to the probe tip, using the endoscopic wheel to obtain optimal images. Figure 6.2 shows how the US plane interacts with the cardiac structures at different

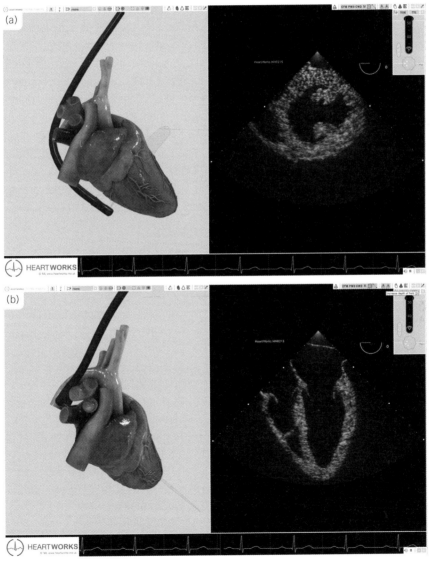

Figure 6.2 Heartworks simulator pictures showing the position of the TOE transducer tip in relation to the heart, and the corresponding 2D image sector obtained. (a) The transgastric mid-papillary view where the probe tip is below the heart, closest to the inferior wall. (b) The four-chamber view where the probe lies behind the left atrium and the sector passes through all four chambers.
Reproduced with kind permission from Heartworks.

positions to produce an image. Guided instruction on one of the echocardiography simulators is proven to be advantageous for the TOE novice, to quickly improve their understanding of this sonoantomy. A comprehensive TOE examination has around 20 planes, depending on which particular guideline one uses, and a significant proportion of these are designed to view the aortic arch and descending aorta. As TTE will usually precede TOE in critical care, a more focused cardiac study may be performed. As TOE views are often superior to those of TTE, with reduced surface artefact, high-quality, accurate Doppler signals may be obtained and the appropriate measurements may be accurately recorded.

The TOE scan planes were originally based on the existing TTE views, and there are some obvious correlations between them. The mid-oesophageal four-chamber can be understood as an 'upside-down' apical four-chamber view. Similarly, the mid-oesophageal two-chamber and long-axis views can be correlated to the other two rotated apical surface views. The TOE transgastric views can be correlated with PSAX views, with the important difference that the inferior wall is closest to the probe, at the apex of the sector, and the anterior wall is furthest away.

Indications for TOE

TOE is well established within cardiothoracic anaesthesia and intensive care practice but is not yet mainstream practice in other branches of perioperative and critical care. The most common indication for TOE in the critical care unit is inadequate TTE views of essential structures in a patient with unexplained instability or failure to progress. The ribs and costal cartilages produce artefact and acoustic shadowing, and increased subcutaneous fat in obese patients attenuates the US signal. Aerated lung is a poor transmitter of US, and this is accentuated in ventilated patients. In the post-cardiac surgery patient, substernal air and subcostal drains limit the windows and utility of TTE. Table 6.1 shows which structures can generally be seen more clearly or measured more accurately with TOE, rather than TTE. There are differences in individual patients, as the orientation of the heart in the thorax is variable. Because of the enhanced views of certain structures, there are a number of well-established indications for TOE for specific pathological conditions that may occur in critical care and some that are specific to critical care. These are detailed in Box 6.1.

Table 6.1 Structures that are best imaged with either TTE or TOE

TTE	TOE
Left ventricular apex	Left atrium and appendage
Tricuspid valve and aortic valve Doppler	Mitral valve
Aortic arch	Aortic valve
Pleura and diaphragms	Aortic root
Inferior vena cava M-mode	Descending aorta
	Atrial septum
	Superior vena cava
	Posterior pericardium
	Left atrium

Box 6.1 Indications for TOE in critical care

- To further investigate endocarditis of the MV and AV
- To exclude LAA thrombus in AF
- To classify the mechanism of, and quantify, MR
- To diagnose aortic dissection and identify complications
- To investigate the causes of failure to wean from the ventilator
- In the patient with severe chest trauma
- In patients with acute respiratory distress syndrome (ARDS) and right ventricular dysfunction
- For semi-continuous, short-term monitoring and management in the haemodynamically unstable ventilated patient
- In the intubated patient on extracorporeal membrane oxygenation

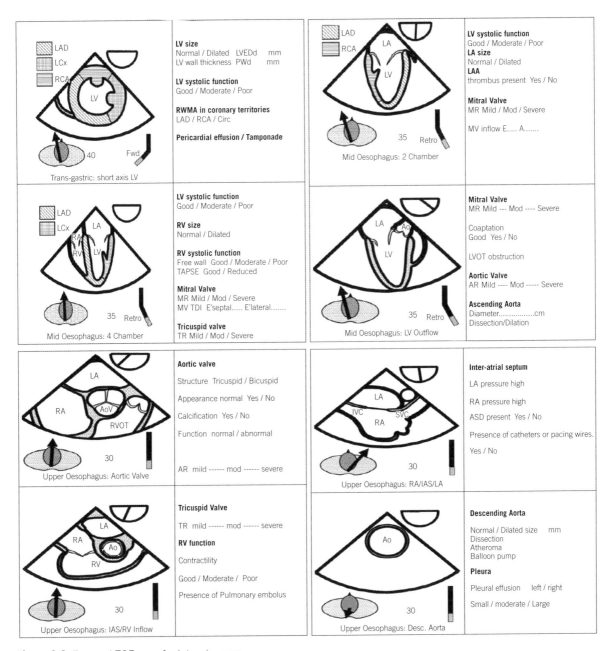

Figure 6.3 Focused TOE scan for intensive care.

Focused TOE

Figure 6.3 sets out a scheme for a focused intensive care scan. The indication for TOE is most likely to be poor TTE views or one from Box 6.1. The critical care clinician will have a specific question in mind, and the views shown in Figure 6.3 should be adequate to identify all significant pathology relevant to the heart. The information relevant to each plane is displayed next to the image of the scan plane. Focused TOE is an appropriate modality to monitor and manage an unstable, shocked patient, as the probe can be left in place for up to 2 hours to obtain sequential imaging. The comprehensive study is structured to give a full evaluation of all cardiac structures, the great vessels, and any coexisting pathology. Findings such as MV prolapse, valvular vegetations, and perivalvular abscesses should be recorded and referred to cardiologists for further imaging and management.

Specific clinical applications

The following are some specific uses of TOE in critical care and relate to the indications in Box 6.1. See also Figure 6.4 and Videos 1.2.1–1.2.4 🔊.

- Assessment of the shock state: excellent views of both ventricles, including all their coronary territories, are possible with TOE, as are views of the pericardium. Dynamic assessment of fluid responsiveness can be made using M-mode of the superior vena cava (SVC). A disposable mini-monoplane TOE probe with a CE mark for 72 hours has recently been described in this context.

- Aortic dissection: TOE is a very good diagnostic tool for dissection in the ascending and descending aorta, with the added value of allowing dynamic assessment of the AV function and the presence of pericardial blood (Figure 6.4a and Video 1.2.1 🔊).

- LAA thrombus: if patients in AF suffer a potentially embolic event, TOE is the cardiac investigation of choice. TOE should also be considered when converting a patient to sinus rhythm (Figure 6.4b and Video 1.2.2 🔊).

- Assessment of the MV: severe MR can occur acutely, mimic adult respiratory distress syndrome, and be a cause of ventilator weaning failure. TOE

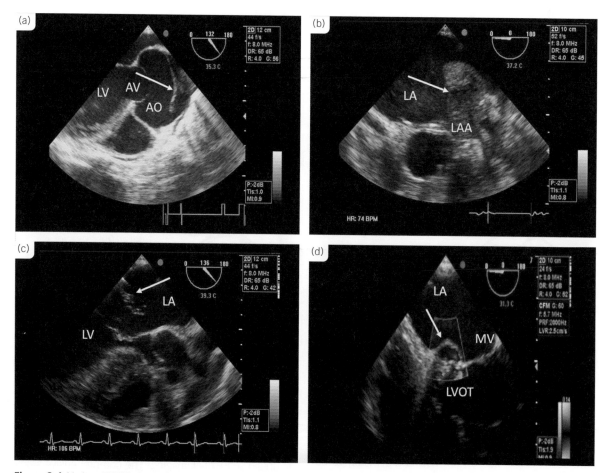

Figure 6.4 Various TOE images. (a) Aortic dissection showing a prominent intimal flap and dilated aortic valve. (b) A large atrial appendage thrombus encroaching on the left atrium. (c) Flail posterior leaflet of the mitral valve. (d) Aortic root abscess with colour Doppler to show its pulsatility. Ao, aorta; AV, aortic valve; LA, left atrium; LAA, left atrial appendage; LV, left ventricle; LVOT, left ventricular outflow tract; MV, mitral valve. For a colour version of this figure, please see colour plate section.

gives optimum views of the MV (Figure 6.4c and Video 1.2.3 ⬤).

- Right ventricular assessment: TTE may not allow optimal imaging of the RV in those with lung disease on mechanical ventilation or oscillation due to signal dropout. TOE can provide good-quality multiplane assessment of the RV in this context, allowing adjustment of ventilator settings (Video 1.2.4 ⬤).

- Pericardial collection: in post-cardiac surgical patients, TTE views may not be adequate to exclude a localized haematoma and tamponade. In particular, the posterior pericardium is particularly difficult to view without TOE.

- Assessment of SVC collapsibility: this is a validated assessment of fluid responsiveness, which can only be utilized with TOE. An observed respiratory collapsibility of the SVC of >36% suggests the patient is likely to be fluid-responsive. The SVC view can be obtained in the upper oesophageal plane.

✔ Multiple choice questions

Interactive multiple choice questions to test your knowledge can be found in the Online appendix at www.oxfordmedicine.com/focusedicu. Please refer to your access card for further details.

Further reading

Charron C, Vignon P, Prat G, *et al*. Number of supervised studies required to reach competence in advanced critical care transesophageal echocardiography. *Intensive Care Medicine* 2013;**39**:1019–24.

Hahn RT, Abraham T, Adams MS. Guidelines for performing a comprehensive transesophageal echocardiographic examination: recommendations from the American Society of Echocardiography and the Society of Cardiovascular Anesthesiologists. *Anesthesia and Analgesia* 2014;**118**:21–68.

Vieillard-Baron A. International consensus statement on training standards for advanced critical care echocardiography. *Intensive Care Medicine* 2014;**40**:654–66.

7

Left ventricular assessment

Marcus Peck

Introduction

Clinical assessment of left ventricular function is challenging in critically ill patients. Coexistent organ failure, systemic inflammation, and intravascular changes in hydrostatic and oncotic pressures all mean that patterns of illness and clinical signs are not as consistent as they are in the outpatient setting and ventricular filling pressure is notoriously difficult to assess. In observational studies, clinical recognition of impaired LVEF by expert intensivists has a sensitivity of 54–60% and specificity of 69–83%. In clinical practice, all too often the true diagnosis is revealed after a chosen treatment strategy has failed and the clinical situation has deteriorated.

FoCUS assessment by non-experts has been shown to be superior to clinical examination for identification of LVEF and structural abnormalities associated with chronic disease, such as left ventricular hypertrophy (LVH) and scarred wall segments, which can impact on immediate management of critically ill patients.

This chapter will outline the relevant structure and function of the LV and its common pathophysiology such as LVH, RWMAs, systolic and diastolic heart failure, and Takotsubo cardiomyopathy. It will describe how FoCUS can be used to assess left ventricular size, shape, wall thickness, and systolic function, including linear, area, and volumetric methods, and how loading conditions impact on these. It will demonstrate how to recognize common left ventricular pathophysiology, and the advanced section will introduce how tissue Doppler can be used to assess systolic and diastolic function.

Relevant anatomy

Shape

The healthy LV is the largest chamber of the heart, with its most muscular walls. Its internal chamber is shaped like a bullet, with a cylindrical base and a hemispheric apex.

Axis

In its short (or 'minor') axis, the normal left ventricular cavity is circular. The LV's long (or 'major') axis varies remarkably between critically ill patients, depending on patient positioning, body habitus, and regional lung volumes. Consequently, the true left ventricular apex may be found anywhere between the lower left parasternal edge and the axilla, and up to two rib spaces below the palpable 'apex beat'.

Axis is important because 'off-axis' imaging can lead to significant error when assessing left ventricular size.

Size

Left ventricular end-diastolic volume depends on a number of factors, including patient size, preload, and the presence of pathology such as valvular and ischaemic heart disease (IHD). A dilated LV indicates adaption to chronic disease and has implications for the immediate clinical management of a haemodynamically unstable patient; hence, it is the subject of a core FoCUS question.

Walls

The left ventricular cavity is lined entirely by compacted trabeculated muscle and contains the anterolateral and posteromedial papillary muscles (PMs).

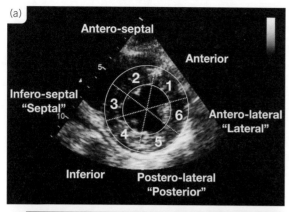

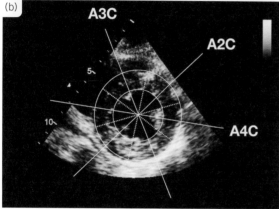

Figure 7.1 A parasternal short-axis view, frozen at end-diastole, demonstrating: (a) the six segments of the LV; and (b) the segments visualized in each apical view.

The normal LV has walls of similar circumferential thickness; any significant asymmetry is pathological.

The basal and mid levels of the LV are each divided into six short-axis segments; the apex has four (plus an apical cap). This model is used in comprehensive echo to describe regional wall thickness and motion. In any true long-axis view, two opposite walls will be seen simultaneously (Figure 7.1).

Blood supply

The LV's blood supply is fairly predictable, with considerable overlap between coronary territories (Figure 7.2).

Whereas the anterolateral PM is supplied by two blood vessels, the posteromedial PM has only one [a branch of the right coronary artery (RCA)], meaning this is the most likely one to rupture post-myocardial infarction (causing a PMVL flail).

Relevant physiology

Global wall motion

Healthy left ventricular walls contract, thicken, and move towards the centre of the cavity equally during systole. The LV shortens longitudinally, radially, and circumferentially in one simultaneous, twisting motion.

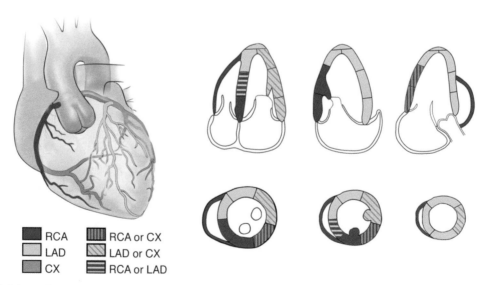

Figure 7.2 Schematic representation of regional left ventricular blood supply.

While each of these components is important, radial shortening contributes the most to left ventricular systolic ejection. This is in contrast to the RV, which contracts almost entirely longitudinally, in a peristaltic fashion, from apex to base.

Visualizing endocardial wall thickening and motion during systole provides the foundation for assessment of RWMAs and LVEF.

Left ventricular function

The LV has two essential functions: to eject blood into the systemic circulation during systole and to fill again during diastole. To pump effectively, it must oscillate efficiently between each of these tasks and accomplish both well.

Systolic function

Systolic ejection depends on four properties: left ventricular preload, afterload, contractility, and geometric shape. Clinical assessment of systolic function is difficult for a number of reasons—the LV's dependence on preload and afterload makes accurate bedside quantification of contractility extremely complex, and most symptoms and signs of heart failure are caused by diastolic dysfunction (DD), which is increasingly prevalent in isolation from systolic dysfunction.

Diastolic function

Diastolic filling of the LV has two distinct phases: 'early' filling associated with myocardial relaxation, and late 'active' filling associated with atrial contraction.

Despite the nomenclature, early filling is, in fact, an active, adenosine triphosphate (ATP)-dependent process, which literally sucks blood into the heart and explains why acute ischaemia causes such a dramatic fall in left ventricular relaxation and compliance. Early filling is the dominant process in the young, but as a patient ages, their LV becomes progressively less compliant, due to increasing viscoelastic properties and filling depends increasingly on atrial contraction (and sinus rhythm).

Relevant pathophysiology

This section will discuss the pathophysiology of conditions commonly seen in ICU. How to image these will be described later in the chapter.

Left ventricular hypertrophy

Left ventricular wall thickness increases with strenuous physical exercise and certain inherited and acquired diseases. In the inherited form, known as hypertrophic cardiomyopathy (HCM), left ventricular hypertrophy (LVH) is asymmetrical and tends to affect the basal septum more than the posterior wall. Acquired LVH usually begins as an adaptive mechanism to protect against wall stress from either pressure (afterload) or volume (preload) overload, and hypertrophy is generally distributed symmetrically.

The terms concentric and eccentric refer to the distribution of increased muscle mass, compared to left ventricular chamber size. Both can be physiological or pathological.

Concentric hypertrophy (small LV with high relative wall thickness) is seen in weightlifters and patients with untreated hypertension or AS due to chronic pressure overload. Concentric LVH is easiest to spot and is strongly associated with DD.

Eccentric hypertrophy (enlarged LV with low relative wall thickness) is seen in runners, swimmers, and patients with chronic valvular regurgitation due to volume overload, which causes the LV to dilate. Eccentric LVH is harder to spot, but a thickened and dilated LV carries the highest risk of cardiovascular death.

Early recognition is important, because LVH has the potential for microvascular ischaemia, DD, and dynamic LVOT obstruction. Patients with LVH need high left ventricular filling pressure to maintain preload and cardiac output; consequently, their therapeutic window for fluid therapy is notoriously narrow.

Systolic anterior motion

Basal septal hypertrophy has the potential to cause life-threatening 'systolic anterior motion' (SAM) of the MV, particularly when the LV is underfilled, hyper-contractile, and exposed to a low afterload. In SAM, high-velocity blood in the LVOT causes low pressure that sucks the anterior MV leaflet into it, producing dynamic LVOT obstruction and functional MR.

Likelihood of SAM increases with inotropic support, abnormal MV attachments (seen in HCM), and right heart failure associated with impaired left ventricular filling. Twenty-five per cent of HCM patients have demonstrable SAM at rest; in the remaining 75%, SAM can be provoked by exercise/stress and acute illness.

If SAM is observed in a FoCUS study, it should prompt immediate fluid resuscitation, introduction of vasopressors, withdrawal of inotropic therapy, and urgent expert referral.

Ischaemic regional wall motion abnormalities

In acute coronary syndrome (ACS), the myocardial territory supplied by the affected vessel demonstrates reduced excursion and thickening, known as an RWMA.

In patients with a high clinical suspicion of ACS but an indeterminate electrocardiogram (ECG), reversible RWMAs confirm the diagnosis. Conversely, in a patient with ECG abnormalities, absence of RWMAs after 45 minutes excludes ischaemia. RWMAs seen with resting echocardiography cannot distinguish between ischaemia and infarction. However, lack of reversibility over serial studies makes the latter more likely.

Non-ischaemic regional wall motion abnormalities

Not all RMWAs are ischaemic in origin. Non-ischaemic RMWAs are characterized by normal wall thickening, but reduced wall motion; causes include:

- Conduction defects:
  - Left bundle branch block (LBBB)
  - Paced rhythm
  - Wolff–Parkinson–White syndrome
- Ventricular interdependence:
  - Right ventricular pressure/volume overload
- Pericardial constriction.

For this reason, all patients with LBBB or ventricular pacing will have at least mild left ventricular systolic impairment.

Heart failure

In a general ICU patient, acute heart failure tends to be associated with a non-dilated, globally impaired LV and shock. Examples include post-cardiac arrest stunning (Chapter 21) and severe sepsis (Chapter 25).

Chronic heart failure can be associated with both reduced and preserved ejection fraction (known as HFrEF and HFpEF, respectively). Regardless of subtype, most symptoms and signs of decompensated heart failure (exertional and paroxysmal nocturnal dyspnoea, orthopnoea, and peripheral oedema) are caused mechanistically by DD.

Heart failure with reduced ejection fraction

Unlike the compliant, thin-walled RV, the LV does not dilate acutely when it becomes overloaded. Remodelling takes time, which is measured in weeks and months, rather than hours and days; therefore, a dilated LV suggests chronic disease.

Heart failure with preserved ejection fraction

When the clinical features of heart failure coexist with an ejection fraction (EF) of >50%, it is known as HFpEF. Epidemiologically, HFpEF is increasingly prevalent and destined to become the most common form of heart failure in western communities. Compared to those with HFrEF, patients with HFpEF tend to be older, female, and have less IHD and more non-cardiac comorbidities such as diabetes, obesity, chronic obstructive pulmonary disease, and peptic ulcer disease. At least 70% of patients with HFpEF have demonstrable DD at rest.

Importantly, a normal FoCUS study does not exclude heart failure from the differential diagnosis.

Takotsubo cardiomyopathy

This is a stress-induced cardiomyopathy that affects predominantly peri-menopausal women, but not exclusively so. Patients present within hours of a stressful experience (emotional or physiological) with chest pain, heart failure, non-specific ECG changes, and reversible RWMAs that do not correlate with coronary territories. FoCUS reveals systolic apical ballooning, resembling a Japanese lobster pot, which gives the condition its name.

To make a diagnosis of Takotsubo cardiomyopathy, coronary angiography must be normal and RWMAs must be completely reversible (although this may take several weeks). Suspected cases require cardiology referral for urgent confirmation, because inotropic agents paradoxically worsen shock and should be withdrawn immediately.

Echo assessment

'Eyeballing' left ventricular size

Knowing at a glance whether any cardiac chamber is large or small comes with experience, but this skill can be readily learnt during FoCUS training programmes.

Visual assessment, or 'eyeballing', involves comparing the optimized 2D image (frozen or moving) with length markers displayed at the edge of the field, to gain an overall impression of chamber size or wall motion.

Advantages of this approach are that it is quick and it can be done to some degree in all views (PLAX, PSAX, and A4C being most useful). However, when multiple cardiac chambers are enlarged, visual assessment can be misleading.

Whether using visual assessment or measurement, care must be taken to obtain optimal images of the correct shape and size. Ellipsoid images in short-axis views usually suggest probe malrotation, which can introduce measurement error.

If the left ventricular cavity is imaged tangentially, off its true long axis, it will be foreshortened and all its internal dimensions will be underestimated (Figure 7.3). A common example is an A4C view with the probe placed too high on the chest wall, which makes both ventricles appear short, rounded, and similar in shape and size.

To find the true apex in A4C, remember that:

1. The normal apex is the thinnest segment of the left ventricular wall. If it appears to have a similar or greater wall thickness than the other visible left ventricular walls, it is likely to be cut tangentially, and not be the true apex.

2. During the cardiac cycle, the true apex does not move and the base of the heart moves up and down relative to it. A mobile apex is unlikely to be the true apex.

In all cases, the probe should be manipulated slowly and carefully to obtain an image with the correct proportions and largest dimensions possible.

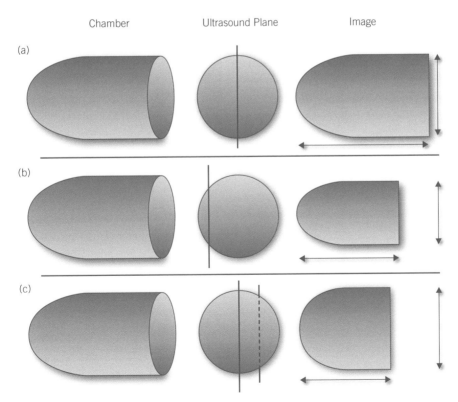

Figure 7.3 A schematic demonstrating foreshortening of the LV. (a) On-axis imaging with correct dimensions. (b) Tangential imaging with all dimensions underestimated. (c) Oblique imaging with correct width but underestimated length.

Measuring left ventricular end-diastolic dimensions

Measurements are not essential in FoCUS, but to be able to recognize significant pathology, it is important to remember some reference values.

'Left ventricular internal dimension in diastole' (LVIDd) defines left ventricular dilatation (Table 7.1) and is measured in the PLAX view (Figure 7.4). An LVIDd of >6.4 cm in a man and >5.8 cm in a woman suggests that the LV is at least moderately dilated.

End-diastole can be defined by any of the following:

1. The frame immediately after MV closure
2. The frame when left ventricular dimension is at its largest
3. The beginning of QRS complex.

End-systole can be defined by any of the following:

1. The frame immediately after AV closure
2. The frame when left ventricular dimension is at its smallest
3. The end of the T wave.

To measure LVIDd, first obtain an optimal PLAX view, with maximum left ventricular basal width, and freeze the image at end-diastole. Find the tip of the open MV leaflets, and bisect the LV at this level, perpendicular to its long axis, using 2D calipers. LVIDd is the distance along this line between the opposing endocardial borders (blood–tissue interface). This process can be repeated at end-systole to obtain left ventricular internal dimension in systole (LVIDs).

Pitfall

When the heart is visibly 'off-axis' in PLAX, M-mode will overestimate left ventricular dimensions, and 2D measurement is preferred.

Wall thickness

Significant LVH is usually obvious when eyeballing any FoCUS view, as long as care is taken not to overestimate wall thickness by oblique imaging. Eyeballing wall thickness is more difficult when chambers are dilated, so measuring it can be useful. Wall thickness of >1.5 cm suggests significant LVH.

End-diastolic dimensions of the interventricular septum (IVSd) and posterior free wall (LVPWd) can be measured in the same way as LVIDd, with calipers placed at the epicardial and endocardial surfaces of each wall (Figure 7.4 and Table 7.2).

Table 7.1 Reference values for LVIDd in men and women

LV size	LVIDd (males)	LVIDd (females)
Small	≤4.1 cm	≤3.9 cm
Normal	4.2–5.9 cm	3.9–5.3 cm
Mildly enlarged	6.0–6.3 cm	5.4–5.7 cm
Moderately enlarged	6.4–6.8 cm	5.8–6.1 cm
Severely enlarged	≥6.9 cm	≥6.2 cm

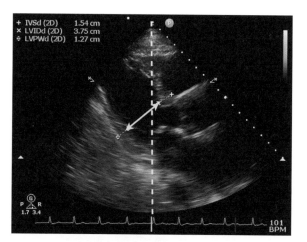

Figure 7.4 A PLAX image demonstrating LVIDd measurement using 2D versus M-mode. This heart's axis lies obliquely to the direction of the US field. The M-mode (large broken white line) would grossly overestimate the LVIDd, so the correct method to assess this is with 2D calipers (oblique arrow).

Table 7.2 End-diastolic LV wall thickness values

Severity of LVH	Wall thickness (males and females)
Normal	0.6–1.2 cm
Mild	1.3–1.5 cm
Moderate	1.6–1.9 cm
Severe	≥2.0 cm

Assessing wall motion

Regional systolic thickening is usually assessed visually, in conjunction with wall motion, and described in terms seen in Table 7.3. PSAX visualizes all coronary territories simultaneously (Figure 7.1).

> **Pitfall**
> Severe LWMAs are usually obvious, but recognizing mild RWMAs is difficult for inexperienced echo practitioners.

Assessment of left ventricular systolic function

Visual estimation of EF is the mainstay of FoCUS assessment of systolic function and will be described in Left ventricular ejection fraction—visual estimation, p. 63. However, other linear, 2D, and volumetric assessments exist and can be useful adjuncts:

1. Fractional shortening (FS)
2. E-point to septal separation (EPSS)
3. Mitral annular plane systolic excursion (MAPSE)
4. Fractional area change (FAC)
5. EF—visual estimation and biplane (Simpson's) method.

Each has limitations, but utility in certain circumstances, and the most accurate assessment will involve a combination of these methods.

Fractional shortening

Once LVIDd and LVIDs are measured, FS is calculated automatically, according to the equation:

$$FS = \left[(LVIDd - LVIDs)/LVIDd \right] \times 100$$

Values of FS corresponding to normal and abnormal left ventricular systolic function can be found in Table 7.4.

FS is quick and easy to perform; hence, it is widely quoted in comprehensive studies. It has low inter- and intra-observer variability and has been widely validated in valvular heart disease and the outpatient setting. However, it is based on a single linear dimension, so it is vulnerable to error in the presence of basal RWMAs and it performs less well in sick hearts. Interventricular delay, paradoxical septal motion, and poor M-mode alignment are other sources of inaccuracy. Consequently, FS is not a useful assessment in critically ill patients.

Once left ventricular dimensions are recorded, many echo machines automatically estimate FS, EF, stroke volume (SV), and even cardiac output, using something called the Teichholz formula. This method is no longer recommended, as it is based on geometric assumptions that are inaccurate in the presence of pathology.

E-point to septal separation

In PLAX, the tip of the maximally opened AMVL is known as the E-point, and the perpendicular distance between this and the left endocardial border of the IVS is known as the EPSS (Video 1.3.1 ⬤).

In the absence of mitral stenosis (MS) or ventriculoseptal defect, the extent to which the AMVL

Table 7.3 Definition of regional wall motion

Description	Definition
Normal	Normal excursion and systolic thickening >50%
Hypokinesia	Reduced excursion and systolic thickening 10–40%
Akinesia	No excursion and systolic thickening <10%
Dyskinesia	Outward motion and systolic thinning

Table 7.4 Relationship of fractional shortening with left ventricular systolic function

Fractional shortening	Degree of LVSD
25–43%	Nil (normal)
20–24%	Mild
15–19%	Moderate
<15%	Severe

opens in diastole correlates with early trans-mitral flow (E wave), and therefore SV. High-output states cause the AMVL to touch the IVS; in extremely low-output states, it hardly moves at all. In addition, LVIDd increases in HFrEF. Consequently, the distance between the E point and IVS correlates with left ventricular systolic dysfunction (LVSD). In a healthy LV, EPSS is <6 mm, and this increases as left ventricular function deteriorates.

EPSS measurement is relatively easy to perform in PLAX, using 2D calipers, but it is poorly validated and interpretation has limitations; it will be underestimated in asymmetrical basal hypertrophy and overestimated whenever AMVL opening is restricted (i.e. MS and severe AR). EPSS may be more useful as an adjunct when eyeballing left ventricular function.

Mitral annular plane systolic excursion

As the LV ejects, it shortens longitudinally, and in A4C, the distance that the lateral MV annulus travels towards the left ventricular apex during systole is known as MAPSE (Figure 7.5). Despite contributing relatively little to systolic ejection, longitudinal function of the LV tends to decline before radial function, so MAPSE is a useful way of detecting early disease.

MAPSE can be eyeballed in 2D or measured using M-mode in A4C. To measure it, obtain a true A4C view

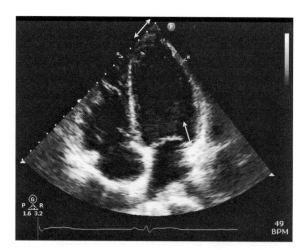

Figure 7.5 An A4C view, demonstrating MAPSE. The arrow at the mitral annulus (representing MAPSE) is duplicated next to the length marker on the top left of the image. Eyeballing would suggest that MAPSE is approximately 2 cm, which is well inside the normal range.

and place the M-mode sampling line over the lateral MV annulus; click again to start the M-mode trace, then freeze it, and place calipers at its lowest and highest points.

MAPSE of >12 mm is a predictor of LVEF of >50%, and MAPSE of <6 mm predicts severe LVSD.

MAPSE is technically easy to learn and has good accuracy for estimating EF when performed by novice observers. Accurate MAPSE requires reasonable 2D endocardial definition, a true A4C view, and correct (longitudinal) M-mode alignment. Basal lateral wall RWMAs will cause MAPSE to underestimate systolic function.

Fractional area change

The assessments described so far rely on linear measurements to estimate LVEF, which is based on volume. FAC is a step closer to LVEF, because it is based on area (not length) and it can take RWMAs into account.

FAC is measured according to the equation:

$$FAC = \left[(LVEDA - LVESA)/LVEDA \right] \times 100$$

where LVEDA = left ventricular end-diastolic area; LVESA = left ventricular end-systolic area.

FAC can be performed serially to assess response to therapeutic interventions such as the addition of inotropic support. FAC is thought to correlate well with LVEF. However, reference values are not widely published.

FAC can be performed in any view, but a mid-papillary short-axis (parasternal or subcostal) view lends itself well to this.

To measure FAC, use the planimetry function to trace the endocardial border, ignoring the PMs, at end-diastole (to obtain LVEDA), then again at end-systole (to obtain LVESA).

> **Pitfall**
>
> LVEF will be overestimated by FAC in PSAX at the apex, because its contraction is entirely radial. FAC should be assessed in PSAX at the mid-papillary level.

Left ventricular ejection fraction

Technically, LVEF is an advanced echo technique because it involves knowledge of apical views beyond the

A4C. However, it is discussed here because it is based on 2D imaging, universally quoted in comprehensive studies, and accurate interpretation is essential for all intensive care echo practitioners.

LVEF is defined as SV, expressed as a percentage of the end-diastolic volume, according to the equation:

$$LVEF = EDV - ESV/EDV \times 100\%$$

where EDV = end-diastolic volume; ESV = end-systolic volume.

In comprehensive echo, LVEF is quantified as 5% bands (i.e. 45–50%). This detail is unnecessary in intensive care where semi-quantitative terms are more useful (Table 7.5).

Left ventricular ejection fraction—visual estimation

In comprehensive echo, visual estimation of LVEF is based on the net effect of wall motion of all six left ventricular segments, seen in three apical views: the A4C and two advanced views, known as A2C and A3C (Figure 7.1b and Chapter 5). The extent of thickening and excursion ('kinesia') of each wall is quantified and assimilated to produce the final estimation in 5% bands (Table 7.3). This method is reliable when performed by experienced operators but can overlook subtle findings.

Novices have been shown to detect significant abnormalities, with considerable accuracy using visual assessment. However, it is well recognized that FoCUS level practitioners have increasing difficulty recognizing less severe abnormalities.

To visually assess left ventricular function, use all available views, and in each one, rest your gaze in the centre of the chamber, and observe how the walls thicken and move in towards it. Then take into account all the adjuncts outlined previously (i.e. FS, EPSS, MAPSE, and FAC), and put all this information together to make your final assessment. The more experienced you are, the better you will become.

Left ventricular ejection fraction—biplane (Simpson's) method

This technique assumes that the left ventricular cavity is divided along its long axis (from mitral annulus to apex) into a stack of 20 parallel discs of uniform height but different radii. After tracing the endocardial border in two orthogonal views (usually A4C and A2C views), frozen at end-diastole and end-systole, the echo machine then calculates LVEF.

International echo societies recommend this technique for comprehensive echo, because it is highly accurate and reproducible. However, it takes time to perform and relies on good endocardial border definition from an apical window, which is rare in an ICU patient.

Foreshortening of ventricles in the A4C view results in underestimation of internal dimensions and overestimation of LVEF.

Interpretation of left ventricular ejection fraction in critically ill patients

LVEF depends on the LV's geometric shape, preload, afterload, and contractility, which are all highly variable in a critically ill patient. All the assessments outlined in Assessment of left ventricular function, p. 61, are loading-dependent, so interpretation must take this into account, as well as the levels of inotropic support and presence of left-sided valve disease.

Commonly encountered clinical scenarios in intensive care include:

1. Septic shock, when high LVEF is commonly caused by vasoplegia and low afterload, rather than increased contractility
2. Septic shock, when low LVEF can be the result of acutely impaired contractility and/or overzealous vasopressor therapy
3. Dilated cardiomyopathy, when large chamber size and low LVEF do not predestine the patient to be unresponsive to fluid challenges

Table 7.5 Semi-quantitative description of LVEF

LVEF	Description
≥70%	Hyperdynamic
55–70%	Normal
45–54%	Mild systolic dysfunction
36–44%	Moderate systolic dysfunction
≤35%	Severe systolic dysfunction

4. Any patient on inotropic support, when a visually 'normal' LVEF indicates that left ventricular systolic function is, in fact, far from normal

5. Severe MR, when high LVEF should be expected due to retrograde flow and does not necessarily indicate good systolic ejection

6. Significant AS, when low LVEF may be caused by outflow obstruction, impaired contractility, or both.

Left ventricular diastolic dysfunction

Detailed assessment of diastolic function is complex and considerably beyond FoCUS-level scanning. However, FoCUS can detect the structural changes associated with chronic DD, be they cause or effect. For example, in a patient with exertional dyspnoea, but no significant left-sided valve disease, left atrial enlargement is strongly associated with chronic DD. 2D evidence of right ventricular dysfunction is also suggestive, but not specific for DD, and some degree of DD can be assumed in any patient with LVH.

Left ventricular hypertrophy

SAX views are good for eyeballing left ventricular dimensions and wall thickness, but not for measurement, because off-axis imaging can cause error. In comprehensive echo, an optimized PLAX view is used to measure left ventricular wall thickness in the same way as LVIDd, as described in Measuring end-diastolic dimensions, p. 60. The upper limit of normal for left ventricular wall thickness is 1.2 cm (Video 1.3.2 ◯)

> **Pitfall**
>
> In patients with significant LVH, the small left ventricular cavity size seen throughout the cardiac cycle can be misinterpreted as hypovolaemia.

Hypertrophic cardiomyopathy

While a prominent basal septal bulge in PLAX is highly prevalent in the older population, echo criteria for the diagnosis of HCM include:

1. Unexplained maximal wall thickness of >15 mm in any myocardial segment, or

2. Septal/posterior wall thickness ratio of >1.3 in normotensive patients, or

3. Septal/posterior wall thickness ratio of >1.5 in hypertensive patients.

HCM has the potential for LVOT obstruction from SAM, so any significant asymmetric LVH seen in a haemodynamically unstable patient should prompt urgent referral for a comprehensive study.

Systolic anterior motion

2D features of SAM include LVOT narrowing, paradoxical motion of the AMVL with abnormal septal contact during systole, and associated MR. Sometimes, only the chordae tendinea are involved, and this milder form is known as chordal SAM (Video 1.3.3 ◯).

Ischaemic heart disease

In acute myocardial infarction, the affected ventricular walls appear similar in 2D to neighbouring healthy ones but don't thicken or move as well, and these associated RWMAs are usually non-reversible (Video 1.3.4 ◯).

In an old myocardial infarction, the affected left ventricular walls may become brightly echogenic and thinned. This is suggestive of scarring (Figure 7.6).

Heart failure

Hallmarks of HFrEF are left ventricular dilatation and reduced EF, which are both readily visible in FoCUS. HFpEF patients are more difficult to spot using 2D US. However, the presence of left atrial

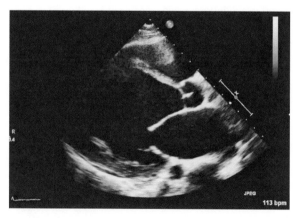

Figure 7.6 Myocardial thinning secondary to previous myocardial infarction. This PLAX view demonstrates a bright, thin-walled septum, consistent with scarring from a previous anteroseptal myocardial infarction. Compare this with the healthy-looking posterior free wall. Note: associated left ventricular dilatation.

enlargement may provide a clue in a patient with typical symptoms of heart failure and no known mitral valve disease.

When LVEF is critically low, as seen in acute heart failure, spontaneous echo contrast (SEC) can be seen as smoky swirls of slow-flowing blood within the left ventricular chamber itself (Video 1.3.5 ⊙). SEC is extremely abnormal in the LV, and its presence exhibits potentially life-threatening cardiogenic shock.

Pitfall

In patients with symptoms and signs of heart failure, a normal FoCUS study cannot rule out this diagnosis—only comprehensive echo can do this—so expert referral must not be delayed.

Takotsubo cardiomyopathy

Takotsubo cardiomyopathy is a difficult diagnosis to make without echo. Typically, the entire LV is akinetic, with the exception of the basal segments, which are usually hyperkinetic (Video 1.3.6 ⊙). However, several variants have been reported with akinesia in any myocardial segment, including the distal RV, which is seen in approximately 25% of cases. Characteristically, in Takotsubo, RWMAs do not correlate with coronary blood supply territories, and the diagnosis can only be confirmed after coronary artery disease has been excluded.

Advanced echocardiography

Systolic function

S-wave velocity

Tissue Doppler imaging (TDI) utilizes PW Doppler with a low-pass filter to exclude high-velocity blood and evaluate tissue motion. When sampled from the medial or lateral annulus in A4C, DTI enables measurement of mitral annular peak systolic velocity, known as S-wave velocity or S′ (pronounced S prime).

Like MAPSE, systolic contraction (movement towards the probe) is displayed above the baseline, and lower values suggest systolic impairment (Figure 7.7).

HFpEF patients with early longitudinal systolic dysfunction typically demonstrate S′ <4.4 cm/s.

S-wave velocity has been shown to be a sensitive marker of impaired longitudinal left ventricular systolic shortening (superior to LVEF in early disease), which increases with dobutamine and exercise and decreases within 15 s of ischaemia. It is afterload-dependent and prone to error in the context of basal RWMAs. However, S′ is emerging as a potentially useful marker of systolic function.

Diastolic function

Diagnosis and grading of DD is complex and evolving. Much of what is known is based on PW Doppler in spontaneously breathing patients with chronic heart failure.

Very little has been validated in critically ill patients, who are challenging to investigate because early trans-mitral blood flow (E velocity) is heavily dependent on loading conditions, which are highly variable in this group.

Updated recommendations (Figure 7.8) now classify normal, abnormal, or indeterminate diastolic function, based on the following echo parameters:

1. e′ velocity
2. E/e′
3. TR velocity
4. Left atrial volume index.

Tissue Doppler imaging (e′ and E/e′)

PW Doppler can be used to measure early trans-mitral blood velocity, known as E′, by placing the sampling volume at the tip of the open MV leaflets in a true A4C view and recording the height of the first positive waveform. E is load-dependent, so it is difficult to interpret in critically ill patients.

The peak velocity of early diastolic basal wall motion (the first negative waveform seen using TDI; Figure 7.8) is known as e′ and provides a load-independent measure of diastolic relaxation. e′ can be measured in a true A4C view, with the TDI sampling volume placed first at the septal, and then lateral, MV annulus. These values should ideally be averaged for interpretation.

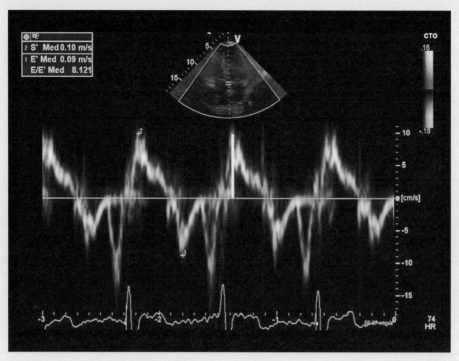

Figure 7.7 TDI waveform demonstrating S-wave velocity, sampled from the medial mitral valve annulus in an A4C view.

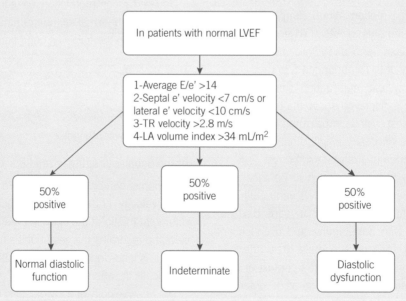

Figure 7.8 Updated guidelines on assessing left ventricular diastolic function in patients with normal LVEF. For a colour version of this figure, please see colour plate section.

Reprinted from *Journal of the American Society of Echocardiography*, **29**, 4, Nagueh, Sherif F., *et al.*, 'Recommendations for the evaluation of left ventricular diastolic function by echocardiography: an update from the American Society of Echocardiography and the European Association of Cardiovascular Imaging', pp. 277–314, Copyright © 2016 with permission from Elsevier.

Conceptually, E relates to the pressure difference between the LA and LV, and e′ to the change in left ventricular volume produced by this pressure, so E/e′ indicates left ventricular elastance (the reciprocal of compliance). Consequently, the lower e′ and the higher E/e′ are, the more likely there is to be DD.

Cut-off values for DD are:

- Septal e′ <7 cm/s
- Lateral e′ <10 cm/s
- Average E/e′ >14.

Tricuspid regurgitation velocity

In the absence of chronic pulmonary or vascular disease, elevated pulmonary arterial systolic pressure (PASP) suggests left ventricular DD.

Calculation of PASP is based on measurement of peak TR velocity using CW Doppler in multiple views (PSAX at the AV level, A4C, S4C, and right ventricular inflow), guided by colour flow Doppler to map TR jets (Chapter 8).

The cut-off value for DD is:

- TR velocity >2.8 m/s.

Left atrial volume

In the absence of chronic MV disease, atrial arrhythmias, and anaemia, left atrial enlargement suggests chronically raised left ventricular filling pressure. Normal left atrial size does not rule out acute increases in left ventricular filling pressure, as remodelling takes weeks to months.

Maximal left atrial volume can be measured by planimetry at end-systole in both A4C and A2C, according to the area–length method (Chapter 9).

The cut-off value for DD is:

- Left atrial volume index >34 mL/m².

✔ Multiple choice questions

Interactive multiple choice questions to test your knowledge can be found in the Online appendix at www.oxfordmedicine.com/focusedicu. Please refer to your access card for further details.

Further reading

Colebourn C, Newton J (eds). *Acute and Critical Care Echocardiography: Oxford Clinical Imaging Guides.* Oxford: Oxford University Press; 2017.

Lancellotti P, Price S, Edvardsen T, *et al.* The use of echocardiography in acute cardiovascular care: recommendations of the European Association of Cardiovascular Imaging and the Acute Cardiovascular Care Association. *European Heart Journal-Cardiovascular Imaging* 2015;**16**:119–46.

Lang RM, Badano LP, Mor-Avi V, *et al.* Recommendations for cardiac chamber quantification by echocardiography in adults: an update from the American Society of Echocardiography and the European Association of Cardiovascular Imaging. *Journal of the American Society of Echocardiography* 2015;**28**:1–39.

Nagueh SF, Smiseth OA, Appleton CP, *et al.* Recommendations for the evaluation of left ventricular diastolic function by echocardiography: an update from the American Society of Echocardiography and the European Association of Cardiovascular Imaging. *Journal of the American Society of Echocardiography* 2016;**29**:277–314.

8

Right ventricular assessment

David Hendron

Introduction

The RV has not always had the kudos it deserves. For a long time, it was perceived as a simple conduit to blood flow, lacking significant contractile performance, when compared to the LV. We now know that haemodynamics of the RV are much more sophisticated than previously thought, and right ventricular function is strongly associated with clinical outcomes in many conditions. Right ventricular function has implications not only for the pulmonary and venous circulations, but also for function of the LV and systemic circulation.

The RV is notoriously difficult to assess clinically. The relationship between right ventricular end-diastolic pressure and volume is complex, inconsistent, and often oversimplified; the same can also be said of pressure and volume relationships between the right and left hearts. Using right atrial pressure (RAP) as a marker of left ventricular preload or potential fluid responsiveness makes a number of unreliable assumptions and has limited clinical utility in critical care. Methods allowing dynamic assessment of right heart size and function are considerably more useful, and TTE is ideal for this purpose. Focused echo has become an invaluable tool that enables rapid assessment of the failing right heart and its response to treatment, all in real time.

This chapter will outline how the RV differs from the LV, in terms of anatomy and physiology, and will describe the concepts of right ventricular pressure and, volume overload, as well as ventricular interdependence. It will describe how 2D echo can be used to detect right ventricular enlargement and systolic impairment, and distinguish between acute and chronic pathophysiology. The advanced section will introduce how to recognize pulmonary hypertension (PHT) and use tissue Doppler analysis to assess right ventricular systolic function.

Relevant anatomy

The RV is unique from the LV in a number of ways—its geometric shape is more complex (crescent-shaped in its short axis; triangular when viewed from the side), and it wraps around the LV at the IVS.

The RV is divided anatomically into three distinct portions:

1. The inlet—a smooth, muscular inflow region consisting of TV, chords, and PMs
2. Trabecular apical myocardium
3. The infundibulum (or 'conus')—the cone-shaped, smooth-walled RVOT.

The walls of the RV are thinner than those of the LV and are mostly trabeculated on their endocardial surface. Another distinguishing feature is the presence of a moderator band that runs from the IVS to the free wall, at the base of the anterior PM. A common misconception about the moderator band is that it acts as a supporting structure for the free wall, moderating over-distension and chamber dilatation in the face of acute rises in afterload. Its actual role is as a conduit for conducting tissue, as it conveys branches of the right bundle of His to the right ventricular free wall.

Owing to its reduced musculature and more compliant walls, the RV can dilate acutely when exposed to volume and pressure overload.

The RV has three PMs (supporting the TV apparatus), and this differentiates it from the LV, which has only two. The TV sits more apically in the RV than the MV does in the LV. Apical displacement becomes pathological in congenital Ebstein's anomaly, which results in 'atrialization' of the RV.

Coronary perfusion of the RV is predominantly via the RCA, which sends marginal branches to its lateral and posterior walls. The left anterior descending artery supplies the right ventricular anterior wall and apex. The posterior descending artery (PDA) supplies the right ventricular inferior wall and the posterior third of the IVS. In 85% of the general population, the PDA arises from the RCA (known as 'right dominant'), and the RCA will therefore supply most of the RV. The remaining 10–15% of people are either 'left dominant' [the PDA is supplied by the circumflex artery (Cx)—a branch of the left coronary artery] or 'co-dominant' (the PDA is supplied by both the RCA and Cx). Importantly, in a left dominant system, >50% of the RV is supplied by the left coronary artery.

Relevant physiology

Unlike the LV, which is perfused only in diastole, perfusion of the healthy RV occurs throughout systole and diastole, and it has generous collateral flow, providing additional protection against ischaemia. In the presence of right ventricular hypertrophy (RVH), the RV begins to mimic the LV, with increasing dependence on diastolic perfusion.

Right ventricular systolic function

Systolic contraction of the RV is sequential, starting with the inlet, followed by the apical myocardium, then finally the outlet (separated by about 50 ms), giving it a characteristic peristaltic appearance. It occurs earlier and finishes later than the LV, and the right ventricular ejection fraction (RVEF) may be up to 10% lower; normal values are 45–60%.

There are three components to RV contraction:

1. Longitudinal shortening—the TV annulus moves towards the apex (the dominant component to right ventricular ejection)

2. Inward motion of the right ventricular free wall—contraction of the IVS produces a bellows-like effect

3. Contraction of the LV—from traction on its free wall at points of attachment (pulling the RV around it).

Continuity of muscle fibres between both ventricles binds them together, structurally and functionally, providing traction on the right ventricular free wall when the LV contracts. In contrast to the LV, twisting and rotational movements do not contribute significantly to contraction of the RV.

Right ventricular loading

The healthy RV adapts well to changes in preload. Increases within the physiological range are accompanied by increases in contractile performance. The 'low-pressure, high compliance' pulmonary circulation can accommodate large increases in blood-flow, without accompanying rises in pulmonary artery pressure, via recruitment and distension of the pulmonary capillary bed. Conditions causing sudden rises in pulmonary artery pressure (eg PE) however, may cause the RV to acutely dilate.

Right ventricular pressure overload

When right ventricular afterload exceeds its ability to cope, as seen in PHT or pulmonary stenosis, the abnormal pressure differential between the ventricles displaces the septum towards the cavity of the LV throughout systole. This state is known as 'right ventricular pressure overload'.

The RV is more sensitive to changes in afterload than the LV. Small rises in pulmonary vascular resistance, such as those caused by the application of positive pressure ventilation, can lead to a marked fall in SV (especially when the RV is also volume-overloaded). Other common causes of increased right ventricular afterload include hypoxaemia, hypercapnia, and acidaemia.

Right ventricular volume overload

When right ventricular preload exceeds its ability to cope, as seen in TR or atrial septal defect (ASD), the RV dilates and excessive diastolic trans-tricuspid blood flow displaces the septum towards the LV, most obviously at end-diastole. This state is known as 'right ventricular volume overload'.

Ventricular interdependence

This refers to the state when changes in the size, shape, and compliance of the RV directly influence filling characteristics of the LV. Severe right ventricular enlargement can squeeze the LV into the corner of the pericardium and compromise its filling. Anatomical connections, septal motion, and the pressure exerted by the pericardium all contribute to ventricular inter-dependence, which becomes most apparent with sudden changes in loading conditions and manifests on echo as distinct septal motion patterns, according to the cardiac (e.g. pressure/volume overload) and re-spiratory (e.g. cardiac tamponade) cycles.

Echo assessment

In short axis, the LV resembles a doughnut, and the RV a more sophisticated croissant stuck on the side.

Views of the right heart

TTE windows can be suboptimal in an ICU popu-lation, especially those receiving positive pressure ventilation. When views are limited, information on right ventricular chamber size, wall thickness, and systolic function must be assimilated from those available.

The PLAX view demonstrates the right ventricular free wall and RVOT. It is useful for measuring right ven-tricular wall thickness and eyeballing radial function.

The PSAX view at the level of the AV demonstrates the basal anterior right ventricular wall and RVOT, as they 'wrap around' the LVOT. This view is useful for detecting TR and measuring its peak velocity if its alignment is parallel to the US beam.

PSAX views at the mitral and mid-papillary levels demonstrate the anterior, inferior, and lateral walls of the RV. Here it appears crescent-shaped beside the round LV. These views are useful for analysing interventricular septal motion patterns.

The A4C view visualizes the RV in its longitudinal axis, alongside the LV. It is useful for assessing right ventricular and atrial chamber sizes and comparing them with corresponding chambers of the left heart. It can also be used to assess right ventricular systolic function via tricuspid annular plane systolic excursion (TAPSE) and FAC, as well as estimating PAP (if TR is present). From an A4C view, the RV can be centred to facilitate assessments of right ventricular function (Videos 1.4.1 and 1.4.2 ▣).

The S4C view is often the most reliably attainable view in mechanically ventilated patients. The lateral wall of the RV is seen clearly in this view, which is used for measuring right ventricular wall thickness. In the presence of a pericardial effusion, 2D features of tamponade physiology (diastolic collapse of the RV, systolic collapse of the right atrium) are often best visualized in this window.

Right ventricular size

What constitutes 'normality' for right ventricular chamber size will vary according to body surface area, height, gender, and ethnicity of the individual. However, a healthy RV will always be smaller than the LV.

Assessment of right ventricular size can be:

- Qualitative—'eyeballing', comparing the size of the right ventricular chamber with that of the LV
- Quantitative—making chamber measurements.

To eyeball

An A4C window visualizes both ventricles in long axis and enables qualitative assessment by comparing chamber sizes of each. When discussing compara-tive ventricular size, the literature is not clear about whether this refers to the area or basal width, and both appear to be interchangeable.

Normal

The LV is the apex-forming ventricle, and the size of the RV should be no more than two-thirds that of the LV.

Mildly dilated

The size of the RV exceeds two-thirds that of the LV.

Moderately dilated

The RV is equal in size to the LV and may occupy part of the cardiac apex (Figure 8.1a).

Severely dilated

The RV is larger than the LV, and it becomes the apex-forming ventricle (Figure 8.1b and Video 1.4.3 ▣).

> **Pitfall**
>
> When the LV is dilated, eyeballing can lead to underestimation of right ventricular size.

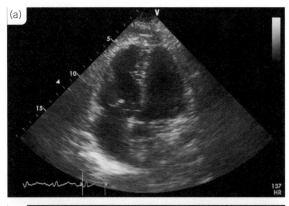

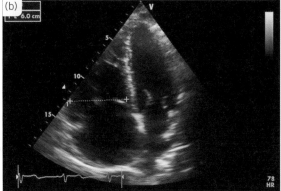

Figure 8.1 Assessing right ventricular chamber size.
(a) A moderately dilated RV, with the RV forming part of the apex (pulmonary embolus). (b) A severely dilated RV, with concurrent right atrial dilatation (portopulmonary hypertension).

To measure

Right ventricular chamber size is measured at end-diastole in an RV-focused A4C window (Figure 8.2). To achieve this from A4C, rock the beam slightly medially to bring the RV into the field, then rotate it about 15° anticlockwise to open it up maximally. The basal diameter (RVD1) is measured as the transverse diameter in the basal third of the RV. The mid-cavity diameter (RVD2) is measured in the middle third, approximately halfway between the basal diameter and apex, at the level of the left ventricular PMs. The longitudinal dimension is measured from the tricuspid annular plane to the apex.

Care must be taken to avoid foreshortening and malrotation, which can both affect the apparent size of the RV, compared to the LV (Figure 8.3).

Reference values for right ventricular chamber size are based on population studies of 'normal' individuals without heart disease and were updated by Lang *et al.* in 2015 (Table 8.1).

Pitfall

In A4C, by foreshortening the ventricles, one can overestimate right ventricular size; by rotation of the beam, one can underestimate it (Figure 8.3).

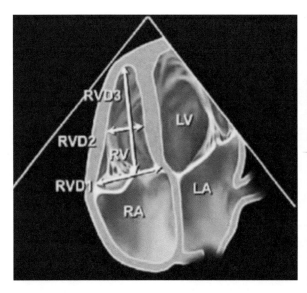

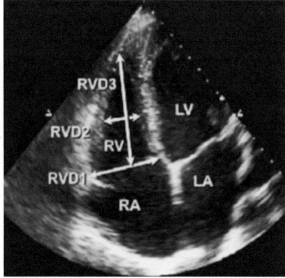

Figure 8.2 Right ventricular cavity dimensions.

Reproduced from Lang, Roberto M., *et al.*, 'Recommendations for chamber quantification', *European Heart Journal-Cardiovascular Imaging*, 2006, **7**, 2, pp. 79–108. Copyright © 2006, by permission of Oxford University Press.

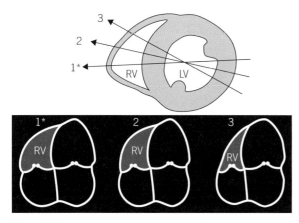

Figure 8.3 Effect of angulation on right ventricular chamber size.

Reprinted from *Journal of the American Society of Echocardiography*, **23**, 7, Rudski, Lawrence G., *et al.*, 'Guidelines for the echocardiographic assessment of the right heart in adults: a report from the American Society of Echocardiography: endorsed by the European Association of Echocardiography, a registered branch of the European Society of Cardiology, and the Canadian Society of Echocardiography', pp. 685–713, Copyright © 2010 with permission from Elsevier. Published by Mosby, Inc.

Right ventricular wall thickness

The walls of the RV are much thinner than those of the LV; as a result, RVH may be a subtle finding and easily missed. RVH is usually the consequence of chronic right ventricular pressure overload.

To measure

Right ventricular wall thickness is the perpendicular distance between the epicardial and endocardial surfaces of its free wall (Figure 8.4). It is measured at end-diastole (just before the onset of the QRS complex) in the subcostal view, at the level of the TV chords.

RVH is present when wall thickness is >5 mm.

Table 8.1 Reference values for right ventricular cavity dimensions

Dimension	Normal limit (cm)
Basal (RVD1)	<4.1
Mid cavity (RVD2)	<3.5
Longitudinal (RVD3)	<8.3

Measurement of right ventricular systolic function

The most accurate 2D methods for quantifying right ventricular systolic function involve measurement of systolic longitudinal shortening and FAC.

Calculation of RVEF using 2D volumetric methods (e.g. area–length or 'Simpson's' disc summation) is possible. However, due to the complex shape of the RV and the geometric assumptions required, these methods are not recommended. Advanced imaging modalities, such as 3D echo and MRI, are more accurate at quantifying RVEF than 2D echo.

A4C is the optimal view for assessing right ventricular systolic function. S4C can be used for eyeballing, but it is often less stable than A4C and interpretation is prone to error in inexperienced hands.

Tricuspid annular plane systolic excursion

This linear measurement is a simple and well-validated technique for quantifying right ventricular systolic function (Figure 8.5). TAPSE measures the distance that the lateral annulus of the TV moves towards the apex during systole, reflecting systolic longitudinal shortening of the RV. Quoted cutoff values for normal/abnormal vary between 15 and 20 mm, depending on age and condition, making it difficult to recommend any one. Conservative reference ranges can be found in Table 8.2.

- Advantages—it is simple and quick, and does not require optimal imaging.
- Disadvantages—it is angle-dependent and will be underestimated in the presence of basal wall motion abnormalities.

To measure

Obtain an optimized A4C view, and ensure that the lateral wall is well aligned. Place the M-mode sampling line through the lateral TV annulus, and measure its vertical displacement by placing calipers at the trace's lowest and highest points.

Pitfall

TAPSE can be remarkably well preserved in association with severe right ventricular dysfunction, so it must be interpreted in the context of right ventricular fractional area change.

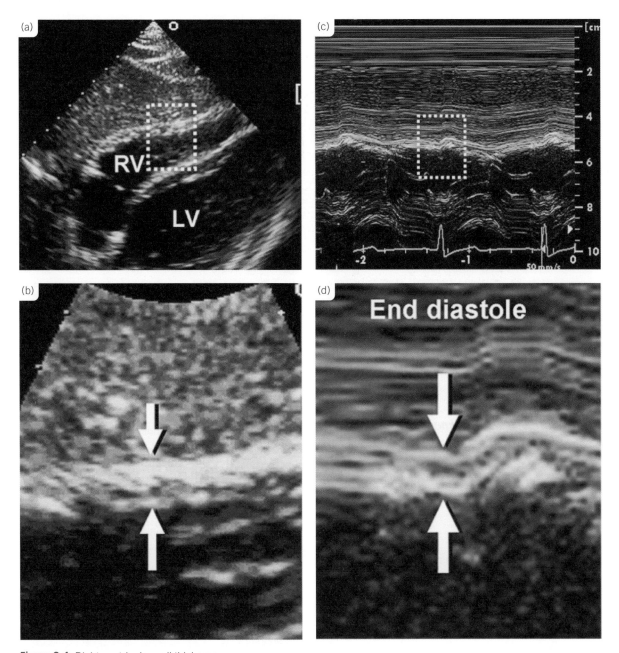

Figure 8.4 Right ventricular wall thickness.

Reprinted from *Journal of the American Society of Echocardiography*, **23**, 7, Rudski, Lawrence G., *et al.*, 'Guidelines for the echocardiographic assessment of the right heart in adults: a report from the American Society of Echocardiography: endorsed by the European Association of Echocardiography, a registered branch of the European Society of Cardiology, and the Canadian Society of Echocardiography' p. 685–713, Copyright © 2010 with permission from Elsevier. Published by Mosby, Inc.

Fractional area change

FAC is a 2D measurement of the percentage change between end-diastolic (EDA) and end-systolic (ESA) areas, according to the equation (Figure 8.6):

$$EDA - ESA/EDA \times 100$$

- Advantages—it correlates well with RVEF calculated by cardiac MRI.

- Disadvantages—it requires good definition of the right ventricular endocardium in both systole and diastole.

FAC of <35% implies right ventricular dysfunction.

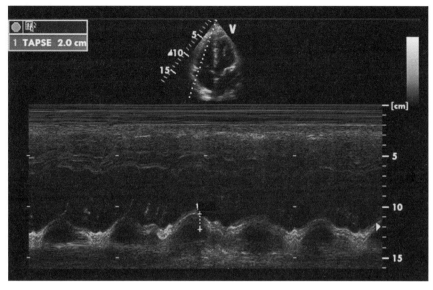

Figure 8.5 TAPSE: calipers set between the bottom and top of the slope demonstrating a TAPSE of 2.0 cm, which is well within the normal range.

Table 8.2 Rough guide to right ventricular function and TAPSE

Right ventricular function	TAPSE (mm)
Normal	>20
Severely impaired	<10

To measure

Trace the endocardial borders of the RV in A4C, at both end-diastole (maximum right ventricular volume) and end-systole (minimum right ventricular volume). Starting at the TV annulus, move along the free wall to the apex, then along the IVS back to the annulus, including all trabeculations within the cavity. The ratio of the ejected area to end-diastolic areas can then be calculated.

$$FAC = \left[(EDA - ESA)/EDA \right] \times 100$$

Normal FAC is >35%.

Pitfall

Assessing RVEF must always take into account the effects of inotropic support.

Spontaneous ventilation, inferior vena cava collapsibility, and right atrial pressure

RAP can be estimated from the IVC diameter and its degree of respiratory variability. The IVC collapsibility index was originally validated for estimating RAP in response to a 'sniff' in spontaneously breathing patients. It performs well when RAP is high or low, but less well for intermediate values, and to reflect this, traditional cut-off values were revised by Rudski *et al.* in 2010.

Revised criteria

An IVC diameter of <2.1 cm that collapses >50% with a sniff suggests a RAP of 3 mmHg (0–5 mmHg).

An IVC diameter of >2 cm that collapses <50% with a sniff suggests a RAP of 15 mmHg (10–20 mmHg).

To measure

In a S4C view centred on the right atrium, rotate the probe in an anticlockwise direction (usually <90° rotation), and the IVC will open up in long axis as it drains into the right atrium (Figure 8.7). Using either calipers or M-mode, measure the IVC diameter (perpendicular to its long axis) just proximal to the entrance of the hepatic veins (usually within 1–2 cm of the IVC junction with the right atrium), and record the maximum and minimum IVC dimensions as the IVC changes with respiration.

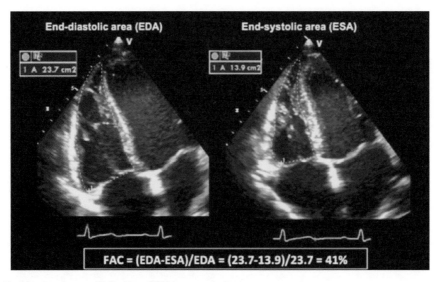

Figure 8.6 Fractional area change. FAC above 35% is normal.

Adapted from *Journal of the American Society of Echocardiography*, **28**, 1, Lang, Roberto M., *et al.*, 'Recommendations for cardiac chamber quantification by echocardiography in adults: an update from the American Society of Echocardiography and the European Association of Cardiovascular Imaging', pp. 1–39, Copyright © 2015, with permission from Elsevier.

Pitfall

The IVC can be pulled out of the imaging plane by deep inspiration. When measuring IVC diameter using M-mode, ensure that it is seen in a true, not tangential or oblique, plane. Bright endothelial signals seen throughout the respiratory cycle suggest a true diameter.

RAP, estimated by IVC size and collapsibility, is used in the calculation of PASP in spontaneously breathing patients. The relationship between RAP and intravascular volume is much less clear.

Mechanical ventilation, inferior vena cava distensibility, and predicting fluid responsiveness

Positive pressure ventilation reverses the phasic collapse observed with spontaneous breathing, such that the IVC distends, rather than collapses, with inspiration. The distensibility index of the inferior vena cava (DIVC) reflects this degree of respiratory variability, and a cut-off of >18% has been found to be a reliable predictor of fluid responsiveness in septic ventilated patients, with a sensitivity and specificity of around 90% (Barbier *et al.*, 2004; PMID: 15034650).

$$DIVC = 100 \times IVC_{max} - IVC_{min}/IVC_{min}$$

In ICU patients receiving mechanical ventilation, fair assumptions would be:

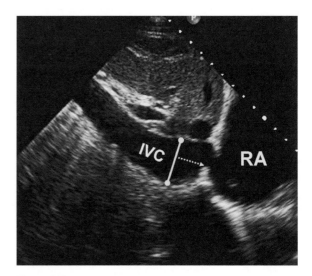

Figure 8.7 IVC dimension and collapsibility.

Reprinted from *Journal of the American Society of Echocardiography*, **23**, 7, Rudski, Lawrence G., *et al.*, 'Guidelines for the echocardiographic assessment of the right heart in adults: a report from the American Society of Echocardiography: endorsed by the European Association of Echocardiography, a registered branch of the European Society of Cardiology, and the Canadian Society of Echocardiography', pp. 685–713, Copyright © 2010 with permission from Elsevier. Published by Mosby, Inc.

- A dilated IVC with low respiratory distensibility reflects high RAP

- A small IVC with high respiratory distensibility with respiration reflects low RAP.

Ventricular septal motion

Under normal conditions, the LV in short axis remains circular throughout the entire cardiac cycle, with the IVS bowed towards the RV. Conditions causing pressure or volume overload of the right heart can change this morphology, causing the IVS to flatten and become D-shaped at various stages during the cardiac cycle (Figure 8.8). This is best appreciated in the PSAX view, although the subcostal SAX view is a good alternative (Videos 1.4.4 and 1.4.5 ▢).

Pressure overload:

- Reversal of the normal septal curvature throughout the cardiac cycle (worse at end-systole)

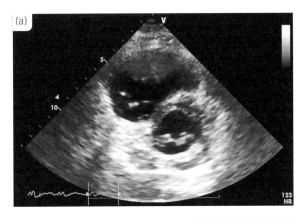

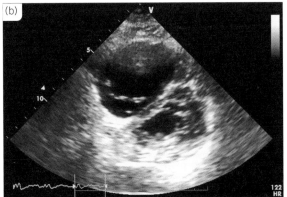

Figure 8.8 PSAX images of a patient with right ventricular volume-overload. (a) Image frozen at mid-systole; (b) image frozen at end-diastole diastole.

- The LV is D-shaped in systole and (relatively) circular in diastole.

Volume overload:

- Septal flattening in mid- to late-diastole

- The LV is D-shaped in diastole and circular in systole

- Paradoxical septal motion, caused by hyperdynamic ventricles, making the septum appear to move anteriorly in systole.

Pressure and volume overload:

- Usual ventricular shapes appear to be reversed

- The RV is circular and the LV is crescentic, throughout the cardiac cycle.

> **Pitfall**
> Abnormal septal motion patterns can be caused by conduction defects, especially LBBB.

Acute pulmonary embolism

An acute pulmonary embolus (PE) results in haemodynamic changes when at least 30–40% of the pulmonary arterial bed is obliterated. Right ventricular dysfunction can be diagnosed with TTE in up to 70% of normotensive PE patients, and its presence increases the risk of short-term death tenfold.

In patients with suspected PE, the main role of echocardiography is to disclose signs of acute right ventricular dilatation and systolic dysfunction. On occasion, it may confirm the diagnosis by visualizing a PE 'in transit' through the right heart, and it can also be used to determine the severity of PHT, which often coexists.

In a collapsed patient, the absence of right ventricular dysfunction effectively rules PE out as the cause of shock. However, it is important to remember that a 'normal' echo cannot exclude PE as a diagnosis.

Echo features consistent with a large PE include right ventricular dilatation, McConnell's sign, septal displacement, elevated PASP, and a dilated IVC with minimal variability. The presence of RVH points towards chronic pathology that may or may not include venous thromboembolism.

McConnell's sign describes severe hypokinesia of the right ventricular free wall, with relative sparing of the apex. This was originally described in 1996, with high specificity (94%) and reasonable sensitivity (77%) for acute PE. However, more recently, its specificity has been challenged.

In an otherwise healthy patient with acute onset of typical symptoms and signs of PE, FoCUS evidence of right ventricular dysfunction should prompt consideration of interventions such as thrombolysis or embolectomy.

Chronic pulmonary hypertension

To identify chronic PHT, look for features that suggest development over a prolonged period such as the presence of RVH or concurrent dilatation of other chambers.

A hypertrophied RV is capable of generating much higher PASP than a normal RV. Patients with PASP of >60 mmHg are highly likely to have a chronic component, as acute rises in PAP of this magnitude are usually fatal in patients with no comorbidity. Conversely, right ventricular dilatation associated with normal PAP is more suggestive of ischaemia than embolism. In chronic disease, hypokinesia of the RV is more likely to be global.

Advanced echocardiography

Additional views

The RVI view is achieved by tilting the beam down slightly towards the right hip from the PLAX position. It visualizes the right atrium, the TV, and both the inferior and anterior walls of the RV (on the left and right sides of the sector, respectively). It is a useful view for detecting TR jets with colour Doppler and using their peak velocity to estimate PAP.

The RVO view is achieved by tilting the beam up towards the left shoulder from the PLAX position. It visualizes the anterior wall of the RV, RVOT, pulmonary valve, and main pulmonary artery.

Estimating pulmonary arterial systolic pressure

TR is present, to some degree, in at least 80% of the population, and providing that there is no RVOT obstruction, this jet enables estimation of PAP. The TR jet velocity is determined by the RV/RA systolic pressure gradient, which can be estimated using the simplified Bernoulli equation:

$$\Delta P_{RV-RA} = 4(TRV)^2$$

where ΔP_{RV-RA} is the pressure gradient between the RV and right atrium, and TRV is the peak velocity of the TR jet.

To estimate PASP, add RAP to this value:

$$PASP = 4(TRV)^2 + RAP$$

In spontaneously ventilating patients, RAP can be estimated from the size and respiratory variability of the IVC (as previously described). However, this relationship is not valid in mechanically ventilated patients. Critical care patients are likely to have central venous access, and in such cases, it is more accurate to use their measured central venous pressure (CVP).

To measure

1. Assess for the presence of TR using colour flow Doppler. Any view where the TR jet aligns with the US beam will be suitable; options include RVI, PSAX at the level of the AV, and A4C.

2. Superimpose CW Doppler onto the colour flow Doppler image, aligning the sampling line through the centre of the TR jet (Figure 8.9). Freeze the trace, and record its peak velocity (TRV).

3. Use the simplified Bernoulli equation to calculate the PASP (built-in software often enables this calculation automatically from the peak TRV). Add estimated RAP (or measured CVP) to calculate PASP.

TR jets can be in any direction, so their peak velocity should be assessed from multiple windows. The view with the best alignment and highest velocity jet should be recorded.

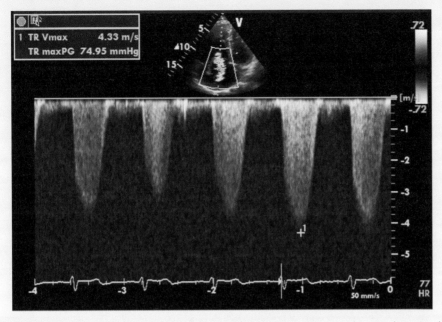

Figure 8.9 CW Doppler trace of TR. The extremely high-velocity TR jet indicates severe pulmonary hypertension that is likely to be chronic. For a colour version of this figure, please see colour plate section.

European guidelines for the diagnosis and treatment of PHT were published in 2016, recommending that, rather than estimating PASP, the probability of PHT is determined by peak TRV and the presence of other echo signs of PHT (RV/LV basal diameter ratio >1, a D-shaped ventricle, a dilated right atrium, and others). High risk for PHT = TRV >3.4 m/s (or 2.9–3.4 m/s with other signs), low risk for PHT = TRV ≤2.8 m/s without other signs. PHT should then be quantified by right heart catheterization, if indicated.

Estimating right ventricular systolic function using tissue Doppler imaging (RV S′)

TDI uses a low-pass filter to exclude blood and measure only tissue velocities. The peak systolic velocity of the right ventricular free wall at the level of the lateral TV annulus (as it moves in its longitudinal plane) is known as S′ (pronounced 'S prime') and can be measured using TDI. RV S′ is analogous to TAPSE, only it measures the tissue velocity, rather than the distance of excursion.

- Advantages—ease of measurement, reliability, and reproducibility

- Disadvantages—it is angle-dependent and assumes that the function of a single segment represents the function of the entire RV, so it is inherently inaccurate in the presence of basal RWMAs.

To measure

It is performed using PW TDI, in an A4C view, with the sampling volume placed at either the lateral annulus of the TV or the middle of the basal segment of the right ventricular free wall. The S′ is read as the peak systolic velocity, represented as an upward deflection (Figure 8.10).

Normal S′ is >10 cm/s.

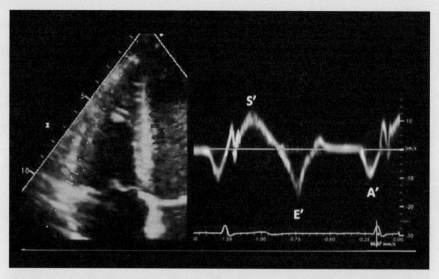

Figure 8.10 TDI calculation of S'. The RV has the same TDI properties as the LV, with an E' and A' wave, and S' wave in the opposite (positive) direction. For a colour version of this figure, please see colour plate section.

Adapted from *Journal of the American Society of Echocardiography*, **28**, 1, Lang, Roberto M., *et al.*, 'Recommendations for cardiac chamber quantification by echocardiography in adults: an update from the American Society of Echocardiography and the European Association of Cardiovascular Imaging', pp. 1–39, Copyright © 2015, with permission from Elsevier.

✔ Multiple choice questions

Interactive multiple choice questions to test your knowledge can be found in the Online appendix at www.oxfordmedicine.com/focusedicu. Please refer to your access card for further details.

Further reading

Anderson B. The two-dimensional echocardiographic examination. In: Anderson B. *Echocardiography: The Normal Examination and Echocardiographic Measurements*, 2nd ed. Brisbane: MGA Graphics; 2007. pp. 35–75.

Colebourn C, Newton J (eds). *Acute and Critical Care Echocardiography: Oxford Clinical Imaging Guides.* Oxford: Oxford University Press; 2017.

Galiè N, Humbert M, Vachiery JL, *et al.* 2015 ESC/ERS Guidelines for the diagnosis and treatment of pulmonary hypertension. *European Heart Journal* 2016;**37**:67–119.

Lang RM, Badano LP, Mor-Avi V, *et al.* Recommendations for cardiac chamber quantification by echocardiography in adults: an update from the American Society of Echocardiography and the European Association of Cardiovascular Imaging. *Journal of the American Society of Echocardiography* 2015;**28**:1–39.

Otto C. Left and right ventricular systolic function. In: Otto CM, Schwaegler RG, Freeman RV. *Echocardiography Review Guide*, 2nd ed. Philadelphia, PA: Elsevier Saunders; 2011. pp. 95–119.

Rudski LG, Lai WW, Afilalo J, *et al.* Guidelines for the echocardiographic assessment of the right heart in adults: a report from the American Society of Echocardiography: endorsed by the European Association of Echocardiography, a registered branch of the European Society of Cardiology, and the Canadian Society of Echocardiography. *Journal of the American Society of Echocardiography* 2010;**23**:685–713.

9

Atrial assessment

Paul Diprose

Introduction

Abnormalities of the atria may arise from a variety of cardiac and non-cardiac pathologies. Standard clinical examination will rarely, if ever, be capable of delineating atrial pathology. While routine radiological examination, including chest radiographs, may identify atrial enlargement, it is less likely to be able to characterize the pathology that led to the enlargement. TTE can provide direct 2D imaging of the walls and cavities of the atria, providing valuable information of the atria themselves and their associated valves. This can be supplemented by colour Doppler imaging that (in particular) may identify inter-atrial shunts.

Although other non-echocardiographic imaging techniques may be of benefit in delineating atrial pathology (including CT and MRI), bedside TTE permits rapid, repeatable, and dynamic assessment of the atria. TOE may, in some circumstances, provide better quality imaging of the atria than TTE, because the high-frequency TOE probe will come very close to the LA, with few other structures intervening.

This chapter will describe the important anatomical features of both atria and how these can be identified using 2D echo. It will explain how to recognize atrial dilatation and how to make inferences about atrial pressure from the position of the atrial septum. It will discuss atrial masses, including thrombus and tumour, and other more commonly seen structures that may be misinterpreted as such. The advanced section will introduce atrial volume assessment, as well as how colour Doppler and bubble contrast can be used to recognize midline septal defects.

Normal sonoanatomy

The atria lie above the level of the atrioventricular valves, with the LA more posteriorly positioned than the right. The LA is relatively oval in shape, with thin walls, and can be identified posterior to the aortic root and superior to the LV. The LA can be readily visualized in a number of different views, including the PLAX view and apical and subcostal views. In most subjects, four pulmonary veins drain blood from the lungs to the LA—two enter from the right, and two from the left into the superior wall of the LA. The entrance of one or two of the pulmonary veins may, on occasion, be seen towards the far field in the A4C view.

The right atrium (also ovoid in shape) receives inflow of blood from the IVC, SVC, and coronary sinus. It can be readily visualized in a number of different echocardiographic views, particularly in the apical and subcostal positions.

The atrial appendages are complex structures that are frequently multi-lobed. These are not usually well visualized with TTE, and TOE is the echocardiographic imaging modality of choice. The LAA is usually around 1.5 cm wide and 4 cm in length, although the anatomy is very variable. Both the right and left atrial appendages are lined with pectinate muscles—these are thickened (usually >1 mm) muscular ridges that may be mistaken for thrombus.

Abnormalities (usually congenital) of the atrial septum are relatively frequently observed. The septum is usually best visualized in the apical and subcostal probe positions.

Relevant physiology

During the cardiac cycle, the LA receives oxygenated blood from the lungs via the pulmonary veins during both systole and diastole. If the patient is in sinus rhythm, then there is a brief period of flow reversal associated with atrial contraction when a small volume of blood flow occurs back through the pulmonary veins. Similarly, the right atrium receives (deoxygenated) blood from the IVC, SVC, and coronary sinus throughout the cardiac cycle, with a short period of flow reversal during atrial contraction.

Ejection of blood from the atria towards the ventricles occurs during diastole, which is a complex process involving both active and passive processes. Atrial contraction (towards the end of ventricular diastole) will usually contribute approximately 20% of total filling, but this fraction may be increased, particularly in circumstances where the ventricular diastolic function is impaired (such as with LVH secondary to AS).

The direction of the atrial septum usually alters during the cardiac cycle, with a normal slight septal movement leading to bowing from right to left in mid-systole, returning to a left-to-right curvature in diastole.

Both atria are relatively compliant structures and will therefore gradually dilate in response to chronic volume or pressure overload. Chronic causes of pressure overload include mitral and (to a rarer extent) tricuspid stenosis, and both systolic and diastolic ventricular dysfunction. Left atrial dilatation (especially when the diameter exceeds 6 cm) is associated with an increased risk of developing AF. However, pre-existing AF may itself lead to progressive atrial dilatation.

Echo assessment

Two-dimensional appearances

The common imaging planes and the location of the left and right atria are demonstrated in Figure 9.1.

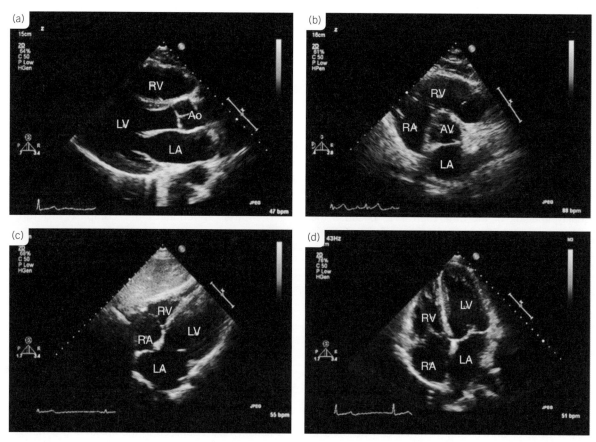

Figure 9.1 The atria visualized in standard TTE views. (a) PLAX view. (b) PSAX view at the aortic valve level. (c) Subcostal view. (d) A4C view. AV, aortic valve; Ao, ascending aorta.

A systematic approach should be taken to the 2D echocardiographic assessment of the atria and atrial septum. This should specifically include an assessment of atrial dimensions, observation for masses and other abnormalities within the atrial chambers, and analysis of the integrity and movement of the atrial septum.

Atrial dimensions

It is important, when measuring atrial dimensions, to set the gain correctly to ensure as good tissue definition as possible, since it may otherwise be difficult to accurately determine the location of atrial walls. This may be a particular issue when attempting to determine the position of the posterior wall of the LA, particularly if there is relatively stagnant blood flow within it.

Atrial dimensions should be measured at end-systole, timed to just before opening of the MV/TV, when the atria will be maximally filled. It is important to avoid 'foreshortening' of the atria, by ensuring that their true axes are identified.

The antero-posterior diameter of the LA is usually measured in the PLAX view; an 'eyeball' estimation of atrial size can be made by comparison with the 1 cm markers on the side of the US display. A caliper measurement can be made either using the standard 2D image or M-mode may be used to estimate this dimension, with the cursor set at the level of the closed AV leaflet tips (Figure 9.2). Care should be taken with any technique to avoid overestimation of the size as a result of gaining an oblique measurement. The normal range for atrial diameter is 3–4 cm for men or 2.7–3.8 cm for women. Severe atrial dilatation is considered present when the diameter is >5.2 cm in men or 4.7 cm in women.

Right atrial size is usually determined in the A4C view. The minor axis dimension (perpendicular to the major axis) of the right atrium extends from the lateral border of the right atrium to the atrial septum. The normal minor axis dimension is 1.7–2.5 cm, with severe dilatation said to be present when the dimension exceeds 3.2 cm.

The atrial septum

The atrial septum should slightly bow during the systolic component of the cardiac cycle, moving from the right atrial to the left atrial side. If the septum remains

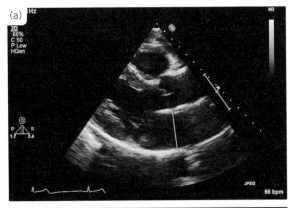

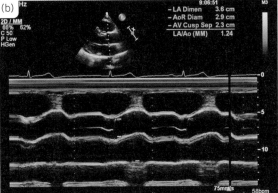

Figure 9.2 Measuring left atrial diameter. (a) Using calipers in the PLAX view, frozen just prior to mitral valve opening. (b) Using the M-mode in PLAX, with the line positioned at the leaflet tips of the aortic valve, when the left atrial diameter is at its maximum.

bowed towards the right or the left side consistently throughout the cardiac cycle, then it will imply significantly elevated pressures within the contralateral atrium.

Common pathophysiology

Atrial dilatation

Left atrial dilatation will occur in response to chronologically elevated pressures within the atrium. This can arise from MV pathology (both regurgitant and stenotic lesions) and from left ventricular systolic and/or diastolic dysfunction. Left atrial enlargement may act as a marker of both severity and chronicity of atrial pressure elevation. Right atrial dilatation (which may occur in acute, as well as chronic, settings) usually arises from TV disease, right ventricular dysfunction, or PHT.

As previously stated, AF may be a cause or a consequence of atrial dilatation.

Spontaneous echo contrast

SEC is the appearance of swirling, 'smoke-like', relatively echo-dense blood within the cavities of the heart. These appearances reflect sluggish flow within the cardiac cavity in question. If seen within the atria, the most common causes will be AF, mitral (or tricuspid) stenosis, or low cardiac output states. There is an association between the presence of SEC and an increased risk of developing atrial thrombus.

Thrombus

The most common cause of a mass within the atria is the presence of thrombus, and the most common location of atrial thrombi are within the LAA. Conditions that predispose to stasis, and thus thrombus formation, include AF, MV stenosis, and hypercoagulable states. As a general rule, and because the LAA is a relatively posterior structure, TTE cannot be relied upon to adequately exclude the presence of LAA thrombus. However, thrombus may occasionally be seen in the LAA in the far field on the right side of an A2C view. This is achieved with an approximate 60° anticlockwise rotation of the probe from the A4C view, so that only the LV is seen in the near field (and the LA in far field).

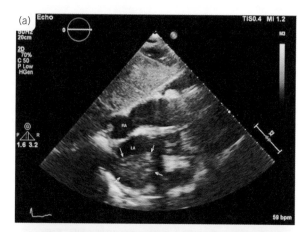

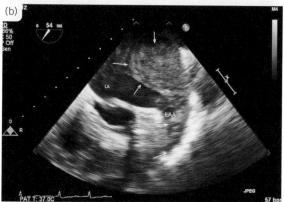

Figure 9.3 Left atrial thrombus. (a) Subcostal view demonstrating a large mass (arrows) in the left atrium—this was, in fact, thrombus. (b) TOE view of the same patient, demonstrating more clearly the left atrial thrombus (arrows) extending from the LAA (see also Video 1.5.1 📷).

Pitfall

One of the difficulties in performing TTE of the atria is that they lie relatively far from the probe. This means that subtle abnormalities within the atria (and the LAA in particular) can be easily missed. Under most circumstances, it is appropriate to use TOE to exclude atrial thrombus because the resolution of the image, particularly for the LAA, is vastly better (Figure 9.3a and b, and Video 1.5.1 📷).

Right atrial thrombi can occur (most frequently in association with AF) but are less common than those on the left side of the heart. Rarely, embolic material (for example, from leg or pelvic vein thrombus) can be seen transiting (or held up within) the right atrium, en route to the pulmonary circulation (Figure 9.4 and Video 1.5.2 📷).

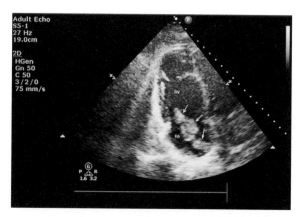

Figure 9.4 Modified A4C view demonstrating a mobile mass in the right atrium prolapsing through the tricuspid valve (arrows)—this was embolic material from a deep vein thrombosis. Note also: the dilated RV, likely related to pressure overload from previous pulmonary emboli (see also Video 1.5.2 📷).

Pitfall

Pectinate muscles are thickened ridges of the myocardium that are present within both the right and left atrial appendages. They may be mistaken for thrombus formation at these sites. A normal ridge of tissue, called the crista terminalis, lying at the opening of the right atrial appendage, close to the orifice of the SVC, may also be mistaken for a pathological mass within the right atrium.

Cardiac tumours

Benign tumours of the heart are considerably more common than malignant varieties. Approximately 30% of all primary heart tumours are myxomas. The

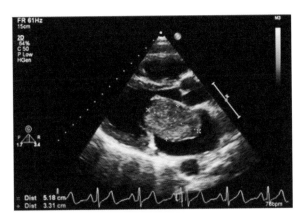

Figure 9.5 A PLAX view demonstrating a large atrial myxoma prolapsing through the mitral valve during diastole (see also Video 1.5.3 ⬤).

majority of these are solitary (5% of cases have multiple lesions), and 75% will arise within the LA, usually from an attachment on the atrial septum (Figure 9.5 and Video 1.5.3 ⬤). They may be large enough to almost fill the atrial cavity and can adversely affect diastolic flow across the MV. In approximately 15% of cases, the tumour will lie in the right atrium (the remaining patients present with myxomas within the RV or LV).

Pitfall

Lipomatous hypertrophy of the atrial septum is an acquired thickening of the atrial septum, secondary to fatty infiltration, that usually spares the region of the fossa ovalis (Figure 9.6). The appearance is classically described as a 'dumbbell'-shaped atrial septum. It is considered a normal variant (associated with obesity and old age) but may be mistaken for thrombus or tumours related to the atrial septum.

Metastatic cardiac tumours may occur from primary sources throughout the body. The atria may be particularly affected by direct extension of tumour material. Renal cell carcinoma can extend via the IVC into the cavity of the right atrium and sometimes has an appearance more in keeping with thrombus. These tumours may be particularly well visualized in the subcostal view where the junction between the IVC and the right atrium can be imaged (Video 1.5.4 ⬤). These tumours may embolize into the pulmonary artery, causing signs and symptoms of right heart failure. More rarely, lung tumours can extend into the LA via the pulmonary veins.

Pitfall

Within the right atrium, as the IVC enters, there is a prominent ridge of tissue that in utero baffled blood across the atrial septum. This may be mistaken as a pathological entity. A Chiari network is a thin filamentous structure that traverses the right atrium from the same position and again is an embryological remnant that rarely causes any clinical issue.

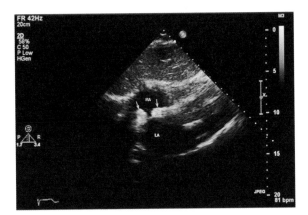

Figure 9.6 Subcostal view demonstrating lipomatous hypertrophy of the atrial septum (arrows).

Presence of wires and catheters

The presence of wires and catheters should be noted when studying the cardiac cavities. Those seen within the right atrium may include pacing wires and pulmonary artery catheters. Thrombus formation or endocarditic lesions may occur around intra-cavity devices, including pacing wires and intra-cardiac catheters. These two conditions may be impossible to differentiate on echocardiographic grounds alone.

Advanced echocardiography

Volume assessment of the left atrium

No single dimension can be used to derive an estimate of the overall volume of the LA, since asymmetric enlargement can occur with or without associated extrinsic localized compression or distortion of atrial walls. An estimation of left atrial volume may be achieved by measuring with planimetry the area of the LA at end-systole in the A4C and A2C views and determining the linear dimension of the LA (in the four- or two-chamber view) from the superior aspect of the LA to the level of the mid point of the mitral annulus [calculated by (0.85*a1*a2)/L]. Alternatively, left atrial volume can be determined by measuring the left atrial diameter in the PLAX view (as previously described) and multiplying by the two diameters seen in the A4C view (calculated by d1*d2*d3*0.523). The normal range for left atrial volume (indexed for body surface area) is 22 ± 6 mL/m². Severe left atrial dilatation is considered present if the atrial volume exceeds 40 mL/m².

Colour Doppler

Colour Doppler interrogation of the atria may identify normal flow into the right atrium from the vena cavae and the coronary sinus, and on the left atrial side from the pulmonary veins. Abnormal flow across the atrial septum, for example with a patent foramen ovale (PFO) or an ASD, may be demonstrated, particularly in the apical and subcostal views.

Patent foramen ovale

PFO is a common finding, occurring in up to 30% of adults, and results from a failure of the primum and secundum atrial septa to fuse following birth. It may be identified by a small right-to-left shunt of blood identified with contrast studies or during colour Doppler study of the atrial septum. Demonstration of a PFO with a right-to-left shunt requires not only the presence of a PFO, but also elevated right heart pressures, which may, for example, be deliberately achieved by a 'Valsalva manoeuvre' or may occur in the chronic situation due to right ventricular dysfunction, PE, or PHT.

> **Pitfall**
>
> PFO is a common finding in healthy patients, so contrast studies should not be performed, unless clinical suspicion is high.

Atrial septal defects

ASDs are usually singular and vary greatly in size. Echocardiography is a standard technique for the

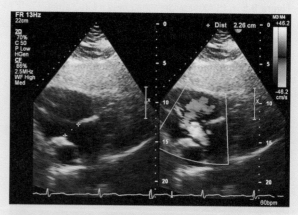

Figure 9.7 Subcostal view (two-dimensional and colour Doppler) demonstrating a large secundum atrial septal defect with a left-to-right shunt. Note: orange flow towards the transducer (see also Video 1.5.5 ●). For a colour version of this figure, please see colour plate section.

visualization of ASDs and any associated cardiac lesions. Colour Doppler study in the subcostal view is particularly helpful to delineate the extent and direction of associated shunting at the atrial level. There are broadly four types of ASDs that arise, following abnormal development of the atrial septum, occurring at specific developmental stages and at specific locations. The most common type is the secundum defect, located in the middle of the atrial septum (Figure 9.7 and Video 1.5.5 ■). An ostium primum defect (approximately 15% of all ASDs) is located at the most inferior part of the septum (close to the atrioventricular valves) and may be associated with defects of the atrioventricular valves or the inlet portion of the ventricular septum (endocardial cushion defects). These defects will be associated with the MV and TV lying in the same plane. The final two (rarer) types of ASD involve either defects in the superior and posterior septa near to the SVC (a sinus venosus ASD) or a defect in the region of the coronary sinus. Evaluation of ASDs requires detailed knowledge and skill set and is best performed by those expert in this area.

Contrast studies of the atria

A simple saline 'bubble' contrast study may be performed by rapid injection of saline that has been agitated (for example, by repeatedly passing 20 mL of saline between two 20-mL syringes via a three-way tap). The most commonly used view is the A4C view to permit simultaneous visualization of all four cardiac chambers. Injection of contrast is followed by the application of a 'Valsalva manoeuvre'—bubbles seen in the LA within 3–4 beats of opacification of the right atrium suggest that there is a connection across the atrial septum. These connections may be from a PFO, any kind of ASD, or pulmonary arteriovenous malformations, although in the latter case, the contrast typically appears in the left side of the heart a few cycles later.

There are other (commercially developed) contrast agents that are designed for different purposes, including endocardial border detection and myocardial perfusion studies. These latter agents are small enough to traverse the pulmonary capillary bed and thus reach the left side of the heart with normal right-to-left connections.

✔ Multiple choice questions

Interactive multiple choice questions to test your knowledge can be found in the Online appendix at www.oxfordmedicine.com/focusedicu. Please refer to your access card for further details.

Further reading

Armstrong WF, Ryan T. Contrast echocardiography. In: Armstrong WF, Ryan T. *Feigenbaum's Echocardiography*, 7th ed. Philadelphia, PA: Lippincott Williams and Wilkins; 2010. pp. 67–90.

Armstrong WF, Ryan T. Left and right atrium, and right ventricle. In: Armstrong WF, Ryan T. *Feigenbaum's Echocardiography*, 7th ed. Philadelphia, PA: Lippincott Williams and Wilkins; 2010. pp. 185–216.

Armstrong WF, Ryan T. Congenital heart diseases. In: Armstrong WF, Ryan T. *Feigenbaum's Echocardiography*, 7th ed.

Philadelphia, PA: Lippincott Williams and Wilkins; 2010. pp. 561–632.

Armstrong WF, Ryan T. Masses, tumors, and source of embolus. In: Armstrong WF, Ryan T. *Feigenbaum's Echocardiography*, 7th ed. Philadelphia, PA: Lippincott Williams and Wilkins; 2010. pp. 711–40.

Lang RM, Badano LP, Mor-Avi V, *et al*. Recommendations for cardiac chamber quantification by echocardiography in adults: an update from the American Society of Echocardiography and the European Association of Cardiovascular Imaging. *Journal of the American Society of Echocardiography* 2015;**28**:1–39.

Lang RM, Bierig M, Devereux RB, *et al*.; Chamber Quantification Writing Group; American Society of Echocardiography's Guidelines and Standards Committee; European Association of Echocardiography. Recommendations for chamber quantification: a report from the American Society of Echocardiography's Guidelines and Standards Committee. *Journal of the American Society of Echocardiography* 2005;**18**:1440–62.

10

Pericardial assessment

Shirjel Alam and Michael Gillies

Introduction

Cardiac tamponade should be considered in the differential diagnosis of any haemodynamically unstable, critically ill patient presenting with elevated jugular venous pressure.

Pericardial tamponade is a clinical diagnosis that is often difficult to make in critical care. Endotracheal tubes and central venous catheters (CVCs) limit the visual assessment of neck veins, and mechanical ventilation can make heart sounds difficult to hear, so diagnosing tamponade using 'Beck's triad' (jugular venous distension, distant heart sounds, and hypotension) is not always feasible.

Echocardiography, performed rapidly at the bedside, is the single most useful tool for identifying pericardial fluid and assessing cardiac compromise.

This chapter will outline the anatomy and physiology of the pericardial space and common causes of pericardial collections seen in critically ill patients. It will explain how to recognize a pericardial collection and answer these important questions—is it definitely pericardial? What is its size? What is its composition? Are there any associated abnormalities? And is it clinically significant? Simple collections will be distinguished from haemopericardium and pyocardium, which require surgical management. Finally, it will discuss the 2D signs of cardiac tamponade that should guide the intensivist towards pericardial drainage in life-threatening cases. The advanced section of this chapter will introduce the spectral Doppler signs of pulsus paradoxus that indicate cardiac tamponade.

Normal anatomy

The pericardium consists of a tough outer fibrous layer and a delicate inner serosal sac. The serosal sac has two reflected surfaces. The inner membrane is called the visceral pericardium and is adherent to the cardiac epicardium. The outer membrane is called the parietal pericardium and is adherent to the fibrous pericardium.

The potential space within the serosal sac normally contains 15–35 mL of serous fluid, which can usually be seen during echocardiography.

The fibrous pericardium is fused to the central tendon of the diaphragm, sternum, and root of the great vessels.

Relevant physiology

In health, pericardial fluid serves to lubricate the visceral and parietal layers of the pericardium. The fibrous pericardium and its attachments protect and stabilize the heart within the chest, and when the heart is exposed to acute volume overload, they help prevent the ventricles from over-distension. In addition, the pericardium has a role in limiting the local spread of infection.

Pathophysiology

Pericardial collections can accumulate for a number of medical and surgical reasons (Box 10.1). In a general ICU setting, common causes include pneumonia, cancer, and catheter laboratory intervention.

Box 10.1 Causes of pericardial disease

- Idiopathic
- Viral infection (echovirus, Coxsackie, adenovirus, human immunodeficiency virus, mumps, Ebstein–Barr virus, cytomegalovirus, varicella, rubella, parvovirus, etc.)
- Bacterial infection (*Pneumococcus, Haemophilus*, tuberculosis, etc.)
- Fungal/parasitic infection (*Candida, Histoplasma/Entamoeba, Toxoplasma*, etc.)
- Uraemia
- Systemic connective tissue disorder (systemic lupus erythematosus, rheumatoid arthritis, scleroderma, etc.)
- Myocarditis
- Post-myocardial infarction (early or late)
- Cardiothoracic surgery
- Acute aortic dissection
- Penetrating trauma
- Malignancy
- Radiation-induced

The clinical effects of a pericardial collection depend on both the volume and rate of accumulation. One that accumulates slowly may become very large before symptoms and clinical signs develop, whereas a rapid collection of smaller volumes (as little as 50–100 mL of fluid) can have marked clinical consequences, including hypotension and shock.

It is not unusual for chronic pericardial effusions to remain clinically undetected until critical illness and then to become an unanticipated finding on focused echo. Uraemic pericarditis is a rare, but potentially fatal, complication of chronic kidney disease (CKD).

Pericarditis and pericardial effusion

Clinical features

Pericarditis may present with fever, malaise, or systemic upset. A common symptom is sharp, stabbing chest pain that is worse on inspiration and classically relieved by sitting forward. It may be severe, substernal, or submammary, and thus be confused with ischaemic chest pain. Radiation to the trapezius ridge is highly specific for pericarditis.

Most signs on clinical examination, such as tachycardia or low-grade fever, are non-specific. However, a pericardial rub is considered to be pathognomonic, and on auscultation, this sounds characteristically like 'crunching snow', best heard at the lower left sternal edge, with the patient leaning forward.

Investigations

Classical ECG findings of pericarditis include: concave, or 'saddle-shaped', upward ST elevation seen in all leads, ST depression in aVR and V1, and a PR segment that deviates in the opposite direction to P-wave polarity. After several days, these changes may resolve and become replaced by flattening and inversion of the T waves. With chronic inflammation, T-wave inversion may persist indefinitely. Low-voltage QRS complexes are seen, sometimes with 'electrical alternans' (beat-to-beat variability in QRS voltage) that is caused by excessive cardiac mobility.

Chest X-ray should be performed to identify pathology, such as consolidation, but it may also reveal an enlarged cardiac silhouette, indicative of pericardial fluid. Blood tests for inflammatory markers, bacterial culture, viral serology, and troponin (myocarditis) should also be sent.

Haemopericardium

Haemopericardium can be fatal due to rapid accumulation of blood in the pericardial space or due to the underlying pathology that caused it. Causes of haemopericardium include aortic dissection, blunt or penetrating trauma, oesophageal perforation, and myocardial infarction. In the hospital setting, cardiac surgery and percutaneous coronary intervention (PCI) are the commonest causes, mediated via direct injury to the coronary arteries or local structures, or generalized ooze from coagulopathy. Haemopericardium is more common after valve surgery than coronary artery bypass grafting alone. Pericardial drains placed at the time of surgery can become blocked or obstructed, and blood can accumulate quickly in the pericardial space; thus, if tamponade is suspected clinically, clinicians should not seek false reassurance from the absence of blood in surgical drains.

In aortic dissection without involvement of the aortic root, a small amount of pericardial (and pleural) fluid may accumulate due to sympathetic activity or obstructed lymphatic drainage. In proximal aortic dissection when the 'flap' extends proximally to involve the aortic root, haemopericardium and tamponade can occur rapidly. Rupture of an aneurysm of a sinus of Valsalva (dilatation of the aortic cusps) has similar effects. In such cases, prompt diagnosis and surgical treatment of haemopericardium are necessary to prevent mortality.

Fortunately, traumatic causes of haemopericardium are rare, but they are associated with high mortality. US has been established as a vital diagnostic tool in the acute assessment of the trauma patient [e.g. Focused Assessment with Sonography for Trauma (FAST) scanning], because tamponade is a life-threatening injury that can be rapidly diagnosed and treated.

Myocardial rupture and haemopericardium can be an acute or late complication of acute myocardial infarction. Occasionally, haemopericardium may also be seen with severe infection (particularly tuberculosis) in anticoagulated patients with pericarditis, and in those with malignancy.

Percutaneous drainage of haemopericardium risks exsanguination, so rapid surgical intervention is the definitive treatment.

Cardiac tamponade

Tamponade occurs when the accumulation of fluid causes intrapericardial pressure to exceed the pressure in the RV. Once this happens, cardiac filling is impeded, and if left untreated, hypotension can progress rapidly to shock and cardiac arrest.

Cardiac tamponade is a clinical diagnosis. However, in this setting, critically ill patients present particular challenges to haemodynamic assessment—haemodynamic instability is often multifactorial, venous pressure can be difficult to assess in the context of mechanical ventilation, and vasoactive drugs can compensate for haemodynamic effects of cardiac tamponade until a late stage.

Echocardiographic assessment of a pericardial collection

This section discusses six questions that should be answered when assessing pericardial collections.

1. Is there a collection?

Pericardial fluid can be seen easily on 2D echo as echolucent (black) areas between the pericardium and myocardium, and should be assessed in all FoCUS views. In normal subjects, only a trace of pericardial fluid should be visible. Occasionally, and especially in patients with high adiposity, epicardial fat collections can mimic the appearance of pericardial fluid. Epicardial fat can be distinguished from fluid, as it typically has a granular appearance, is of low volume, and tends to move with the myocardium.

PSAX can reveal the distribution of pericardial fluid around the LV (Figure 10.1). The A4C view can reveal pericardial fluid around the lateral wall of the LV and the right ventricular free wall (Figures 10.2 and 10.3, and Video 1.6.1 ●). The subcostal view allows excellent visualization of fluid adjacent to the right ventricular free wall and any associated right ventricular wall motion abnormalities; in addition, assessment for a subcostal approach to drainage can be made (Video 1.6.2 ●). The IVC diameter should be assessed by direct visualization and M-mode, as significant pericardial collections cause a dilated IVC, with little or no respiratory variation.

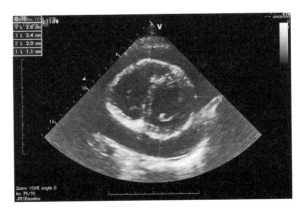

Figure 10.1 A PSAX view, indicating the circumferential depth of a large pericardial effusion.

(a)

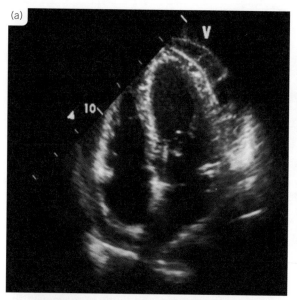

(b)

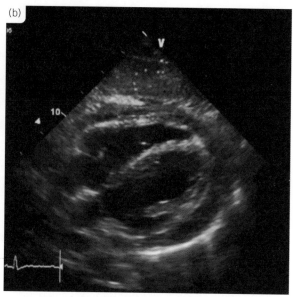

(c)

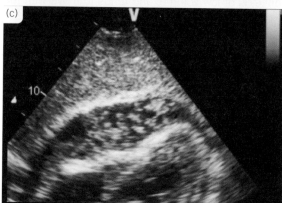

Figure 10.2 Different pericardial collections: (a) fibrinous (with stranding due to acute pericarditis); (b) simple; and (c) purulent (organized, heterogenous appearance).

2. Is the collection definitely pericardial?

Distinguishing pericardial fluid from pleural fluid can be challenging. A useful technique is to use the PLAX image; pleural effusions are visualized posterior to the descending aorta, whereas pericardial collections are visualized anterior to it (Figure 10.4).

3. What is the size of the collection?

The depth of the effusion can be measured at end-systole, perpendicularly between the pericardium and epicardial surface of the heart. A pericardial effusion is classified as small when its depth is <0.5 cm, moderate when 0.5–2 cm, and large >2 cm. Maximal measurements of pericardial fluid around each regional wall should be made.

4. What is the composition of the collection?

The composition of pericardial fluid can be assessed by echocardiography. Simple effusions are serous and will appear as a uniform echo-free space. However, fibrinous, exudative effusions are common, and stranding may be seen on echocardiographic examination (Figures 10.2 and 10.3). Loculation or septation of the fluid suggest that percutaneous drainage may be difficult, and in such cases, a surgical approach may be necessary. Old blood appears more echogenic and grainy, due to thrombosis. Acute haemorrhage into the pericardium will not and thus may have a similar appearance to serous effusions.

A purulent effusion, known as pyocardium, may also be echogenic and accumulate quickly, causing

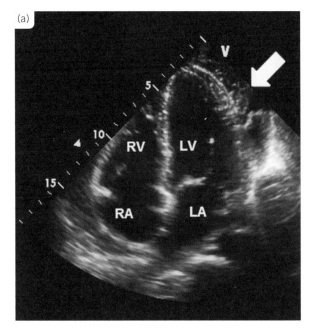

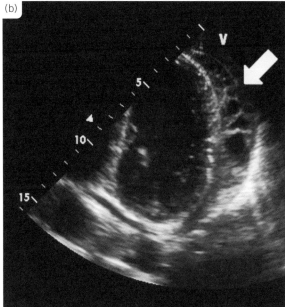

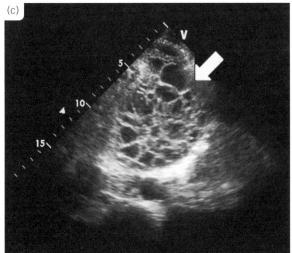

Figure 10.3 A progressively modified A4C view (tilted downwards), revealing a fibrinous exudate (white arrows).

compromise. In such cases, frequent monitoring with echocardiography is appropriate, and although percutaneous drainage may be useful for diagnostic purposes or relief of acute tamponade, surgical management is usually necessary.

5. Are there any associated abnormalities?

Assessment of the pericardium, myocardium, and aorta is essential to exclude surgical causes of pericardial effusion such as aortic dissection or myocardial rupture.

6. Is the collection clinically significant?

Depending on their clinical setting, any critically ill patient presenting with signs of shock, elevated venous pressure, and a pericardial collection should trigger immediate referral to a cardiologist or cardiac surgeon. Deviation from this pathway is risky. However,

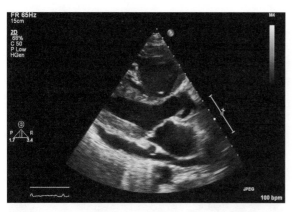

Figure 10.4 A small posterior pericardial effusion, seen anterior to the descending aorta. Note: due to the improved acoustic window that this produces, the coronary sinus is visible in the posterior atrioventricular groove. Note also: B lines to the left of the descending aorta indicate the lung. If a pleural effusion were present, this is where it would be seen.

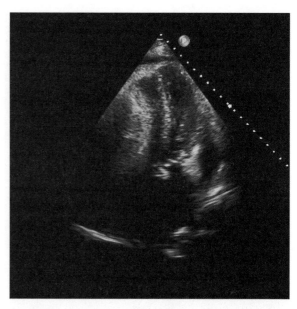

Figure 10.5 Right ventricular collapse due to a large local pericardial collection.

it is useful for non-specialists to appreciate the echo signs of tamponade because in extreme cases, lifesaving immediate drainage may be necessary.

> **Pitfall**
>
> The use of vasoactive drugs in intensive care patients can mask the marked hypotension that cardiac tamponade induces.

Echo signs of tamponade

Chamber collapse

This is best assessed in the A4C and subcostal views. As pericardial pressure increases, the first chamber to become affected is the right atrium, which is at its lowest pressure as it relaxes and is pulled downwards during ventricular systole. Hence, right atrial systolic collapse is an early sign of tamponade (Video 1.6.3 ⏺). Right ventricular diastolic collapse occurs next, which indicates impaired ventricular filling and usually heralds significant haemodynamic compromise (Figures 10.5 and 10.6). Left ventricular collapse occurs very rarely, as a late sign of cardiac tamponade.

Inferior vena cava

In cardiac tamponade, the IVC is dilated and unreactive during spontaneous ventilation, as a result of increased RAP (Figure 10.7).

> **Pitfall**
>
> In a mechanically ventilated patient, a dilated and unreactive IVC is common, so this finding is not specific for tamponade.

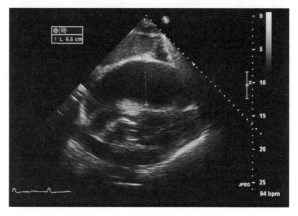

Figure 10.6 A massive (6.6 cm) pericardial effusion compressing the RV.

(a)

(b)

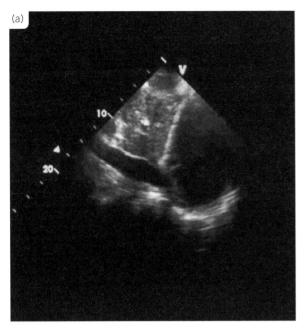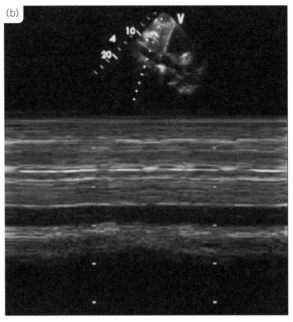

Figure 10.7 A dilated IVC with no respiratory variation. (a) A subcostal IVC view. (b) M-mode across the IVC.

Advanced echocardiography

Pulsed wave Doppler

During spontaneous inspiration, venous return is augmented, and in cardiac tamponade, this causes ventricular interdependence (right ventricular enlargement with corresponding pressure discordance and compromise of left ventricular ejection), manifest by the displacement of the IVS towards the LV and pulsus paradoxus.

By placing the sampling volume just distal to the open MV or TV leaflet tips in A4C, PW Doppler can measure inflow velocities at those points. In the context of a spontaneously breathing patient with a pericardial effusion, >25% of respiratory variation in peak early inflow (E wave) velocity (decreased during spontaneous inspiration) suggests tamponade physiology (Figure 10.8).

Pitfall

Positive pressure ventilation reverses the direction of E wave variability in tamponade and significantly attenuates this response; therefore, this is an unreliable method to attempt to diagnose tamponade in ventilated patients.

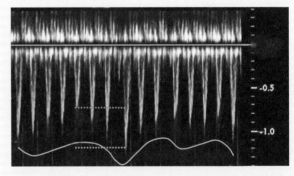

Figure 10.8 PW Doppler of mitral valve inflows in a patient with a large pericardial effusion. Note: there is >50% respiratory variation in peak E wave velocity.

Reproduced with permission from Colebourn C. and Newton J., *Acute and Critical Care Echocardiography*. Figure 6.6. Copyright (2017) with permission from Oxford University Press.

Multiple choice questions

Interactive multiple choice questions to test your knowledge can be found in the Online appendix at www.oxfordmedicine.com/focusedicu. Please refer to your access card for further details.

Further reading

Beck C. Two cardiac compression triads. *JAMA* 1935;**104**: 714–16.

Brathwaite CE, Rodriguez A, Turney SZ, *et al*. Blunt traumatic cardiac rupture. A 5-year experience. *Annals of Surgery* 1990;**212**:701–4.

Colebourn C, Newton J (eds). *Acute and Critical Care Echocardiography: Oxford Clinical Imaging Guides*. Oxford: Oxford University Press; 2017.

Masud KH, Espinosa RE, Nishimura RA. Pericardial disease: diagnosis and management. *Mayo Clinic Proceedings* 2010;**85**:572–93.

Peebles CR, Shambrook JS, Harden SP. Pericardial disease– anatomy and function. *British Journal of Radiology* 2011;**84** Spec No 3:S324–37.

11

Aortic valve assessment

Marcus Peck and Michaela Scheuermann-Freestone

Introduction

Clinical recognition of significant AV disease can be challenging, even in a controlled environment with plenty of time for detailed assessment.

AS, for example, can be asymptomatic even when it is severe, and as the disease progresses, the murmur it produces may become quieter, not louder. In such cases, a thorough clinical history and physical examination may not always detect life-threatening disease, especially in the context of an acutely deteriorating patient, and FoCUS can provide useful insight.

Quantitative AV assessment is a complex task that should be reserved for fully trained practitioners performing comprehensive echocardiography. However, being able to recognize severe AV disease and knowing when to escalate out of hours to a cardiologist or a cardiac surgeon is a lifesaving skill all intensivists should know.

This chapter will cover in detail the 2D sonoanatomy and pathophysiology of common AV lesions and explain step by step how to image the AV and detect significant disease. The advanced section will introduce how to use colour and spectral Doppler to recognize acute/severe pathology that requires immediate management.

Normal anatomy

The AV is a complex, but reliable, structure consisting of three cusps, separated by three commissures contained within a fibrous annular ring, all of which are readily visible with 2D TTE (Figure 11.1).

The normal AV has three delicate, crescent-shaped leaflets, fixed securely within the annulus and aortic root. These are known as the left coronary, right coronary, and non-coronary cusps, according to their relationship with the coronary ostia.

Each cusp has a thin and highly mobile free edge, the midline and upper rim of which are slightly thickened. During coaptation in diastole, these edges overlap significantly with those of the neighbouring cusps, ensuring that the valve closes tightly; together with a large leaflet coaptation zone, this design makes the AV very effective.

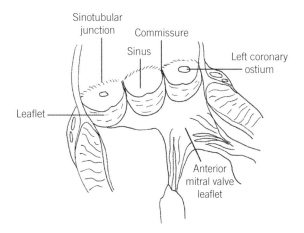

Figure 11.1 Schematic drawing of aortic root structures after longitudinal opening of the root.

Reproduced from Figure 4, Misfeld, Martin, and Hans-Hinrich Sievers. 'Heart valve macro-and microstructure.' *Philosophical Transactions of the Royal Society of London B: Biological Sciences* **362**.1484 (2007): 1421–1436. © 2007 The Royal Society.

Commissures

The base of each AV cusp anchors securely into the aortic media, and the hinge-points between neighbouring cusps are known as commissures.

When closed in diastole, the AV cusps and commissures form a characteristic Y-shape in the short-axis view, sometimes referred to as the (inverted) 'Mercedes Benz' sign (Figure 11.2).

In the PSAX view, the normal AV orifice at mid-systole is typically shaped like a large triangle with curved sides, like a guitar pick (Figure 11.3).

Sinuses of Valsalva

Adjacent to each cusp is a sinus of Valsalva, which bulges laterally, enabling the cusp to open fully, in parallel with the LVOT and aortic walls, to allow unobstructed systolic ejection of blood into the aorta. The sinuses also provide a continuous supply of blood to the right and left coronary ostia, which are located within their respective sinuses. The right coronary cusp lies anteriorly, and the non-coronary sinus lies adjacent to the IAS.

Together with the AV cusps, the sinuses of Valsalva form the aortic root, which narrows at their distal

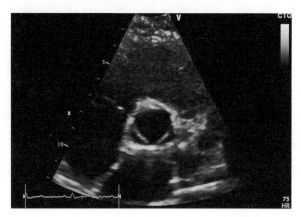

Figure 11.3 A normal AV, seen open at mid-systole in a PSAX view.

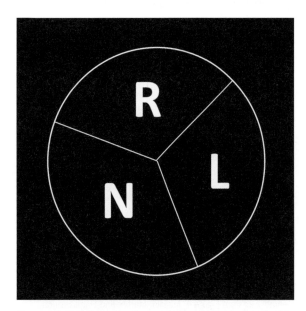

Figure 11.2 Schematic of normal AV cusps, as seen at mid-diastole in a PSAX view. The right coronary cusp (R) abuts the RV; the left coronary cusp (L) contains the origin of the left main stem, which is mostly visible in short-axis views; the non-coronary cusp (N) abuts the inter-atrial septum.

margin to form the sinotubular junction (STj) (the origin of the proximal aorta).

Annulus

The AV annulus provides essential structural support to the valve complex. It is shaped like a three-pointed crown, with its fibrous ring encircling the cusps and its points extending distally into the aortic root, supporting each commissure.

The MV lies very close to the AV and shares some of its cytoskeleton. Consequently, the left and non-coronary cusps and the AMVL are all directly adjacent to each other. This relationship can be seen most clearly in the PLAX view.

Normal physiology

A normal AV enables unobstructed systolic ejection of blood, unidirectional flow, and preserved coronary perfusion throughout a wide range of loading conditions.

Pathophysiology of aortic valve obstruction

Narrowing of the left ventricular outflow can occur at any anatomical level, from subvalvular (fixed subaortic membrane or dynamic obstruction seen in HCM) to supravalvular stenosis, but the most common cause, by far, is chronic valvular AS.

As a consequence of reduced valve area, the pathophysiology of AS involves a sequence of chronic left ventricular pressure overload, adaptive concentric hypertrophy, diastolic dysfunction, raised left ventricular filling pressure, maladaptive eccentric hypertrophy, left ventricular dilatation, systolic dysfunction, and right ventricular involvement.

The onset of left ventricular dysfunction is an important indication for AV replacement surgery.

Aortic stenosis

AS is a progressive disease that usually follows a long subclinical period and presents with typical symptoms, including dyspnoea, chest pain, and syncope.

AS may be the primary reason for ICU admission, but it is also a common finding in FoCUS studies performed in the elderly population. As with all imaging, the pre-scan probability improves the diagnostic accuracy of echocardiography, so understanding the different pathologies involved will help the practitioner get the most from the echo assessment.

Common causes of AS include:

- Calcific (80% of cases in Europe/United States)
- Bicuspid—both congenital and functional (becoming increasingly prevalent)
- Rheumatic (rare in industrialized countries, commonest form of AS worldwide).

Calcific aortic stenosis

Twenty-five per cent of patients over the age of 65 have leaflet calcification without stenosis (so-called aortic sclerosis), and about a third of this group will progress to significant calcific AS, usually before they reach their 70s.

Calcific AS presents in patients between the ages of 70 and 85, and given the rising age of the general population, its prevalence is destined to increase. It appears to be more than just a degenerative process. Risk factors include age, male sex, smoking, hypertension, hyperlipidaemia, and diabetes, suggesting that atherosclerosis may play a role in its development.

On 2D echo, the tri-leaflet valve demonstrates increased echogenicity, first at the base of its cusps, and then more extensively as disease progresses. Progressive thickening and failure of separation in systole are seen best in PLAX. However, PSAX can be useful, particularly for identifying functional or congenital bicuspid disease. In PSAX, the calcific AS orifice seen at mid-systole is typically stellate (Figure 11.4c and Video 1.7.1 ⏺).

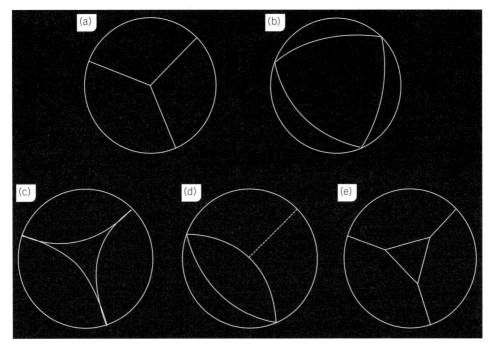

Figure 11.4 Schematic diagram of the AV, as seen in a PSAX view, in both diastole (a) and systole (b–e). (a) Normal AV during diastole. (b) Normal AV during systole. (c) Calcific AS (stellate orifice). (d) Functional bicuspid AV (ovoid orifice; the dotted line represents a raphe). (e) Rheumatic AV (triangular orifice, commissural fusion).

Bicuspid aortic stenosis

The congenitally bicuspid AV characteristically presents between adolescence and early adulthood, affecting males most commonly. It is the most prevalent form of congenital heart disease (1–2% of the general population) and is commonly associated with aortic root dilatation and aortic coarctation. Associated abnormalities of the MV are common. Not all cases will need valve replacement, but many do, and these tend to be required earlier in life than in other aetiologies.

Congenital absence, fusion (often between the right and left coronary cusps, causing a functional bicuspid valve), or dysplasia of one or more commissures become progressively flow-limiting due to inflammation and fibrosis. Associated AR is common.

Functionally, the bicuspid valve has only two cusps and commissures, and when cusps are fused, a raphe can usually be seen throughout systole in PSAX. In PLAX, diastolic bowing of the leaflets (back towards the LVOT) can sometimes be seen. As disease progresses, the leaflets become increasingly calcified and these features are more difficult to identify.

In PSAX, the bicuspic AS orifice, seen at mid-systole, is typically ovoid (Figure 11.4d and Video 1.7.2 📹).

Rheumatic aortic stenosis

Acute group A streptococcal infection ('rheumatic fever'), usually seen in adolescence, can cause acute cardiac inflammation and chronic scarring of all heart valves—the MV in particular. Thus, isolated AV disease is rare.

Rheumatic AS is characterized by fibrosis, minimal calcification, commissural fusion, and restricted leaflet opening, causing AS and sometimes AR.

In PLAX, increased echogenicity of the free cusp edges can be seen, associated with systolic bowing (towards the aorta). These features make it difficult to distinguish rheumatic from calcific AS, and the diagnosis is based on coexisting changes seen in other valves, usually the MV.

In PSAX, the rheumatic AS orifice seen at mid-systole is typically triangular (Figure 11.4e and Video 1.7.3 📹).

Adaptive changes in chronic aortic stenosis

AS has chronic upstream and downstream effects that are readily visible with 2D echo.

Post-stenotic dilatation

Dilatation of the aortic root is associated with most forms of AS, but bicuspid disease in particular. Turbulent, high-velocity blood flow has been postulated as a cause but abnormal remodelling of the extracellular matrix within the walls of the proximal aorta is more likely.

For further discussion about aortic assessment, see Chapter 18.

Left ventricular hypertrophy

Any chronic obstruction to flow throught the LVOT has the potential to cause left ventricular pressure overload and myocardial wall stress. LVH is a healthy initial response to AS, which eventually becomes maladaptive.

In AS, fractional shortening may be supranormal, and LVH is usually reversible if it is corrected surgically.

For further information about LVH, see Chapter 7.

Left ventricular failure

Disease progression can lead to dilatation of the left ventricular cavity, with only modest wall thickening, which is known as eccentric LVH.

The onset of eccentric LVH in AS suggests the beginning of decompensation, and once left ventricular systolic dysfunction becomes established, mortality increases dramatically. Reversibility, by way of AV replacement, is possible at this stage, but not guaranteed.

Aortic regurgitation

AR is caused by abnormalities of the AV cusps and/or the aortic root.

Regurgitation of blood back into the LV during diastole requires it to eject this volume forward again, while coping with the extra distension that it causes. When compensation fails, the state is known as volume overload.

Causes of acute/severe AR include:

- Endocarditis
- Proximal aortic dissection.

Endocarditis

Endocarditis is characterized by infection of the endocardial layers of the heart, including the surface of the valves. This causes formation of vegetations, which are mobile masses that usually originate on the upstream (ventricular) side of a cusp and are seen to move with it but travel excessively, thus appearing to move independently of the valve itself.

Vegetations can cause impaired leaflet coaptation and regurgitation. Leaflet destruction is also possible, and major perforations can cause acute/severe AR, which is usually life-threatening and an indication for emergency valve replacement.

Vegetations on the AV are usually seen as irregular, echogenic masses, extending from one or more of the cusps, moving independently into the aortic root during systole and prolapsing back into the LVOT in diastole, fluttering in a stream of AR.

While the initial assessment of endocarditis is usually by TTE, this cannot rule out vegetations, especially in the presence of chronic valve disease or echogenic artefacts, and TOE remains the gold standard investigation. If any valvular mass is seen on transthoracic FoCUS, or if it appears normal but clinical suspicion is high, cardiology referral is required to exclude endocarditis.

Proximal aortic dissection

Chronic AR is commonly associated with aortic root dilatation, due to loss of leaflet support and failed coaptation. However, in acute dissection of the proximal aorta, retrograde extension can strip the commissures completely off the aortic wall, causing flailing leaflets and acute/severe AR (Video 1.7.4 📷). This is an indication for immediate surgery.

Acute proximal aortic dissection can cause a pericardial collection and tamponade. For further information about pericardial assessment, see Chapter 10.

Volume overload in acute/severe aortic regurgitation

Acute/severe AR into a normal LV causes a marked increase in left ventricular end-diastolic pressure (LVEDP), leading to acute pulmonary oedema, as the ventricle has no time to adapt and dilate. The additional volume momentarily increases left ventricular preload, but the circulation is rapidly overwhelmed by retrograde flow, leading to decreased SV, systolic and pulse pressures, and shock.

Mortality is extremely high in cases of acute/severe AR, and immediate surgery is the only effective treatment.

Common causes of chronic AR include:

- Long-standing systemic hypertension (annular dilatation)

- Marfan's disease (annular dilatation)
- Connective tissue diseases (aortitis)
- Myxomatous disease.

Diseases that cause valvular AS (detailed in Aortic stenosis, p. 99) can also cause AR by restricted leaflet movement and coaptation.

Myxomatous disease is a degenerative process involving a build-up of glycosaminoglycans in the valvular extracellular matrix, the cause of which is not fully understood. It is seen mainly in the MV and is a common cause of MV prolapse, but it can also involve the AV.

Thickened, misshapen AV leaflets are seen with redundant tissue that sags back into the LVOT in diastole, causing them to appear falsely in PSAX, as if they contain masses.

Adaptive changes in chronic aortic regurgitation

In contrast to acute AR, chronic AR is usually well tolerated for a long period of time, with low LVEDP and increased systemic pulse pressure.

Early in the disease progression, LVEF is often normal or augmented by the increased left ventricular preload. Chronic volume overload increases wall stress in the LV, which responds by remodelling with eccentric hypertrophy. As disease progresses, the LV dilates and LVEF deteriorates.

Clinical decompensation is usually heralded by the development of exertional dyspnoea. Valve replacement is recommended at the onset of systolic dysfunction and/or left ventricular dilatation, which requires comprehensive echocardiographic surveillance.

Echo assessment

STEP 1: Ask yourself—what pathology are you expecting to see?

FoCUS should always follow clinical assessment and build on what is already known or suspected. Patient age, clinical history, physical signs, and ancillary investigations all affect the pre-scan likelihood of different pathology, and FoCUS information should relate back to each of these.

If you discover more than you expected at 2D assessment, you will then be able to ask yourself another important question—are these findings consistent with the clinical picture?

Reporting in FoCUS is all about referring back to the clinical setting. If in doubt, refer.

STEP 2: Optimize the 2D image

Paying attention to patient positioning, probe handling, and the setting of depth, gain, compression, focus, and sector width (described in Chapter 3) will all produce significant improvements to your image and will help with your assessment. Autogain functions can be useful, so utilize them, whenever possible.

Activating the zoom function, by laying a box over just the valve and clicking the zoom button, enlarges the image, with more pixelated detail, and optimizes the frame rate to get the most from slow-motion review.

STEP 3: inspect the aortic valve with 2D

In comprehensive echo, spectral Doppler techniques (introduced in Chapter 3 and the advanced section of this chapter) play an important role in grading the severity of AV disease. However, considerable diagnostic information can also be gained from 2D images, which contribute significantly to making a diagnosis.

Sweep slowly through the entire valve in both PSAX and PLAX by tilting the phased array probe along its long edge.

2D assessment involves the following:

1. Number of cusps
2. Degree of thickening/calcification
3. Degree of leaflet mobility
4. Inspection of the AV orifice
5. Associated pathology.

Number of cusps

In PSAX, a normal AV is visibly tricuspid (with three leaflets of equal size), so if a bicuspid valve—functional or congenital—is obvious, it is likely to be pathological. In functional bicuspid disease, the most common line of fusion is the commissure between the right and left coronary cusps (usually visualized near the '2 o'clock' position).

Degree of thickening/calcification

Normal AV leaflets are so thin and move so quickly that they are often hard to see. By contrast, diseased leaflets are usually more visible. However, calcification can make these structures hard to visualize with 2D echo.

Calcification is seen as brightly echogenic areas within the cusps or annulus that can be severe enough to cause acoustic shadowing (seen as signal 'dropout' in the far field, behind the valve).

The degree of thickening and/or calcification may suggest a possible aetiology (i.e. calcific versus rheumatic), but alone these are not good indicators of stenosis.

Degree of leaflet mobility

This is key to making the diagnosis of AS.

Normal leaflets open parallel to the aortic wall in systole and move so quickly that they are usually seen only in their fully open or closed positions. By contrast, diseased leaflets move slowly and fail to open fully in systole, instead pointing towards the centre of the aortic root in PLAX.

In severe AS, the leaflets can move so little that they are almost indistinguishable from each other.

If severely restricted mobility is seen in all but one heavily calcified leaflet, which moves normally, severe AS can be excluded.

Orifice observation and planimetry

While attempting to trace the AV orifice area in mid-systole is possible using 2D echocardiography, it is often hampered by difficulty getting the angle correct and not cutting the valve at its narrowest point. Also, as the disease progresses, calcification and acoustic shadowing make this task more difficult. Consequently, planimetry is not a routine measurement in comprehensive 2D TTE assessment. TOE and/or 3D investigation is much better for detailed AV examination and are usually reserved for specialist investigations.

For reference, the normal AV orifice area is between 3 and 4 cm². AS is severe when this area is reduced to <1 cm² (approximately 25% of normal).

Associated cardiac pathology

The presence of adaptive structural changes on 2D echo can provide useful supportive information; these include:

1. LVH without systemic hypertension—suggests significant AS

2. Dilated aortic root—suggests the potential for AR or AS

3. Other valvular abnormalities—may provide clues to a rheumatic aetiology.

Aortic regurgitation

Unfortunately, 2D assessment provides little useful information relating to the presence or absence of AR. In the presence of significant regurgitation, AV leaflets can appear completely normal, so 2D assessment cannot be relied on to exclude it. Indirect 2D evidence of significant AR includes:

1. 'Reverse doming' of the AMVL. Normally, the AMVL is seen to open in PLAX as a straight line during diastole. Reverse doming describes an abnormal concavity, towards the IVS, caused by pressure of the AR jet.

2. Diastolic fluttering of AMVL in PLAX, caused by the AR jet

3. Increased EPSS—described in Chapter 7.

Aortic root dilatation and AR often coexist. Aortic assessment is discussed in Chapter 17.

Advanced echocardiography

So far, AV assessment has involved only qualitative 2D assessment. It may have produced a diagnosis of suspected AS and even suggested an underlying cause. However, to determine the presence of significant AS or AR, Doppler assessment is required.

Our focus now is on recognizing life-threatening AV disease, to expedite timely referral and enable a fully qualified echo practitioner to perform a comprehensive assessment.

STEP 4: Turn on and optimize colour Doppler imaging

For accurate interpretation of colour Doppler, getting the Doppler settings right is essential. This involves optimization of the following:

1. Doppler box—set just large enough to contain the valve and immediate area of interest (i.e. aortic root in AS, LVOT in AR)

2. Doppler gain—set just below the point at which speckles appear all over the image

3. Nyquist limit—set at 50–60 cm/s.

STEP 5: Colour Doppler assessment

Aortic stenosis assessment

Turbulence

Systolic ejection through a normal AV is usually laminar, and the LVOT runs across the field in PLAX so aliasing is not usually seen. By contrast, in the LVOT may be seen in the A5C of a healthy patient as it is

better aligned with blood flow. Seeing aliasing in the proximal aorta in PLAX indicates turbulent, high-velocity flow and possible AS.

Proximal flow acceleration

Blood flow accelerates towards peak velocity at its narrowest point, which is usually the AV orifice. In AS, systolic proximal flow acceleration is visualized with colour Doppler as a hemispheric area of aliasing on the upstream (LVOT) side of the AV, centred on the valve orifice (Figure 11.5).

The presence of significant flow acceleration in the LVOT suggests the possibility of AS, but it can be also caused by elevated global blood flow seen

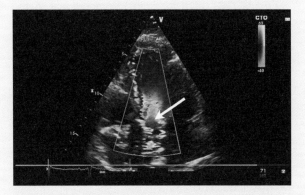

Figure 11.5 An A5C view demonstrating proximal flow acceleration, with aliasing of the colour Doppler jet seen proximal to the aortic stenosis. Note: the red mosaic jet (arrowed) represents abnormally high-velocity blood in the LVOT. For a colour version of this figure, please see colour plate section.

in hyperdynamic states, such as sepsis, or in hypertrophic obstructive cardiomyopathy.

Confirmation of significant AS requires spectral Doppler assessment, which will be introduced in Step 6.

Aortic regurgitation assessment

Colour Doppler is useful for detecting AR. High-velocity retrograde blood flow causes aliasing, which enables semi-quantative assessment using the shape of the turbulent jet.

Jet width

The area of aliasing indicates the origin and vector of the AR jet, which may be central (e.g. diseases with annular dilatation) or eccentric (e.g. diseases that restrict leaflet mobility).

AR flows from one high-pressure chamber to another, and the degree of aliasing is affected by loading conditions well as the pathology itself. Typically, central jets are overestimated, and eccentric jets are underestimated by jet area. Consequently, using jet area (relative to the left ventricular cavity) is not recommended for quantifying AR. However, AR severity does appear to correlate with jet width (relative to the LVOT), mild being <25% and severe being >65%, so if the LVOT is visualized full of regurgitant flow, AR is likely to be significant.

Vena contracta

AR jets converge to their narrowest point immediately after the valve orifice, and then diverge again. The narrowest point of the regurgitant jet is called the vena contracta (VC), and its width is proportional to the severity of AR.

VC is a useful technique to assess severity in ICU, because it is load-independent and less affected by machine settings.

Accuracy of colour Doppler assessment relies on visualizing the whole AR stream in one image, and non-standard imaging planes may be required for this. The whole AR stream includes flow convergence (seen in the aortic root), VC, and jet turbulence (seen in the LVOT) (Figure 11.6).

VC values can be so small that it is important to use the zoom mode and freeze and caliper functions. The probe should be tilted gently, until the jet is at its narrowest; the VC is measured at this point, perpendicular to the direction of regurgitant flow (not the LVOT).

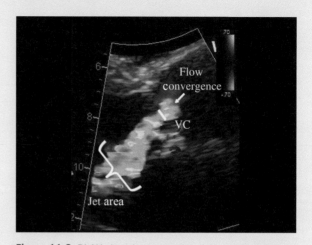

Figure 11.6 PLAX view demonstrating the vena contracta and proximal flow convergence caused by AR. For a colour version of this figure, please see colour plate section.

Adapted from Lancellotti, Patrizio, *et al.*, 'European Association of Echocardiography recommendations for the assessment of valvular regurgitation. Part 1: aortic and pulmonary regurgitation (native valve disease)', *European Heart Journal-Cardiovascular Imaging*, 2010, **11**, 3, pp. 223–244. Copyright © 2010, by permission of Oxford University Press.

Severe AR has a VC width of >0.6 cm; mild AR has a VC of <0.3 cm.

> **Pitfall**
>
> Acute/severe AR may be associated with such severe turbulence in both directions that it becomes very difficult to visualize with colour Doppler. Clinical correlation is always advised.

STEP 6: Spectral Doppler assessment

Aortic stenosis assessment

CW Doppler enables measurement of blood velocity across the AV, which is increased by the narrowed valve orifice in AS. It has important technical limitations in terms of image acquisition and interpretation that must be fully understood, before this information is used in a clinical context. These include (but are not limited to):

• Doppler alignment. The Doppler beam must be aligned as closely as possible in the direction of blood flow, which, in AS, can be eccentric, requiring non-standard views for accurate assessment. Any other angle of imaging will underestimate its velocities.

- Range ambiguity. CW measures all velocities along the sampling line (not at a certain point, as in PW), so it cannot determine at which point the peak velocity was produced. In this way, eccentric MR can be easily misdiagnosed as AS, as they are closely related in phase and location.

- Cardiac output. Increased transvalvular blood flow increases pressure gradients equally on both sides of the valve. In high cardiac output states, the simplified Bernoulli equation, which does not take LVOT pressure into account, will overestimate the severity of AS.

- Left ventricular systolic dysfunction. Low flow states can cause reduced AV leaflet opening, which may overestimate the severity of AS by 2D assessment. It can also cause a reduced AV gradient, which may underestimate the severity of AS by spectral Doppler assessment. In these situations, expert referral is essential to accurately quantify AS, which usually requires stress echocardiography.

Remember—solutions exist to each of these problems, but they require considerable expertise to perform reliably. Quantifying AS is a complex task, particularly in critically ill patients, and all suspicious cases should be referred for urgent comprehensive echo.

Peak velocity

Detecting a raised transvalvular peak velocity should raise suspicion of AS. In the A5C and A3C views, the LVOT, AV, and proximal aorta are usually well aligned for spectral Doppler.

Placing the CW Doppler sampling line across the AV will produce a parabolic trace below the baseline, because blood flow is travelling away from the probe. The lowest point on this curve is the peak velocity (PV), and once this is measured, the echo machine automatically produces a maximum peak gradient (Max PG), according to the simplified Bernoulli equation:

$$\text{Max PG} = 4 \cdot \text{PV}_{AV}^{2}$$

where PV_{AV} = peak velocity across the AV during systole.

Ideally, this should be averaged over three cycles (at least five in the presence of AF).

Normal peak velocity is <2.6 m/s. Severe AS has a peak velocity of >4 m/s.

Dimensionless index

Confounding by cardiac output can be overcome by estimating the AV area using the continuity equation or proximal isovelocity surface area (PISA). However, these are complex and time-consuming methods that require considerable experience to perform accurately. A simpler method to screen for reduced valve area is the dimensionless index (DI), which is obtained by dividing the peak velocity in the LVOT by that in the AV.

In A5C, a well-aligned CW Doppler trace contains two parabolic curves superimposed on each other (Figure 11.7)—one generated by flow through the AV (the highest velocity curve); the other by flow through the LVOT (a denser, lower velocity curve). Peak velocities can be recorded from this single trace.

A normal DI is 1. Severe AS has a DI of 0.25 or less.

The DI is quick and easy to obtain, accounts for cardiac output and body surface area, and does not involve measurement of LVOT diameter (used in the continuity equation), which is prone to error.

Importantly, information from all assessments (clinical, 2D, colour and spectral Doppler) must be assimilated before any conclusions can be drawn. If any of these create suspicion, expert referral is required.

Recognition of aortic replacement valves

The assessment of aortic replacement valves—both tissue valves or mechanical valves—needs to remain

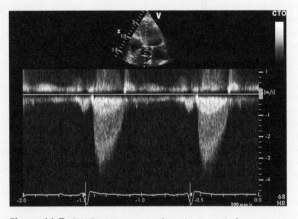

Figure 11.7 CW Doppler trace of aortic stenosis from an A5C view. Note: the superimposed, denser trace with lower peak velocity, caused by flow through the LVOT. The peak velocity is high, suggesting significant AS, and a DI of just over 25% confirms this suspicion. Expert referral is now required for confirmation.

in expert hands, and various valve types will be associated with characteristic appearances on 2D echo, as well as on Doppler assessments. However, it is helpful to realize the presence of a replacement valve early on in the investigation, as the measurements outside the normal range could easily trigger unnecessary alarm when missed.

Tissue aortic valves have a characteristic thickening and a brighter echo contrast at the annulus, as most come mounted on an artificial ring or on a stent. However, stentless valves do exist. Often, the cusps can be seen as thin and mobile structures, just like a native aortic valve (Video 1.7.5a and c 🎥). Transvalvular flow is normally slightly higher than in a native valve, and minor regurgitation is within normal limits.

Mechanical valves have a much brighter appearance overall than tissue valves, and there is usually a characteristic acoustic shadowing seen behind the valve (Video 1.7.5b and d 🎥). The cusps may be seen on either PLAX or SAX, and transvalvular peak velocity is also higher than in a native valve. On spectral Doppler assessment, a characteristic bright vertical line is seen just before the valve opens, and again when it closes; these are not seen with a tissue valve.

✅ Multiple choice questions

Interactive multiple choice questions to test your knowledge can be found in the Online appendix at www.oxfordmedicine.com/focusedicu. Please refer to your access card for further details.

Further reading

Baumgartner H, Hung J, Bermejo J, *et al.*; American Society of Echocardiography; European Association of Echocardiography. Echocardiographic assessment of valve stenosis: EAE/ASE recommendations for clinical practice. *European Heart Journal-Cardiovascular Imaging* 2009;**10**:1–25.

Colebourn C, Newton J (eds). *Acute and Critical Care Echocardiography: Oxford Clinical Imaging Guides.* Oxford: Oxford University Press; 2017.

Lancellotti P, Tribouilloy C, Hagendorff A, *et al.*; European Association of Echocardiography. European Association of Echocardiography recommendations for the assessment of valvular regurgitation. Part 1: aortic and pulmonary regurgitation (native valve disease). *European Heart Journal-Cardiovascular Imaging* 2010;**11**:223–44.

12

Mitral valve assessment

Thomas Clark and Stefanie Bruemmer-Smith

Introduction

Acute MV disease is an important cause of shock, and clinical recognition is not always straightforward. For example, acute severe MR is typically accompanied by haemodynamic instability, causing it to be easily missed on initial examination, and MR can be 'silent' (i.e. with no audible murmur), so echocardiography is sometimes necessary to make the diagnosis.

Diagnostic MV assessment is a complex task that requires comprehensive 2D and Doppler examination. However, a more basic assessment of the MV is a useful tool for the FoCUS-level echocardiographer because it provides valuable information in the shocked, critically ill patient.

The benefits of using FoCUS MV assessment, as a part of your echo skill set, include:

1. Identification of MV obstruction (MVO) or acute MR
2. Determination of MVO/MR aetiology
3. Interpretation of effective cardiac output in the presence of MV disease.

This chapter will describe normal and abnormal 2D sonoanatomy of the MV and explain how FoCUS can be used to screen for haemodynamically significant MV obstruction or regurgitation. It will discuss the acute and adaptive changes that occur with these conditions and explain how to recognize them. The advanced section of this chapter will introduce how colour Doppler can be used to support the diagnosis in acute/severe disease.

FoCUS is limited in its diagnostic capabilities, and this must be kept in mind at all times. If significant pathology is suspected, timely referral for a comprehensive echocardiogram is essential.

Normal anatomy

The MV apparatus is a complex 3D saddle-shaped structure that includes an annulus, and two leaflets and PMs, connected by multiple chordae tendinae. A brief assessment of all constituent parts of this apparatus is essential, so that important diagnoses are not missed.

Mitral valve leaflets

There are two leaflets: the AMVL and the PMVL (Figure 12.1a). The AMVL, being quadrangular in shape, is the thicker and longer of the two, while the PMVL is shorter and thinner. For descriptive purposes, each leaflet is divided into three scallops, numbered 1 (anterior or lateral), 2 (middle), and 3 (posterior or medial) (Figure 12.1b). During systole, the leaflets close along a point of contact called the 'coaptation line', and where the leaflet edges overlap, it is called the 'coaptation zone'.

Commissures

At either end of the leaflets are the commissures, which are tissue continuities between the AMVL and PMVL at their insertion into the annulus. They are labelled as the anterolateral commissure (associated with A1/P1) and the posteromedial commissure (associated with A3/P3).

Annulus

The MV leaflets are attached at their bases to the MV annulus (a fibromuscular ring). The annulus itself is

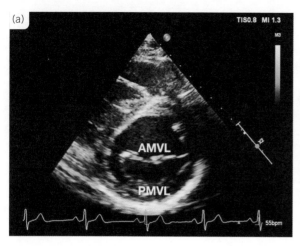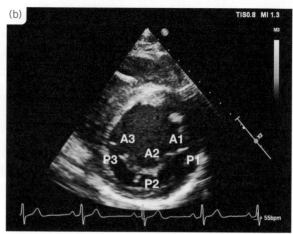

Figure 12.1 PSAX view at the MV level: a) frozen at mid diastole; b) frozen at mid-systole, with annotations describing the three scallops of each leaflet.

saddle-shaped, and it contracts/expands with systole/diastole. The annulus is in continuity with its surrounding structures—anteriorly lies the fibrous trigone (with the non-coronary and left coronary cusps of the AV); posteriorly lies the coronary sinus, and laterally lies the circumflex artery.

Chordae tendinae

Chordae tendinae are the fibrous strands that originate from the PMs and act as scaffolding on which the MV leaflets hang. They play an essential role in maintaining the MV structure during systole, ensuring correct leaflet coaptation. Rupture of primary chords may cause acute MR, as discussed in Mitral regurgitation.

Papillary muscles

There are two PMs in the LV: the anterolateral and the posteromedial. These originate from the left ventricular free walls, and each PM gives rise to chordae tendinae that attach to both MV leaflets. In the LV, there are no septal PMs, which is one way of differentiating it from the RV. Via the chordae tendinae and PMs, the MV is effectively in continuity with the left ventricular posterior and lateral walls, which means that any changes in left ventricular geometry and function can potentially impact upon MV function (e.g. posteromedial PM ischaemia leading to acute MR).

Normal physiology

In health, the MV opens during diastole and closes during systole (with around 20–40% reduction in annular area). Diastole may be subdivided into four phases:

1. Isovolumetric relaxation (prior to MV opening)

2. Rapid, early passive ventricular filling

3. Diastasis, or mid-diastolic, low-flow passive filling

4. Active, late, rapid filling secondary to atrial contraction.

Pathophysiology

Mitral valve obstruction

The MV must open during diastole to allow blood to fill the left ventricular cavity. Any dysfunction of the MV apparatus can result in restricted flow.

Causes of MVO include:

1. Rheumatic MS

2. Prosthetic valve obstruction

3. Left atrial tumours (e.g. an atrial myxoma that 'plugs off' the valve)

4. Severe mitral annular calcification (associated with old age and renal failure)

5. Left atrial thrombus

6. Systemic conditions, e.g. systemic lupus erythematosus, left-sided carcinoid disease

7. Congenital abnormalities.

Rheumatic MS is, by far, the most common cause (at least 80% of cases), and this occurs due to thickening and immobility of the MV leaflets and subvalvular apparatus.

Mitral valve replacements (MVRs) can become obstructed either by thrombus (usually an acute event potentially leading to complete MVO and loss of cardiac output) or 'pannus' formation (a chronic process caused by fibrin deposition).

Acute MVO will lead to haemodynamic collapse and acute pulmonary oedema. Chronic MVO is better tolerated due to a series of adaptive changes.

Mitral regurgitation

MR is the flow of left ventricular SV backwards into the LA through an incompetent MV, and it can be subdivided according to chronicity (acute versus chronic) or severity (trivial, mild, moderate, or severe). Correct systolic closure of the MV requires complete coaptation of the AMVL and PMVL along the full length of the coaptation zone. Dysfunction of any component of the MV apparatus (leaflets, annulus, chordae tendinae, PMs, or the free ventricular wall) may result in failure of this process.

Acute MR has two key lesions: chordae tendinae/PM rupture and infective vegetations. Chordae tendinae/PM rupture can produce a 'flail' leaflet. A patient's history and clinical examination may provide important clues to its aetiology.

Causes of chordae tendinae/PM rupture include:

1. Acute myocardial infarction (acute, common)

2. Infective endocarditis (acute, common)

3. Trauma (acute, common)

4. Spontaneous (acute)

5. Myxomatous disease (acute-on-chronic)

6. Rheumatic disease (acute-on-chronic).

PM rupture secondary to myocardial infarct is a rare, but usually catastrophic, event. The posteromedial PM is most commonly affected, as it has a single-vessel blood supply. Rupture is typically seen a few days after an inferior or posterior infarct.

Endocarditic vegetations may also cause acute MR by preventing leaflet coaptation, destroying the leaflets themselves, or causing annular leaks/abscesses.

Acute mitral regurgitation adaptive changes

In acute/severe MR, much of the left ventricular SV is preferentially ejected into a previously normal, non-compliant LA. This has two consequences:

1. A large rise in left atrial pressure (LAP), resulting in acute cardiogenic pulmonary oedema

2. A drop in left ventricular afterload as blood flows backwards into the LA, rather than forwards into the systemic arterial tree.

The resulting 'off-loading' of the LV causes a 'hyperdynamic' state (high EF), but loss of effective cardiac output, and cardiogenic shock follows. The extent of haemodynamic compromise is dependent on both the severity and acuity of regurgitation.

Chronic mitral regurgitation adaptive changes

In chronic MR, the LA becomes more compliant and has time to dilate gradually in response to its increased load; therefore, regurgitation will cause a more gradual rise in LAP. The LV also dilates in response to its own increased volume load (in comparison to acute MR when the LV is typically small and hyperdynamic). Due to these adaptive changes, a patient may remain asymptomatic, without evidence of pulmonary oedema or heart failure (compensated phase). However, with disease progression, MR transitions into a decompensated phase, heralded by the development of left ventricular dilatation, reduced EF, PHT, and right ventricular pressure/volume overload.

Causes of chronic MR include:

- Primary or valvular:
  1. MV prolapse from degenerative disease
  2. Rheumatic valve disease
  3. Congenital causes (e.g. a cleft)
  4. Infective endocarditis
  5. Mitral annular calcification.
- Secondary or functional:
  1. Ischaemic cardiomyopathy (restricted leaflet movement)

2. Dilated cardiomyopathy (functional MR secondary to annular dilatation ± tethering)

3. HCM (SAM of AMVL).

Mitral regurgitation and left ventricular assessment

MV assessment is a final step in accurate left ventricular function assessment. When estimating LVEF, visually or by measuring it, knowledge that the MV is competent is important. If there is significant MR, a large proportion of the SV will be ejected backwards, and a 'normal LVEF' does not necessarily equate to effective SV or cardiac output. In acute, severe MR, 'normal' left ventricular function equates to a high LVEF. If LVEF is normal in the presence of significant MR and normal left ventricular size, LVSD is highly likely.

FoCUS mitral valve assessment

In the haemodynamicaly unstable patient, we are only interested in acute, severe MR and MVO, and wish to differentiate these from non-acute, non-severe MR and MVO. It is not the remit of FoCUS to differentiate between mild, moderate, and severe disease. Instead, it screens for significant MVO/MR that has meaningful impact upon a patient's clinical state and management plan—if positive, referral for further investigation must always follow.

The MV may be examined in all of the FoCUS views. As the MV is a complex structure, it is difficult to know for certain which part of the valve you are seeing. It is useful to be able to identify the AMVL from the PMVL, but knowing which scallop you are examining does not help you beyond this. As a rule, the AMVL is nearer to the probe in the PLAX and PSAX views, and septal in the A4C and S4C views.

The process of examining the MV needs to be a methodical one. Figure 12.2 is a flow chart illustrating how to complete a step-by-step MV screening examination.

Steps 1 and 2 involve optimizing your 2D image and undertaking a careful assessment of valvular morphology by looking for red flags that suggest severe valvular dysfunction. In cases of severe MR/MVO, the operator should already be highly suspicious that

something is afoot after the first two steps. Steps 3, 4, and 5 involve the use of Doppler and help to merely confirm your suspicions. These are advanced echo skills, which should only be attempted with appropriate training and supervision. Step 6 looks for associated cardiac abnormalities to determine the acuity of any potential MV disease.

It cannot be overemphasized that if any pathology is seen, it is your responsibility to organize a complete echocardiogram to confirm or refute your findings.

Step 1: Optimization of 2D image

Optimizing your image is key, and it is good practice to do so continuously as you scan. Optimization can turn a difficult image into a clear one and make pathology more obvious. Change the depth, focus point, and gain. Consider reducing the sector angle width to blinker 'unwanted' structures. Your aim is to maximize the frame rate, optimize the temporal resolution, and remove distracting signals. Scan through the valve to obtain the correct image, as appropriate to your view.

Step 2: 2D inspection of the mitral valve

Freeze and scroll through your image, frame by frame. It becomes far easier to see pathology as you do this.

Mitral valve obstruction

Rheumatic MS produces a classical picture of an immobile, shortened PMVL, and a doming AMVL with a 'hockey-stick' appearance during diastole, caused by fusion of leaflet tips at the commissures (Video 1.8.1 ⚫).

2D red flags of significant MVO include:

1. Thickened, bright, immobile MV leaflets that simply fail to open during diastole

2. Any mass within the LA that occludes the MV during any part of diastole.

3. A prosthetic MVR.

Prosthetic mitral valve replacements

Prosthetic MVRs are difficult to assess. Mechanical MVRs are more obvious than tissue valves, as their structure causes significant image distortion and dropout. Indeed, when imaging a patient with a

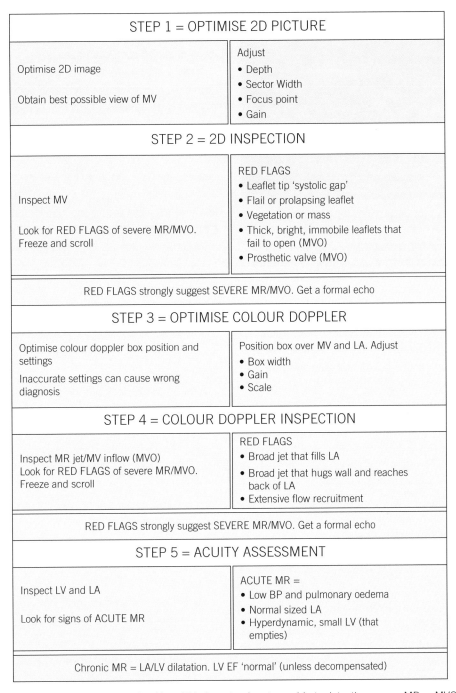

STEP 1 = OPTIMISE 2D PICTURE	
Optimise 2D image Obtain best possible view of MV	Adjust • Depth • Sector Width • Focus point • Gain

STEP 2 = 2D INSPECTION	
Inspect MV Look for RED FLAGS of severe MR/MVO. Freeze and scroll	RED FLAGS • Leaflet tip 'systolic gap' • Flail or prolapsing leaflet • Vegetation or mass • Thick, bright, immobile leaflets that fail to open (MVO) • Prosthetic valve (MVO)
RED FLAGS strongly suggest SEVERE MR/MVO. Get a formal echo	

STEP 3 = OPTIMISE COLOUR DOPPLER	
Optimise colour doppler box position and settings Inaccurate settings can cause wrong diagnosis	Position box over MV and LA. Adjust • Box width • Gain • Scale

STEP 4 = COLOUR DOPPLER INSPECTION	
Inspect MR jet/MV inflow (MVO) Look for RED FLAGS of severe MR/MVO. Freeze and scroll	RED FLAGS • Broad jet that fills LA • Broad jet that hugs wall and reaches back of LA • Extensive flow recruitment
RED FLAGS strongly suggest SEVERE MR/MVO. Get a formal echo	

STEP 5 = ACUITY ASSESSMENT	
Inspect LV and LA Look for signs of ACUTE MR	ACUTE MR = • Low BP and pulmonary oedema • Normal sized LA • Hyperdynamic, small LV (that empties)
Chronic MR = LA/LV dilatation. LV EF 'normal' (unless decompensated)	

Figure 12.2 The FoCUS MV assessment algorithm. This is a step-by-step guide to detecting severe MR or MVO.

mechanical MVR, you will be unable to 'see' anything 'behind' the valve, e.g. the LA from an A4C view.

Detailed MVR assessment is considerably beyond the remit of FoCUS. If you see an MVR in a shocked patient, get an urgent comprehensive echocardiogram.

Mitral regurgitation

The 2D red flags for severe MR include:

1. A large leaflet tip 'systolic gap', i.e. during systole, you can see a gap between the AMVL and PMVL, indicating significant incompetence

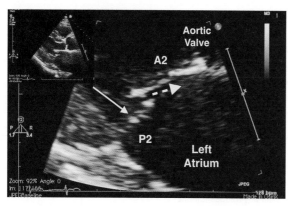

Figure 12.3 PLAX view of the MV at end-systole. P2 is seen slipping behind A2 (solid arrow), leaving a clear gap. The associated jet of MR would be directed forward in the direction of the anterior fibrous trigone and AV (broken arrow).

2. A prolapsing or flail leaflet

3. A vegetation sitting on the MV apparatus. In such cases, look closely for a leaflet perforation. These can be difficult to see but clearly reflect severe pathology.

Prolapse or flail?

A prolapsing scallop or leaflet can be seen to coapt beyond the annular plane, leaving a large gap (Figure 12.3 and Video 1.8.2). During systole, the prolapsing leaflet 'falls' into the LA, but the tip direction remains pointing towards the left ventricular apex.

A flail leaflet appears as a wildly chaotic leaflet that 'flips' and points into the LA during systole. Commonly, the flail is the posterior leaflet. Severe or torrential MR will almost certainly accompany a flail leaflet.

Infective endocarditis

Vegetations will appear as leaflet thickenings, or highly mobile masses on the atrial side of the leaflets that oscillate within the MR stream (Video 1.8.3). This pattern helps to differentiate vegetations from other masses of other types. They may be hard to see as they flip in and out of view, and it can be very helpful to freeze your image and scan through frame by frame. It is also useful to sweep your scan plane through the MV in real time, and then freeze when you see something. If the history fits, be extra careful; remember the low sensitivity of TTE, and consider referral for TOE.

A para-valvular leak around an MVR must always be seen as suspicious and could indicate infective endocarditis, especially if perivalvular abscesses are seen/suspected. A 'rocking' prosthetic valve is another red flag of prosthetic MV endocarditis.

Advanced echocardiography

Step 3: Turn on colour Doppler imaging and optimize the box

This chapter does not aim to teach diagnostic-level colour Doppler techniques. What we want you to recognize is severe or torrential MR. Anything less is unlikely to be clinically relevant in the ICU setting and requires comprehensive echocardiogram to grade.

When activating colour Doppler imaging, a box will appear that corresponds to a colour Doppler map. Using this technology is very processor-heavy, and you will notice degradation in 2D image quality. It is very important to optimize your colour image, not only to ensure the best picture possible, but also to avoid incorrect diagnosis and assessment. You can always make MR look worse or better, depending on your settings. Below is the correct process.

1. Optimize your colour Doppler box position. This is essential.
   a. Move the colour Doppler box, so that it is centred over the MV and LA.
   b. Adjust the colour Doppler sector width, so that it covers only what you want to examine (i.e. the MV leaflets throughout systole and diastole, and the LA). You do not want to miss any of the MR jet or miss an MV leaflet abnormality (e.g. a perforation from which the MR originates). It is best to keep the box as small as possible to optimize the temporal resolution, but large enough to include all the relevant structures.

2. Optimize your colour Doppler gain. Turn this up, so you see 'speckles' of colour across the

image, and then turn it down until they just disappear.

3. Using the 'scale' button on your machine, ensure that your Nyquist limit or 'scale' is set at 50–60 cm/s. Any lower and you will overestimate the size and severity of the MR jet; any higher and you may underestimate it. Check that the baseline is central (velocity equal above and below the line), using the 'baseline' button nearby. Most machines set both of these automatically.

Step 4: Colour Doppler assessment

Mitral valve obstruction assessment

MVO will be highly suspected from the 2D images, and colour Doppler often has little to add. However, on the left atrial side of the MV, you may just see a brightly coloured hemisphere of proximal flow 'recruitment' or 'convergence' throughout diastole. The larger this hemisphere is, the higher the blood velocity, and the more severe the MVO. Other features of severity include a narrow jet of high-velocity blood that fills the LV during diastole.

Depending on your machine, speckled, multicoloured, or green jets indicate turbulent, high-velocity flow. This is usually the case with flow into and out of a narrow orifice. See Chapters 2 and 3 for further discussion about aliasing.

Mitral regurgitation assessment

As with AS, you should be expecting to see bad MR after your 2D assessment of the MV. Colour Doppler inspection is the final piece of the puzzle. Once you have shown that there is an MR jet, you need to decide if it is severe or not, which means looking for the red flags of severe MR. Severe MR red flags include:

1. A broad, large MR jet—this will often be associated with a 2D 'systolic gap'

2. A jet that fills the LA

3. A jet that hugs the wall and reaches the back of the LA, before swirling forward again

4. Obvious proximal flow recruitment at a 'scale' of 50–60 cm/s—this is seen as a hemisphere of bright colour on the left ventricular side of the valve

5. A jet that is seen throughout systole

6. Multiple 'significant' jets—this is difficult to quantify, so get a formal TTE!

Mitral regurgitation jet appearance

The MR jet will appear as a burst of colour flowing back into the LA during systole. The colour change of the MR jet is an indication of direction and velocity.

It is very important to separate MV inflow from MV regurgitation by freezing and scrolling your image. In the tachycardic, hyperdynamic heart, this may be difficult to do in real time.

> **Pitfall**
>
> Confusing forward flow with backward flow, mistaking MV inflow for MR, or vice versa, is easier than you think. Your friend in overcoming this error, once again, is the freeze button. Pause your image, and scroll slowly; take note of where you are in the cardiac cycle; do this by looking at MV movement and the ECG.

Mitral regurgitation jet features—width and flow recruitment

At the origin of the MR jet, colour Doppler will demonstrate a narrow neck, called the vena contracta (VC), and the broader this neck, the more severe the MR (Figure 12.4). Upstream, on the ventricular side of the MV, you may also see a domed hemisphere of 'proximal flow recruitment' during systole (Figure 12.5). Generally speaking, the larger this hemisphere, the more severe the MR. Before commenting on this,

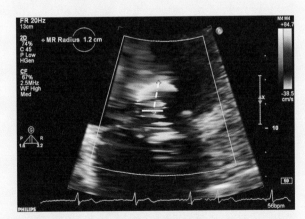

Figure 12.4 A zoomed A4C view of MR with proximal flow recruitment. The vena contracta (solid white line) of the MR jet is wide, with extensive (>1 cm) proximal flow recruitment (dashed white line). These are both markers of severe MR. For a colour version of this figure, please see colour plate section.

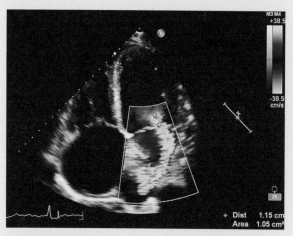

Figure 12.5 An A4C still image of severe MR, with a large hemisphere of proximal flow recruitment. Here you can see an eccentric jet of swirl down the side of the left atrium, reaching all the way to the back of the chamber, before washing forward again. These are red flags of severe MR. For a colour version of this figure, please see colour plate section.

make sure that your scale is set as it should be and your baseline is central. Quantifying both the VC and flow recruitment is used in severity assessment, but simply eyeballing these MR features should give you more confidence in your diagnosis.

A VC of <3 mm suggests mild MR, and >7 mm suggests severe MR.

> **Pitfall**
>
> Underestimating MR severity is easy to do in a critically ill patient. Vasodilatation of any cause reduces afterload, promotes forward flow, and reduces regurgitation through the MV.

Mitral regurgitation jet features—area and direction

The jet itself may be directed centrally (often in functional MR caused by annulus dilatation) or towards a particular side of the LA (eccentric MR caused by leaflet prolapse or restriction). The jet area and the percentage of the LA that it fills are both markers of severity. The MR may hug the left atrial wall, known as the Coanda effect (Video 1.8.4 ◯). In such cases, the jet area will be reduced and you may underestimate the severity of the MR. You must also remember that in MR, the regurgitant volume (volume of MR) is

dependent on both the size of the MR orifice, the compliance of the LA, and the pressure gradient between the LV and LA.

> **Pitfall**
>
> The jet area can underestimate severity if there is:
>
> 1. A high Nyquist limit (>60 cm/s)
> 2. An eccentric jet that hugs the wall (Coanda effect)
> 3. Elevated LAP (e.g. in acute MR)
> 4. Left atrial enlargement.
>
> The jet area can overestimate MR severity by simply turning down your scale (e.g. by changing the Nyquist limit from 50 cm/s to 20 cm/s, you can make mild MR look severe).

In leaflet prolapse or flail, the MR jet is directed away from the side of pathology. In leaflet restriction (functional MR secondary to leaflet tethering and tenting or post-posterior myocardial infarction), the MR jet is directed towards the side of pathology. In symmetric bi-leaflet tethering (dilated cardiomyopathy or large anterior myocardial infarction), there is a central jet or regurgitation.

Step 5: Acuity assessment

In acute MR, left atrial pressure rises rapidly. Because the LA has no time to remodel and become more compliant, pulmonary oedema occurs soon afterwards. The combination of shock, pulmonary oedema and high LVEF should warrant close inspection of the MV, and if MR is significant, immediate expert advice should be sought.

In chronic MR, progressive left atrial enlargement enables lower left atrial, and pulmonary venous, pressure. Increased preload causes left ventricular dilatation and eccentric hypertrophy. Cardiac systolic function is initially well maintained, but as dilatation progresses, wall stress increases and LVEF falls, eventually causing decompensated MR.

As a rule, the presence of left-sided chamber enlargement suggests chronic disease and other causes of shock should be excluded. However, acute on chronic MR may well present as acute pulmonary oedema. Typically, this results from a sudden change in MR morphology (e.g. a snapped chordae tendinae in a patient with chronic PMVL prolapse, or infective endocarditis).

✅ Multiple choice questions

Interactive multiple choice questions to test your knowledge can be found in the Online appendix at www.oxfordmedicine.com/focusedicu. Please refer to your access card for further details.

Further reading

Colebourn C, Newton J (eds). *Acute and Critical Care Echocardiography: Oxford Clinical Imaging Guides.* Oxford: Oxford University Press; 2017.

European Association of Echocardiography recommendations for the assessment of valvular regurgitation. Part 2: mitral and tricuspid regurgitation (native valve disease). *European Journal of Echocardiography* 2010;**11**:307–22.

Rana B, Allen J, Chambers J, *et al. A Guideline Protocol for the Assessment of the Mitral Valve With a View to Repair.* London: British Society of Echocardiography Education Committee; 2011. Available from: https://www.bsecho.org/mitral-valve-repair [accessed 4 September 2018].

13

Intravascular volume and cardiac output assessment

Prashant Parulekar and Tim Harris

Introduction

Both hypovolaemia and hypervolaemia compromise tissue oxygenation and are associated with morbidity and mortality. Under-resuscitation leads to shock, while overzealous volume expansion can cause interstitial oedema and increased compartment pressures. The challenge for any clinician is to assess accurately whether adequate fluid resuscitation has been achieved and to stop before it becomes injurious.

In critically ill patients, signs of tissue hypoperfusion (such as cold, clammy, or pale skin, oliguria, and altered mental status) can coexist with peripheral oedema and both extremes of intravascular volume. Clinical examination is neither sensitive nor specific for identifying changes in circulating volume resulting from fluid therapy. In a shocked patient, accurate diagnosis, haemodynamic evaluation, and correction of intravascular volume are all cornerstones of early management; FoCUS can help with each of these.

This chapter will focus on 2D echo techniques that can detect potential hypovolaemia (small ventricles, high caval variability) and hypervolaemia (dilated, poorly functioning ventricles, low caval variability, and fixed IAS). It will discuss both dynamic and static parameters and how these may help to predict fluid responsiveness and fluid tolerance, respectively. The advanced section will then introduce established Doppler-based echo techniques that can be used to estimate SV and guide volume resuscitation, as well as novel approaches currently under investigation.

Relevant physiology

The Frank–Starling relationship

Ventricular preload is defined as the myocardial stretch imposed by ventricular filling at the end of diastole. Thanks to Starling's work, it is widely appreciated that if contractility and afterload are fixed, a steady increase in venous return and preload results in increased SV until a point, represented by the beginning of the flat section of the Starling curve, after which SV increases no more (Figure 13.1).

Starling curves cannot be easily 'drawn' for individual patients, and which point should be considered 'optimal' in different clinical settings is increasingly less clear. However, this relationship remains the foundation of fluid resuscitation, as knowing whether or not the patient is preload-dependent determines whether or not fluid therapy will improve SV, cardiac output, and oxygen delivery—a state known as 'fluid responsiveness'.

Volume, pressure, and flow

Technically, preload is a linear measurement that translates in vivo to end-diastolic volume. Before the advent of 2D echo that enabled volumetric assessment of the LV, LAP was used as a surrogate, fraught with error, not least because chamber compliance is affected by common cardiac pathology.

The ideal haemodynamic assessment tool needs to assess chamber volume, filling pressure, and blood flow on both sides of the heart; uniquely, echo can achieve all of these.

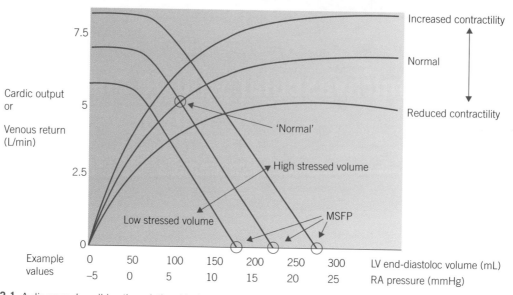

Figure 13.1 A diagram describing the relationship between LVEDP and stroke volume.

Static versus dynamic parameters

CVP and pulmonary artery occlusion pressure were once considered to be reasonable surrogates of right and left ventricular preload, respectively. However, these static parameters are now well known to be poor predictors of fluid responsiveness and require the potentially injurious insertion of a central line or pulmonary artery catheter, so they are rarely used as targets for fluid resuscitation today. That said, both can be qualitatively assessed using TTE and have some clinical utility by indicating ventricular compliance, which informs the risk of developing hydrostatic oedema from fluid loading, a concept increasingly known as 'fluid tolerance'.

In terms of predicting fluid responsiveness, dynamic indices, such as vena caval variability, stroke volume variation (SVV), and changes following passive leg raising (PLR), are more accurate than static parameters. With the exception of PLR, these rely on heart–lung interactions and so can only be utilized in apnoeic, mechanically ventilated patients.

Fluid responsiveness

Approximately half of all shocked patients in ICU are responders to a fluid challenge. However, such studies are heterogenous, and there is no universally agreed definition of what a fluid challenge actually is. According to the FENICE study, contemporary practice varies widely worldwide. Generally speaking, a fluid responder is someone whose SV increases by >12–15% after 250–500 mL of crystalloid fluid is administered over 15 minutes. Fluid responsiveness can be predicted using various 2D and Doppler-based techniques (described in the advanced section of this chapter).

Hypovolaemic versus distributive shock

Hypovolaemic and septic shock can look very similar with 2D echo, and these conditions often coexist. As with all focused US, it is important to integrate echo findings with the clinical picture, which can generally distinguish between the two—hypovolaemia typically being associated with a vasoconstricted state, and sepsis with a vasodilated state.

When to start fluid resuscitation

The 2D echo appearances of gross hypovolaemia in spontaneously ventilating patients include small ventricles, tachycardia, and a small IVC that collapses completely with inspiration.

Left ventricular preload

An LVEDA index of <10 cm² (or 5.5 cm²/m² when indexed for body surface area) indicates an underfilled ventricle. LVEDA is measured in the mid-papillary PSAX view by tracing the endocardial border at end-diastole (excluding PMs), using the planimetry function.

A simpler approach is to eyeball the heart in any view; a small LV is usually obvious. As a general rule, in a shocked patient, a left ventricular end-diastolic dimension of <3 cm, seen in PLAX, suggests that fluid therapy is indicated.

In hypovolaemia, as well as being small in diastole, the walls of the LV are often closely opposed at end-systole, and PMs can appear to touch each other. This is sometimes described as 'kissing' PMs or, more formally, as a 'hyperdynamic' LV with 'end-systolic cavity obliteration'. One caveat to this is the presence of LVH, when the internal dimensions of the LV can be small, independently of preload (Video 1.9.1 ⬤).

A hyperdynamic LV is defined by an LVEF of >70%, and although this is not specific, it is a common finding in hypovolaemia. A small, hyperdynamic LV that normalizes with successful fluid resuscitation, is strongly suggestive of hypovolaemia.

Hyperdynamic left ventricular function on admission to critical care has been associated with increased 28-day mortality, when compared to patients admitted with normal LVEF. The reason for this is unclear, but it suggests that a hyperdynamic state is not benign.

Pitfall

A small, hyperdynamic LV seen in the context of a clinically low cardiac output state is not always indicative of systemic hypovolaemia (Videos 1.9.1 and 1.9.2 ⬤). Acute cor pulmonale (ACP) can also produce these clinical findings; the key difference is the presence of massive right ventricular dilatation, indicating that further fluid resuscitation may, in fact, be harmful.

Right ventricular preload

The RV is a low-pressure, high-volume chamber that varies dramatically in size, according to its loading conditions (afterload, in particular). A small RV at both end-diastole and end-systole strongly suggests low right ventricular preload. In systemic hypovolaemia, the RV and LV are usually both small.

In health, the venous capacitance system contains 60% of the entire intravascular volume. The SVC and IVC are its largest vessels, and when visualized, these can be used to estimate RAP.

The IVC should be visualized in its long axis from the subcostal window, with the probe rotated anticlockwise from an S4C view, centred on the right atrium. Once in SSAX, the IVC diameter should be measured within 2 cm from its entry into the right atrium, immediately proximal to its junction with the hepatic veins (Figure 13.2). Care must be taken to ensure that its maximal width is recorded at all times, because the respiratory cycle can displace the heart, causing error.

As a general rule, the IVC diameter decreases in low intravascular volume and increases in high intravascular volume states. However, a number of non-preload-related factors also affect this. IVC diameter increases with pathology that causes downstream occlusion such as pericardial tamponade, tension pneumothorax, valvular heart disease, and PHT. It also varies with changes in intrathoracic and intra-abdominal pressure. In addition, athletic training, patient habitus, force of respiration, pressure of the US probe, and the site of measurement can all affect IVC size. Each of these factors must be taken into account when interpreting IVC size.

There are no large, high-quality trials to date. However, based on a number of small studies, an IVC of <11–12 mm in spontaneously breathing patients appears to suggest hypovolaemia.

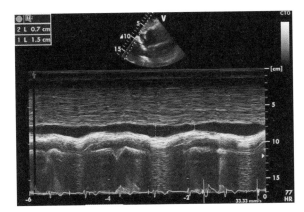

Figure 13.2 M-mode of the IVC in a SC view. Note: respiratory variation of 53%.

Spontaneous ventilation and inferior vena caval collapsibility

IVC compliance is inversely proportional to RAP, and IVC collapsibility, caused by respiratory changes in intrathoracic pressure during spontaneous ventilation, suggests low preload.

Studies combining IVC diameter and variability have predicted RAP with reasonable accuracy in spontaneously breathing patients. The American Society of Echocardiography (ASE) guidelines state that an IVC diameter of <2.1 cm with collapsibility of >50% indicates a RAP of 3 mmHg. Conversely, a dilated IVC (>2.1 cm) with <50% respiratory collapse indicates an RAP of 15 mmHg.

These values are used mainly in comprehensive echo for calculation of PASP, and using them to assess volume status has a number of limitations. They are not well supported by clinical studies in critically ill patients and do not translate to patients on mechanical ventilation. More importantly, as previously stated, CVP is known to be a poor predictor of fluid responsiveness. However, a very small, collapsing IVC does suggest that a shocked patient will be fluid-responsive, but with lower sensitivity and specificity than other measures. By contrast, a dilated, non-collapsing IVC does not predict the patient will always be a non-responder, but it should be regarded as a sign of potential fluid intolerance (i.e. an indicator of risk that fluid therapy could be harmful).

Mechanical ventilation and inferior vena caval distensibility

Mechanical ventilation affects IVC size in an underfilled patient, but in contrast to spontaneous ventilation, its diameter increases during inspiration due to transmission of increased pleural pressure. Several small, but well-designed, studies have outlined this relationship and concluded that the more distensible the IVC is with mandatory ventilation, the more likely the patient is to be fluid-responsive. Barbier and colleagues (2004; PMID: 15034650) produced an IVC distensibility index (IVCDI), which at 18% has 90% sensitivity and 90% specificity for fluid responsiveness, with an AUROC (area under the curve of the receiver operating characteristic) of 91%.

$$IVCDI = \left[(Dmax - Dmin)/Dmin\right] \times 100\%$$

where Dmax = IVC diameter at end-inspiration and Dmin = IVC diameter at end-expiration.

As with all studies predicting volume responsiveness from heart–lung interactions, this has important prerequisites, including that the patient is in sinus rhythm and on mandatory ventilation (i.e. no spontaneous effort) with a tidal volume of >8 mL/kg.

Mechanical ventilation and superior vena caval collapsibility

In a preload-dependent, mechanically ventilated patient, the SVC collapses during inspiration due to raised intrathoracic pressure. SVC collapsibility is potentially more accurate that IVC variability, because it is not affected by intra-abdominal pressure. However, its utility is limited by the fact that it can only be assessed using TOE.

The SVC diameter can be examined using TOE at 0° via the upper/middle oesophageal SAX view of the ascending aorta (Asc Ao). SVC Dmax and Dmin can be measured over one respiratory cycle, using M-mode, in a similar way to IVC.

An SVC collapsibility index of >36% is suggestive of fluid responsiveness.

When to stop fluid resuscitation

As previously mentioned, over-resuscitation with fluids can have detrimental consequences on patient outcome. Below are FoCUS signs of overloaded, stressed ventricles, indicating that further fluid administration may be harmful (Videos 1.9.3 and 1.9.4 ▶).

Signs of an overloaded LV with a potentially raised LAP include:

- High LVEDA (>20 cm²)
- Low LVEF
- Fixed IAS to right (acutely raised LAP)
- Left atrial enlargement, in the absence of significant MV disease (chronically raised LAP)
- Interstitial syndrome on LUS (upstream, pulmonary congestion).

Signs of an overloaded RV include:

- Right ventricular dilatation and systolic dysfunction
- A small, D-shaped LV (ventricular interdependence)

- A dilated IVC, with no variability (high RAP)
- Deranged liver function tests (LFTs) and/or dilated hepatic veins (upstream, hepatic congestion).

Estimating left atrial pressure

Decision-making regarding fluid therapy in patients with biventricular failure is challenging because increasing preload in patients with raised left ventricular filling pressure is not without risk. However, in a patient with known cardiac disease and undifferentiated shock, this is usually the correct initial course of action. Raised LAP does not preclude fluid responsiveness, but it does indicate potential fluid intolerance.

LAP is usually higher than RAP, and the position of the IAS is dependent on the trans-atrial pressure gradient. Consequently, normal LAP causes the IAS to bow towards the right atrium, apart from at mid-systole when it briefly demonstrates 'mid-systolic reversal'. High LAP produces a 'fixed curve' of the IAS, from left to right, throughout the entire cardiac cycle. Similarly, high RAP causes a fixed curve of the IAS from right to left.

Left atrial remodelling takes weeks/months to occur. In the absence of MV disease, left atrial dilatation is a sign of chronically raised LAP. However, it does not rule out acute rises in LAP. This subject is discussed further in Chapter 9.

Right ventricular preload

Acute right ventricular dysfunction is a common finding on ICU. Physiological challenges, such as hypercapnia, hypoxaemia, acidaemia, and mechanical ventilation all raise right ventricular afterload, but the main pathological causes are PE and ARDS.

Severe ACP and hypovolaemic shock can both cause low left ventricular preload, tachycardia, and shock. The only bedside clues to ACP might be a suspicious history and raised jugular venous pressure. Volume-loading a patient with ACP can worsen shock, which is why early identification of right ventricular dilatation is essential in all haemodynamically unstable patients.

The more dilated the RV becomes, the less well it tolerates fluid administration. Massive right ventricular dilatation and a small, D-shaped LV are signs of severe pressure–volume overload, which is an absolute contraindication to fluid therapy (Video 1.9.5). Ventricular interdependence is discussed further in Chapter 8.

Patients with chronic PHT and right ventricular impairment may still be responsive, and SV monitoring is advisable in such cases. A clue to chronic PHT is the presence of right ventricular hypertrophy (>5 mm), which is best seen in the S4C view. This is discussed further in Chapter 8.

> **Pitfall**
>
> Right ventricular failure produces false-positive SVV and pulse pressure variation, so these parameters should not be used to predict fluid responsiveness in ventilated patients with ACP.

Advanced echocardiography

Measuring stroke volume and cardiac output

TTE can be used for assessment of cardiac output. To calculate this, one needs to know the cross-sectional area of the LVOT and the velocity–time integral (VTI) of blood flow at this point, using the following equations:

Cardiac output = heart rate · stroke volume

Stroke volume = LVOT area · LVOT VTI

$$= \pi \cdot (\text{LVOT diameter}/2)^2 \cdot \text{LVOT VTI}$$

Left ventricular outflow tract diameter

LVOT diameter is measured in a PLAX image, frozen in mid-systole, with calipers placed at the white/black interface, perpendicular to the long axis of the LVOT ideally at the same point flow is measured.

The LVOT area is assumed to be fairly constant, because it is part of the cardiac skeleton. However, inaccurate measurement of the LVOT diameter is common and causes significant error when estimating the cardiac output, because its value is squared in the calculation.

Left ventricular outflow tract velocity–time integral

This essentially measures the distance that blood is ejected from the LVOT during systole. It is measured using PW Doppler in a well-aligned A5C (or A3C) view, with the sampling volume placed in the LVOT, as close to the AV as possible, taking care to avoid the opening artefact (seen as a sharp spike on the Doppler trace) caused by AV opening (Figure 13.3). If the sampling volume is placed too close, proximal flow acceleration can cause PW Doppler to overestimate flow.

A fast sweep speed enhances the area of the PW velocity–time display; once this is traced (manually or by the machine), VTI values are calculated automatically, using installed software. Ideally, VTI should be measured at end-expiration and averaged over at least three readings (five in the presence of AF).

Normal values for LVOT VTI are between 15 and 25 cm.

To avoid potential error in LVOT measurement, VTI alone can be used as a surrogate assessment for SV.

Left ventricular outflow tract velocity–time integral variation

LVOT VTI variation predicts fluid responsiveness in mechanically ventilated patients, in the same way that SVV does.

By reducing the horizontal sweep speed, one can capture velocities from all ejections seen over one respiratory cycle (Figure 13.4). After freezing the image, one can scroll through to identify the largest

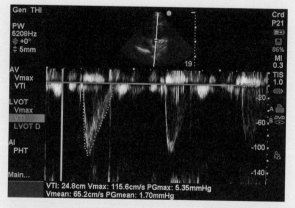

Figure 13.3 An LVOT VTI trace with high sweep speed, using PW Doppler from an A5C view. The VTI measurement is 24.8 cm.

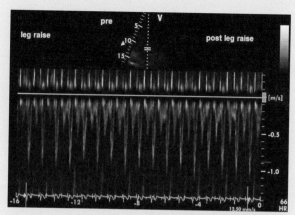

Figure 13.4 An LVOT VTI trace with low sweep speed, using PW Doppler from an A5C view. Pre-leg raise VTI measurements are shown on the left of the image, and post-leg raise measurements on the right. In this case, LVOT VTI variation was <12%, indicating that the patient was not fluid-responsive. For a colour version of this figure, please see colour plate section.

and smallest LVOT VTIs (during mechanical inspiration and expiration, respectively). After tracing these two ejections, the VTI variation can be calculated as follows:

$$\text{LVOT VTI variation} = \frac{(\text{VTImax} - \text{VTImin})}{(\text{VTImean})} \cdot 100$$

A value of >12% predicts fluid responsiveness.

Peak velocity variation

LVOT VTI measurement is time-consuming and becomes increasingly inaccurate with smaller traces, seen at low sweep speeds. An alternative technique involves measuring peak velocities and substituting these values (instead of VTI) into the equation above. In peak velocity variation, values >12% also predict fluid responsiveness.

Passive leg raising and LVOT VTI assessment

PLR is a manoeuvre that provides a transient and reversible fluid challenge (approximately 300 mL) by translocating venous blood from the legs and splanchnic reservoir into the intrathoracic compartment. When both ventricles are preload-dependent, the increased venous return this causes results in increased SV; when they are not, SV does not increase. In this way, TTE and PLR can be used to safely predict fluid responsiveness. LVOT VTI is a good surrogate for SV, particularly in serial assessment, so combining these two methods provides a good bedside test for predicting fluid responsiveness.

PLR is a useful technique because, unlike others, it can be used in spontaneously breathing patients and in the presence of arrhythmias, and it avoids lasting (potentially harmful) effects of fluid administration. PLR is invalid in patients with intra-abdominal hypertension, and pain can cause false positive results in post-operative or trauma patients. It has not been well studied in hospital settings outside ICU, and no outcome studies have been published to date.

Before performing a PLR, the patient should have appropriate analgesia and the procedure explained to them. LVOT VTI is measured initially with the patient in the semi-recumbent position (head up at 45°). The patient is then laid supine, with their legs elevated to 45°, and their LVOT VTI is re-measured after 1 minute. Lamia and colleagues demonstrated that an increase in VTI of at least 12.5% following a PLR predicted an increase in SV of at least 15% following volume expansion, with a sensitivity of 77% and a specificity of 100%.

Pitfalls

There are certain pitfalls to bear in mind when using PLR. These are:

1. Adequate A5C or A3C windows are required
2. Misalignment of the PW Doppler in the LVOT can lead to underestimation of velocities and, in turn, SV. A 15° error in the angle of insonance induces a 5% underestimation in peak velocity or VTI
3. Deep breathing causes displacement of the heart, which can cause false positives in LVOT VTI variation
4. PLR requires three people to perform (the physician performing echo and two people to elevate the legs), which is time-consuming and may be impractical
5. Intra-observer variability is a consideration.
6. In severe hypovolaemia, PLR can be falsely negative due to reduced blood volume in the legs.

Estimating left atrial pressure

High LAP indicates potential fluid intolerance, rather than absence of volume responsiveness. In the absence of MV disease, LAP can be estimated semi-quantitatively, using the same PW Doppler and TDI parameters used in the evaluation of left ventricular diastolic function.

PW Doppler, recorded at the tip of the MV leaflets in A4C, can be used to measure peak early trans-mitral blood flow (E). TDI at the lateral and medial mitral annuli in A4C can be used to measure the peak velocity of early longitudinal left ventricular stretching (e') as it fills. Dividing one by the other produces E/e', which increases with rising LAP. Correlation is not strong enough for quantitative assessment, but it can detect 'low' versus 'high' LAP. More detailed discussion of E/e' can be found in Chapter 7.

Dokainish and colleagues (2004; PMID: 15123522) demonstrated that an E/e' value (averaged) of >15 accurately estimated raised LAP (>15 mmHg), measured invasively, in a mixture of patients from ICU and coronary care. Further validation is needed in mechanically ventilated patients. However, E/e' is non-invasive, relatively easy to obtain, and almost unaffected by loading conditions; as such, it is the subject of considerable interest within the critical care echo research community.

Experimental

Carotid Doppler flow

Studies have shown that common carotid artery (CCA) blood flow can be used to assess fluid responsiveness. CCA blood velocity can be measured using PW Doppler, placed in the centre of the left CCA, 2 cm proximal to the carotid bulb, using angle correction technology to minimize the angle of insonation (Figure 13.5).

Marik and colleagues investigated haemodynamically unstable ICU patients, some mechanically ventilated, before and after a PLR manoeuvre, and observed that a 20% change in carotid arterial minute blood flow ($\pi \times Diam_{CA}^2/4 \times VTI_{CA} \times$ heart rate) predicted volume responsiveness [defined by a 10% rise in stroke volume index (SVI)], with a sensitivity of 0.94 and a specificity of 0.86.

Song and colleagues (2014; PMID: 24722322) demonstrated a strong correlation between an 11%

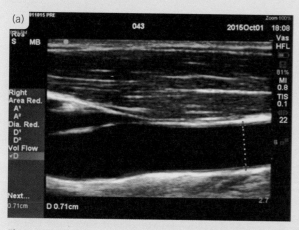 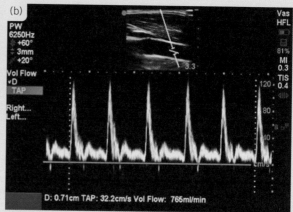

Figure 13.5 Imaging of CCA blood flow. (a) The CCA in long axis. (b) PW Doppler of the CCA, with the sampling volume placed in the centre of the artery, 2 cm proximal to the carotid bulb.

increase in carotid artery peak velocity index {100 × [(maximum peak velocity – minimum peak velocity)/ mean peak velocity]} and volume responsiveness (defined by a 15% rise in SVI after a 6 mL/kg fluid challenge) in mechanically ventilated patients with coronary artery disease, with a sensitivity of 0.85 and a specificity of 0.82.

Whether CCA variability becomes a validated means to determine volume responsiveness in all critically ill patients remains to be seen. However, it is an easily accessible target for non-invasive assessment and is the subject of ongoing research interest.

Micro-fluid challenge

Wu and colleagues (2014; PMID: 24886990) investigated mechanically ventilated patients with sepsis and revealed that a 6% increase in LVOT VTI following a 50 mL challenge, given over 10 s, predicted a 15% increase in cardiac output following a 450 mL challenge, given immediately afterwards over 15 minutes (sensitivity 0.93; specificity 0.91; AUROC 0.91). This technique is currently far from being a validated tool, but this is not the first paper of its kind, and it represents a novel approach for future investigation.

✔ Multiple choice questions

Interactive multiple choice questions to test your knowledge can be found in the Online appendix at www.oxfordmedicine.com/focusedicu. Please refer to your access card for further details.

Further reading

Cecconi M, Hofer C, Teboul JL, et al.; FENICE Investigators; ESICM Trial Group. Fluid challenges in intensive care: the FENICE study. *Intensive Care Medicine* 2015;**41**: 1529–37.

Colebourn C, Newton J (eds). *Acute and Critical Care Echocardiography: Oxford Clinical Imaging Guides.* Oxford: Oxford University Press; 2017.

Godfrey GEP, Dubrey SW, Handy JM. A prospective observational study of stroke volume responsiveness to a passive leg raise manoeuvre in healthy non-starved volunteers as assessed by transthoracic echocardiography. *Anaesthesia* 2014;**69**:306–13.

Lamia B, Ochagavia A, Monnet X, et al. Echocardiographic predication of volume responsiveness in critically ill patients with spontaneously breathing activity. *Intensive Care Medicine* 2007;**33**:1125–32.

Marik PE, Levitov A, Young A, et al. The use of bioreactance and carotid Doppler to determine volume responsiveness and blood flow redistribution following passive leg raising in hemodynamically unstable patients. *Chest* 2013;**143**: 364–70.

Wu Y, Zhou S, Zhou Z, et al. A 10-second fluid challenge guided by transthoracic echocardiography can predict fluid responsiveness. *Critical Care* 2014;**18**:R108:1–8.

14

Lung ultrasound, sonoanatomy, and standard views

Ashley Miller

Introduction

This chapter outlines the technique for performing a systematic assessment of the lung using US that ensures that significant pathology can be identified. A 3-point scan is described, and the appearances of normal lung are reviewed.

Limitations of clinical assessment and the role of ultrasound

The clinical assessment of a patient with acute respiratory failure using a stethoscope has a poor sensitivity and specificity in identifying the correct diagnosis. In experienced hands, point-of-care LUS outperforms conventional chest radiography and can have an accuracy approaching that of CT scanning. LUS can be an extremely powerful tool in the management of critically ill patients with acute respiratory failure, including assessing the underlying diagnosis, identifying the cause of an acute deterioration in gas exchange during ventilatory support, and investigating failure to wean from ventilatory support. LUS provides a rapid bedside test that does not involve exposure to ionizing radiation, has minimal revenue costs, and can be repeated, whenever indicated, without any significant risks to the patient.

LUS has a steep learning curve and can largely obviate the need for the majority of chest X-rays that are undertaken in ventilated patients. However, correct use and interpretation only come with appropriate knowledge, training, and experience.

Anatomy

The lungs are cone-shaped structures situated in the thoracic cage on either side of the mediastinum, to which they are connected by their roots. The shape and positioning of the heart mean that the left lung is different in shape to the right lung, thus differing in their surface projections. The right lung comprises an upper, middle, and lower lobe, while the left lung has an upper and lower lobe. Each is suspended in its pleural cavities and surrounded by visceral and parietal pleura. The pleura are invaginated sacs and so are continuous around the hilum. The serous pleural membranes are closely opposed (except at their recesses), with a tiny amount of fluid between them, allowing them to slide over one another with respiration. The parietal pleura lines the thoracic wall, diaphragm, and mediastinum. The ribcage encases the pleural cavities. Below the lungs, the diaphragm separates the thoracic and abdominal cavities. It is dome-shaped, with its highest point (deep in the thorax) extending as high as the fourth intercostal space anteriorly. The liver on the right and the spleen and stomach on the left are located immediately below the diaphragm in the peritoneal cavity.

Surface anatomy

The surface anatomy of the lungs is shown in Figure 14.1. Anteriorly, the lungs extend to the sixth costal

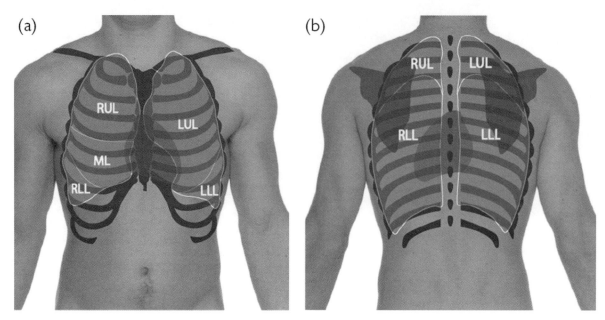

Figure 14.1 Surface anatomy of the lung. For a colour version of this figure, please see colour plate section.

Reproduced from James Thomas and Tanya Monaghan, *Oxford Handbook of Clinical Examination and Practical Skills* 2Ed., © Oxford University Press 2014, Figure 6.1, p. 141. By permission of Oxford University Press. https://global.oup.com/academic.

cartilage on the right and the fourth on the left (because of the heart). Because the ribs run in a caudad direction as they extend around the thorax from the spine, posteriorly, both lung bases can be identified by the level of the tenth thoracic vertebrae. The fact that the lungs can only be visualized down to the horizontal level of the anterior fifth intercostal space catches many novices out—most are surprised by how cephalad the lung bases are situated. The parietal pleural extends significantly lower than the visceral pleura, so pleural effusions may be seen extending caudad to this.

On the right, the border of the upper and middle lobes is located at the third intercostal space anteriorly. The oblique fissure runs roughly in the fifth intercostal space between the posterior and anterior axillary lines, and the pleura of the middle lobe can be visualized with US anteriorly in the fourth and fifth intercostal spaces. The lower lobe can be located in the fifth to eighth intercostal spaces in the posterior axillary line. Posteriorly, the upper and lower lobes meet under the fifth intercostal space.

On the left, the interlobular fissure is steeper than the right. The surface anatomy of the upper lobe is located anteriorly, while in the axilla, the lower lobe is located under the seventh and eighth intercostal spaces. Posteriorly, the upper and lower lobes join in the fourth intercostal space.

Technique

Probe selection

Scans can be performed with a linear (high-frequency vascular access), curvilinear (low-frequency abdominal), or phased array (low-frequency echocardiography) probe. Each has advantages and disadvantages that are outlined in Table 14.1. The curvilinear probe is the best single probe to use, as it can be used to perform a comprehensive scan and elicit all the signs of LUS with the best overall resolution. The high-frequency linear array probe will provide the highest-resolution images of the pleura and can be used if there is difficulty with identifying pleural sliding.

Probe positioning

By convention, the left side of the US display as you look at it must be either cephalad or the right-hand side of the patient. It is therefore essential for the probe's marker dot to be in the correct orientation. A number of different approaches to undertaking a systematic LUS examination have been described. Each lung may be scanned in six regions—upper and lower anterior, mid-axillary, and posterior positions (see figure 23.1). A simpler approach is to use only three points on each hemi-thorax that appears to have a diagnostic accuracy that is as high for most pathologies as using more examination points. Scanning at 28 points in the anterior and axillary areas has also been described to quantify a pulmonary oedema 'score'. For most situations, the simple 3-point approach is appropriate. It is imperative that the operator has a consistent standardized method for each scan performed.

Table 14.1 Ultrasound probes and their merits

	Advantages	Disadvantages
Linear	High frequency allows the superficial pleura to be easily visualized with good appreciation of lung sliding	High frequency and narrow sector width mean lung bases cannot be visualized
Curvilinear	Can be used to perform a comprehensive exam and demonstrate all signs	Lower frequency means lung sliding is slightly harder to appreciate than with a linear probe
		Large footprint means some angulation is needed to eliminate rib shadows
Phased array	Can be used to perform a comprehensive exam and demonstrate all signs Its small footprint is useful for getting in between the ribs	Resolution is less good than the other two probes

In the 3-point scan, the probe is placed in the second intercostal space, mid-clavicular line for the upper anterior point. It lies over the upper lobe. The lower anterior point is located at the fourth intercostal space at the outer edge of the nipple (in a man). This point will miss the heart on the left. It lies over the middle or lingular lobe (Figure 14.2). The postero-lateral point is located by moving laterally and posteriorly, from the lower anterior point, until limited by the mattress of the bed and then going caudad by one or two rib spaces, so the diaphragm is located. It lies over the lower lobe.

The 28-point scanning technique examines the second to fifth intercostal spaces at the parasternal, mid-clavicular, anterior axillary, and mid-axillary lines (without the fifth intercostal space exam on the left due to the position of the heart). As this was designed to evaluate pulmonary oedema specifically, it is necessary to add postero-lateral points inferior to the posterior axillary line in each rib space down to the level

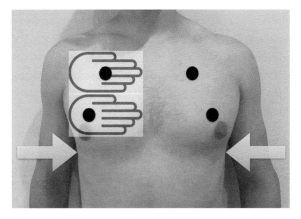

Figure 14.2 Surface anatomy for the 3-point scan. The upper and lower anterior points are highlighted. To identify the correct positions, apply two hands side by side (without your thumbs) over the anterior chest, with your wrists in the anterior axillary line and your upper little finger resting along the clavicle. Your lower little finger will be aligned with the lower border of the lung (the phrenic line). The upper anterior point corresponds to the base of the middle and ring fingers on the upper hand. The lower anterior point lies under the middle of the palm on the lower hand. The postero-lateral point is located laterally and posteriorly from the lower anterior point as far as possible behind the posterior axillary line (limited by the bed).

of the diaphragm, in order to examine for consolidation and pleural effusions. It should be noted that a comprehensive exam can be performed on critically ill supine patients without needing to move them. It is possible to get posterior to the posterior axillary line by pushing the heel of the probe into the bed.

Probe orientation

When scanning anteriorly, the probe should be placed in a longitudinal (cephalad–caudad) orientation. This ensures that the rib and pleural lines are both captured in a single image and clearly differentiated. If the probe is placed transversely, the immobile rib line may be mistaken for a non-sliding pleural line by a novice sonographer, resulting in an erroneous diagnosis of pneumothorax. However, temporarily siting the probe transversely can help in examining a larger area of the pleura and in finding the lung point in a pneumothorax (Chapter 15). When scanning postero-laterally, it is advised that while a cephalad–caudad orientation should be maintained, it is desirable to rotate the probe approximately 30° posteriorly in order to get the probe's footprint in the intercostal space and eliminate the rib shadows from the image. Be aware here that the cephalad portion of the image will then often be slicing through soft tissue posterior to the lung, particularly the more posterior you are.

Machine settings

Whatever you are looking at should fill your screen. Having too great a depth reduces the frame rate and thus the image quality. For most subjects, a depth setting of around 10 cm is appropriate when using the curvilinear probe. The frequency should be set to its highest setting with curvilinear and phased array probes when assessing anterior lung sliding. The default setting should be used when imaging the lung bases. If the focus point(s) are not preset, these should be at the level of interest. The gain setting may need to be changed during the examination. Anterior lung sliding may be best seen with the gain setting low, which is then increased to improve the image of a consolidated lung base or pleural effusion. Contemporary machines often have a number of image processing settings to minimize artefact generation. As artefacts are a core component of LUS, it may be necessary to disable these options in order

to obtain optimal images. However, A-lines and B-lines (see p. 129) are usually visible (if present) in all settings.

Normal sonoanatomy

Anterior

Immediately in the near field, the soft tissue above the ribs will be seen. Deep to this will be the rib line and then approximately 0.5 cm below this, the thin, bright white pleural line will be visible. Centre the pleural line between two ribs in the image, and the 'bat sign' is demonstrated with the rib shadows looking like the wings of a bat (Figure 14.3). In a normal aerated lung, only shadow and artefact will be visible deep to the ribs and pleural line.

Lung sliding

The pleural line should be closely examined for the phenomenon of lung sliding. The two pleural layers slide over one another with respiration, which is demonstrated by the pleural layers moving backwards and forwards. Little blebs (white or black) are seen within the pleural line or just below it that will move to and fro with the respiratory cycle (Video 1.10.1 ⬤). The space below the pleura will shimmer. Lung sliding is easiest to appreciate with the depth reduced, the gain turned down, and the probe on the highest-frequency setting.

Lung sliding can also be demonstrated with M-mode. Placing M-mode through the pleural line will demonstrate the 'seashore' sign. The relatively immobile soft

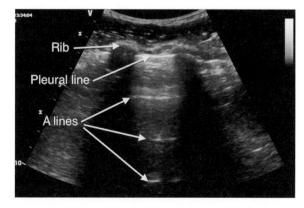

Figure 14.3 Normal 'bats wing' appearance. The bright pleural line is visible between two ribs. A lines are seen as deeper replications of the pleural line.

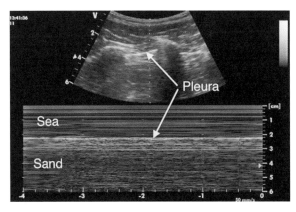

Figure 14.4 M-mode appearance of normal lung sliding: seashore sign.

tissue above the pleura will yield clear horizontal lines (the sea), while the moving pleura will generate a chaotic 'sandy' appearance below the pleural line (Figure 14.4).

The presence of lung sliding immediately excludes a pneumothorax at that point in the chest with 100% specificity. The absence of sliding signifies that the pleura are either separated (pneumothorax, effusion), stuck together (infection, ARDS, pleurodesis), or that there is no respiration (one-lung intubation, pneumonectomy). In M-mode, absent sliding appears as a series of horizontal, straight lines above and below the pleural line that has been termed the barcode or stratosphere sign (Figure 14.5 and Video 1.10.2 ▢). Present, but diminished, sliding will be seen with low tidal volumes, hyperinflated lungs, and ARDS. The lungs expand more at their bases than their apices, and so sliding is easier to visualize at the lung bases.

A-lines

The acoustic impedances of soft tissue, bone, and air are very different. When US hits a boundary of differing acoustic impedances, it will be reflected back to the transducer. This explains why nothing can be visualized deep to the ribs and the pleura (assuming there is no fluid in or around the lung). The transducer itself will reflect some of the returning US waves, and these will bounce backwards and forwards between the probe and the pleura. This causes reverberation artefacts below the pleural line that appear as exact copies. Their spacing will be the same as between the probe and pleural line. These are termed A-lines and signify that there is air below the parietal pleura. Hence, they are present both in normal lungs and when there is a pneumothorax. Sometimes there are highly echogenic interfaces between soft tissue layers, which can cause artefactual lines to appear below the pleura. These can be differentiated from A-lines by their spacing.

B-lines

These artefacts are laser-like lines resembling comet tails, which extend from the pleural line to the depths of the image. They move backwards and forwards with lung sliding and obliterate A-lines when they pass across them (Figure 14.6). Their aetiology is debated, but it has been suggested that they result from the juxtaposition of thickened interlobular alveolar septa and air within the alveoli producing a reverberation artefact. When looked at carefully, B-lines are seen to be composed of closely repeating horizontal lines. The

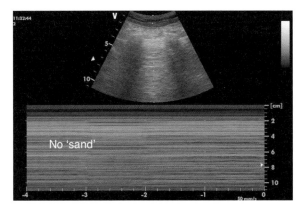

Figure 14.5 M-mode appearance of no lung sliding: stratosphere sign.

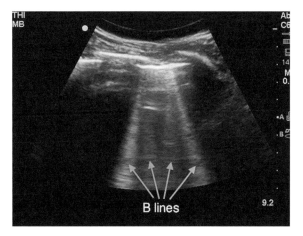

Figure 14.6 2D mode: B-lines.

generation of B-lines requires that the parietal and visceral pleura layers are in opposition, and their presence therefore excludes a pneumothorax.

B-lines are present in any disease affecting the interstitium and are therefore seen in pulmonary oedema, ARDS, and lung fibrosis. Their location can be unilateral, bilateral, disseminated, localized, homogenous, or non-homogenous, depending on the pathology. The most common cause is pulmonary oedema. Increasing severity yields more B-lines, which become closer together. When severe, B-lines will coalesce, yielding a 'white lung' appearance below the pleural line that can be misinterpreted as B-lines being absent. Importantly, no A-lines will be seen and the pleural space will be much whiter than usual.

Up to two B-lines between ribs can be considered normal (particularly at the lung bases), while three or more, or B-lines close together in a transverse image, are considered pathological. It should be noted that whenever there is a juxtaposition of air and fluid within the lung, comet artefacts are generated and they are therefore seen bordering consolidation and atelectasis. Although they look similar, they are only termed B-lines if they originate from the pleural line.

Lung pulse

If the pleura are apposed to one another, then the cardiac pulsation will be transmitted through the lung to the parietal pleura. This can be seen with US as a small amount of lung sliding in time with the heartbeat. It can be visualized in 2D and M-mode. It can be appreciated as separate from the sliding of respiration by asking a subject to hold their breath while examining the pleura. The use of this sign is that in instances where there is no sliding due to lack of lung ventilation, it demonstrates that there is no pneumothorax, as by definition the pleural layers have to be touching. If unsure whether lung pulse is present on the 2D image, M-mode may be used which yields the lung pulse as 'T lines' (Figure 14.7). Lung pulse is seen over areas of atelectatic lung and over the non-ventilated lung following endobronchial intubation.

Postero-lateral

In the postero-lateral zones, the same signs should be looked for as with anterior scanning. The difference is that the diaphragm is now an important component

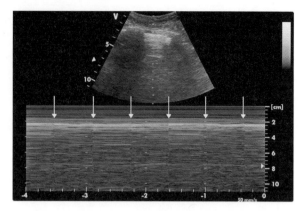

Figure 14.7 M-mode appearance of the lung pulse. T lines (highlighted with arrows) represent pleural movement from transmitted cardiac pulsation on the background of a motionless lung, which produces a stratosphere sign appearance in between.

of the exam. Locating it and differentiating between supra- and sub-diaphragmatic structures are vital. The depth will need to be great enough to extend to the mediastinum (around 15 cm is appropriate). The diaphragm is highly reflective to US waves and produces a bright, curved line that moves with respiration. The left of the image, as you look at it, will be the lung; the diaphragm should be right of centre, and the liver or spleen will be on the right (Figures 14.8 and 14.9). When scanning the left side, it is important to ensure that the spleen, rather than the stomach, is visualized in order to allow proper

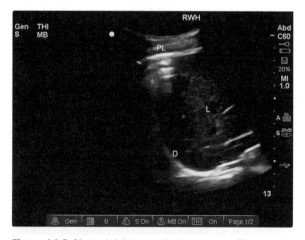

Figure 14.8 Normal right posterior lateral scan. PL, pleural line; L, liver; D, diaphragm identified. Superior diaphragm not visible as obscured by normal aerated lung (veil sign).

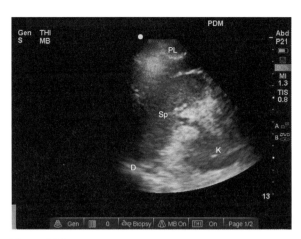

Figure 14.9 Normal left posterior lateral scan. PL, pleural line; Sp, spleen; K, left kidney; D, part of diaphragm identified. Limited view of the diaphragm as the majority obscured by normal aerated lung.

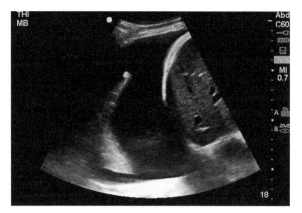

Figure 14.10 Effusion and collapsed lung with clear view of the diaphragm.

assessment of the diaphragm and any effusions. The spleen lies behind the stomach and will be revealed by either moving or angling the probe posteriorly. The depths of the image will be the mediastinum or spine, which will only be seen if an acoustic window from fluid is present.

With a normal air-filled lung, only the posterior portion of the diaphragm will be seen. Air in the costophrenic angle obliterates any structures below it. With respiration, the artefact of an air-filled lung will be seen coming across the screen like a curtain obliterating the view of the diaphragm and liver or spleen during inspiration. This has been termed the curtain or veil sign (Videos 1.10.2).

When there is a pleural effusion or a consolidated lung base, then the diaphragm is easy to visualize due to the US window provided (Figure 14.10). Diaphragmatic muscle thickness and excursion with respiration can be measured.

A collapsed or consolidated lung base has a very similar US appearance to the liver and spleen, and it is vital to differentiate the two by their relationship to the diaphragm. Similarly, it is easy to confuse ascites with a pleural effusion. Moving the probe around and looking from different angles is useful to clearly define what is what.

Pitfalls

The bright, motionless rib line may be mistaken for a lack of pleural sliding by having the probe in the transverse plane. Scanning in the longitudinal plane is recommended to produce the typical bats wing appearance that clearly differentiates the rib and pleural lines.

Use of too great a depth setting will make pleural sliding difficult to visualize.

Subcutaneous emphysema prevents transmission of US waves and visualization of the pleural line. It may be possible to massage the air out of the way using the probe in order to obtain images.

A full stomach may be misinterpreted as left basal consolidation or effusion. It is essential to identify the diaphragm to confirm that the lung is being imaged when scanning in the postero-lateral zones.

The spleen may be hypoechoic, which can be misinterpreted by novices as a pleural effusion. The position of the diaphragm must be identified to confirm an effusion.

✅ Multiple choice questions

Interactive multiple choice questions to test your knowledge can be found in the Online appendix at www.oxfordmedicine.com/focusedicu. Please refer to your access card for further details.

15

Pleural assessment

Jennie Stephens

Introduction

This chapter describes the use of US to assess pleural disease in the ICU setting. The US signs of pneumothorax are described and the specificity reviewed, with the pitfalls highlighted. The assessment and quantification of pleural effusions are outlined, together with the limitations and pitfalls.

Benefit of ultrasound

Thoracic US is a very powerful tool for the assessment of pleural pathology. US is the gold standard method for the assessment of pleural effusions and is more sensitive than chest radiography for the diagnosis of pneumothorax. US is very sensitive in the diagnosis, assessment, and quantification of pleural effusions, as well as guiding safe diagnostic aspiration and therapeutic drainage. US is the imaging modality of choice when it comes to identifying complex loculated effusions. Pneumothorax can be accurately and rapidly ruled out or diagnosed using specific US signs in a time frame that is impossible to achieve with chest radiography or CT scanning.

Normal sonoanatomy

Pleural sliding

The adjacent parietal and visceral pleura can be visualized directly, even in the absence of pathology (Video 1.11.1 📹). Lung sliding or gliding describes the US appearance of the movement of the two adjacent pleural layers seen throughout the respiratory cycle in normal lung. It is a shimmering back-and-forth movement seen at the pleural line and is an important US sign to recognize. The presence or absence of pleural sliding can provide useful and accurate information about the underlying lung.

With a postero-lateral scan at the level of the hemidiaphragm, pleural sliding is easy to visualize because, during inspiration, the curtain of aerated lung appears to 'slide' over the hemidiaphragm, obliterating it and the underlying structures. During expiration, the lung 'slides' back, once again, revealing the hemidiaphragm (Video 1.11.2 📹). When scanning above the hemidiaphragm or over the anterior chest wall, sliding may be harder to identify. In these circumstances, reducing scan depth and changing probe will make pleural sliding easier to appreciate. The high-frequency linear array probe is better placed to visualize more shallow structures, and it will give a more detailed view of the pleura.

Seashore and stratosphere signs

M-mode can be used to confirm or rule out lung sliding, as it makes the presence or absence of movement at and below the pleural line easier to visualize. The seashore sign (Figure 15.1) confirms the presence of lung sliding at the rib space being visualized. This is compared to the stratosphere sign (Figure 15.2), which reflects the absence of lung sliding at the rib space being visualized. The differentiation between these two M-mode signs can be demonstrated by asking a normal model to hold their breath in inspiration while you scan their anterior chest wall. In normal respiration, the seashore sign should be apparent, and during a breath-hold, the stratosphere sign should be seen.

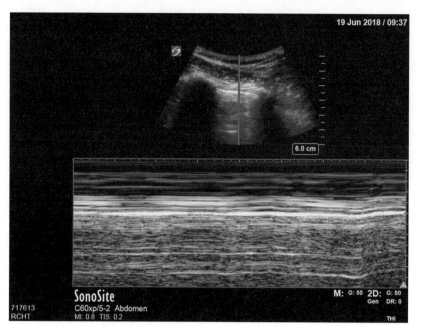

Figure 15.1 The seashore sign. Normal lung sliding. The subcutaneous tissue and musculature create straight lines representing the 'sea'. Below the pleural line, the continually moving aerated lung creates the speckled 'sand'.

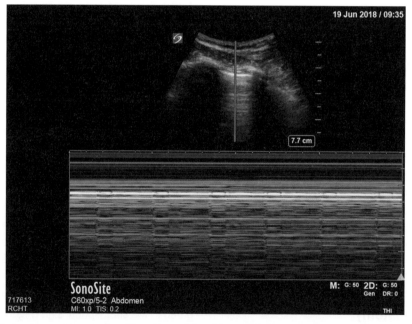

Figure 15.2 The stratosphere or barcode sign. Absent lung sliding. The straight lines created by the static subcutaneous tissue and musculature continue beyond the pleural line. The absence of movement deep to the pleural line creates multiple straight lines.

Ultrasound assessment of the pleura

The pleura is visualized over the entirety of the chest wall, excluding subscapular and substernal areas. Particular pleural pathologies are more likely to be found in specific areas of the thoracic cavity, which will influence where you prioritize your scanning. A pneumothorax is most often present in the apical region of the thoracic cavity in a seated or semi-recumbent patient and can be identified by scanning the anterior chest wall. In contrast, pleural effusion, unless loculated or confined by tethered lung, is affected by gravity and is most usually seen in the postero-lateral areas. There are, of course, exceptions to these rules of thumb, and you are encouraged to take a systematic and thorough approach to scanning the lungs for pleural pathology.

Common pathophysiology

Pneumothorax

The optimum place to scan for a pneumothorax is the anterior aspect of the chest wall. Usually the collapsing lung will move down and in, towards the mediastinum as the pneumothorax expands, meaning the US signs of a pneumothorax are first found anteriorly. When the diagnosis of a pneumothorax is suspected, the scan should start with the upper and lower anterior points bilaterally. Perform a full assessment of the pleura beneath the anterior chest wall, before moving to the lateral and posterior areas.

The US signs of a pneumothorax are:

- Absence of pleural sliding
- Absence of sliding B-lines
- Absence of a lung pulse
- Presence of a lung point.

The presence of pleural sliding, sliding B-lines, or a lung pulse reliably rules out a pneumothorax in the area of the lung being scanned. A lung point (described in Presence of a lung point, pp. 135–7) identifies the boundary between the empty, but air-filled, thoracic cavity and inflating and deflating lung and is a sign that rules in a pneumothorax. The combination of absence of pleural sliding, absence of B-lines, and presence of a lung point has been shown to have a specificity and positive predictive value approaching 100% in diagnosing a pneumothorax.

Absence of pleural sliding

This identifies that there is no movement of the visceral pleura over the parietal pleura with respiration (Video 1.11.3 ◉). It occurs in any condition that prevents ventilation of the lung immediately underlying the area being visualized and is not a sign that is specific to a pneumothorax. Absent pleural sliding is therefore seen in atelectasis, consolidation, endobronchial intubation, and breath-holding, in addition to pneumothorax. Pleural sliding may also appear to be absent in severe parenchymal lung disease that prevents lung expansion. Lung hyperinflation as a result of obstructive airways disease or application of high levels of positive end-expiratory pressure (PEEP) may also make pleural sliding difficult to identify, particularly in the apical and anterior regions.

> **Pitfall**
>
> Absence of pleural sliding does not diagnose a pneumothorax; the presence of pleural sliding excludes a pneumothorax in the underlying lung.

Absence of sliding B-lines

B-lines arise from subpleural interlobular septa and will only occur if the visceral and parietal pleura are directly adjacent. Multiple B-lines are a pathological finding, but a single B-line excludes the presence of a pneumothorax in the area of the lung being scanned.

Absence of a lung pulse

A lung pulse describes movement of the pleural line as a result of transmission of the cardiac pulsation through underlying static lung tissue (Video 1.11.4 ◉). Subtle pleural movement is seen to occur at the same frequency as the heart rate, while no movement is seen in time with respiration. For the phenomenon to occur, the parietal and visceral pleura must be adjacent and the lung tissue must be stationary. It is best demonstrated with M-mode, which reveals an underlying 'stratosphere' appearance with superimposed intermittent bursts of a 'seashore' appearance in time with the heartbeat (Figure 15.3). A lung pulse occurs with atelectasis, endobronchial intubation, and breath-holding. The presence of a lung pulse excludes a pneumothorax in the area of the lung being scanned.

Presence of a lung point

A lung point is a US sign specific to pneumothorax. It requires the US probe to be placed over a point on the chest wall where the border of the lung and pneumothorax crosses under the footprint of the US probe during the respiratory cycle (Figure 15.4).

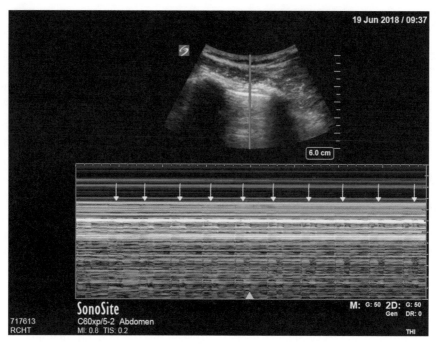

Figure 15.3 Lung pulse. The cardiac pulsations (see arrows) transmitted through static lung are clearly visualized using M-mode. This ultrasound sign is known as the 'lung pulse'.

The boundary between the air-filled thoracic cavity and lung is identified by the presence of pleural sliding moving into and across the rib space with inspiration and back with expiration (Video 1.11.5 🎦). The US probe needs to be placed exactly, so that at the end of inspiration, the boundary of the inflated lung does not reach the upper rib. This is the lung point and is highly specific to the diagnosis of a pneumothorax. The lung point can occur at any point over the anterior chest wall and requires a systematic approach to ensure that it is identified. If the other three signs of a pneumothorax have been identified, the lung point is

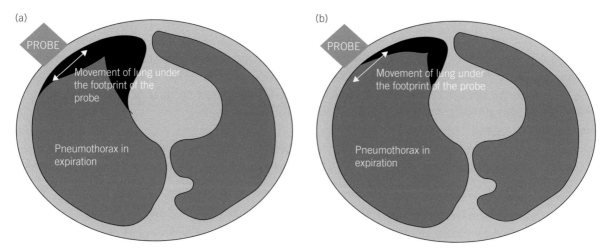

Figure 15.4 The lung point. When the probe is placed over the lung point, the aerated lung will move under the probe on inspiration and back on expiration. This can be seen as intermittent pleural sliding in 2D mode or as a transition between the seashore and stratosphere sign in M-mode. For a colour version of this figure, please see colour plate section.

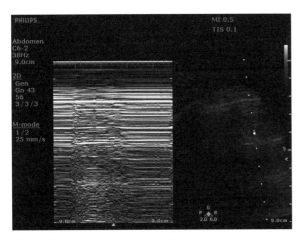

Figure 15.5 Lung point (M-mode). Transition between seashore and stratosphere signs seen using M-mode at the lung point.

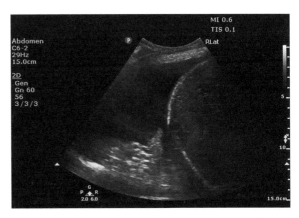

Figure 15.6 Pleural effusion. Large anechoic area with atelectatic lung seen lying deep within the effusion. The diaphragm is clearly visualized in its entire length.

searched for by slowly moving the probe laterally and observing the point where lung sliding comes and goes with respiration.

M-mode is a useful modality to help with the identification of a lung point. Once a lung point has been confirmed using the 2D mode, M-mode can be used to identify the boundary between sliding and non-sliding pleura. By placing the scan line directly over the lung point, the M-mode trace will switch from the seashore sign to the stratosphere sign and back again as the lung slides through the scan line (Figure 15.5). The US features of a pneumothorax are summarized in Box 15.1.

Pleural effusion

Pleural effusions are normally found in the most dependent part of the thoracic cavity, relative to the position of the patient; therefore, the search for pleural fluid should start at the most postero-lateral point possible in the semi-recumbent patient. It is important to note, however, that tethered lung and loculations mean that effusions can be found anywhere, and a systematic approach to scanning the whole lung is important.

Ultrasound features of effusion

The key US sign that identifies a pleural effusion is an echo-free space that is clearly above the diaphragm and shows dynamic change with respiration (Box 15.2, Figure 15.6, and Video 1.11.6). Fluid within the pleural cavity can be a transudate, an exudate, or frankly purulent, each with characteristic US findings. Fluid, on the whole, is anechoic and is seen as a black space separating the parietal and visceral pleura. It is not uncommon to see a small pleural effusion at the costo-phrenic angle of critically ill ventilated patients without known respiratory pathology.

Lung sliding is no longer present because the pleura are no longer adjacent. When the pleural effusion is large, the lung can be collapsed and seen freely

---

Box 15.1 Ultrasound signs of a pneumothorax

- Absent lung sliding
- A-lines present
- No B-lines
- Absent lung pulse
- Visible lung point

Box 15.2 Ultrasound characteristics of a pleural effusion

- Echo-free space
- Dynamic signs
  - Change in shape during respiratory cycle
  - Atelectatic or consolidated lung
  - Swirling motion in echo-free space
- Positive identification
  - Diaphragm
  - Liver/spleen

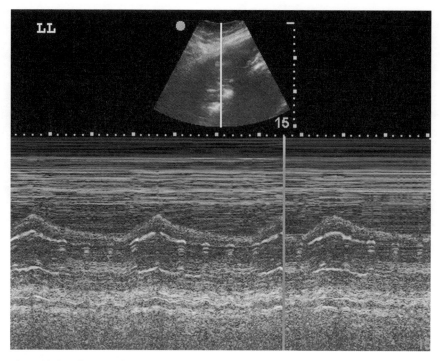

Figure 15.7 The sinusoid sign. By using M-mode, a pleural effusion can be seen to change in size with respiration, forming a sinusoid wave moving towards and away from the pleural line. This is in contrast to pleural thickening, which does not change in size with respiration.

floating as a non-aerated structure within the pleural fluid. The hemidiaphragm is clearly visualized, often in its entirety, if there is adjacent pleural fluid. A large effusion that contains collapsed consolidated lung transmits US waves and allows visualization down to the mediastinum, including cardiac structures lying closer to the surface than originally suspected.

Pleural effusions will vary in shape and size with respiration. The lung within a pleural effusion will move closer to the chest wall with inspiration and away with expiration. This can be demonstrated using M-mode by the sinusoid sign (Figure 15.7), which can be useful for differentiating small effusions from pleural thickening.

Assessment of size

The decision of whether to drain a pleural effusion should depend more on the clinical condition of the patient, rather than the size of the effusion. Infected effusions will need to be drained, independent of size. Uncomplicated effusions are frequently seen in critically ill patients, and the majority do not require drainage as they will resolve spontaneously. Large simple effusions (e.g. >800 mL) should be drained

if there is evidence of respiratory compromise such as impaired gas exchange or ventilator dependence. Pleural US can provide information about diaphragmatic movement, the possible nature of the effusion, and the lung within the effusion. The depth of the effusion measured at the lung base in expiration can be used to provide an approximate estimate of the effusion size. A number of formulae have been published of varying complexity, with the simplest being:

Estimated volume (mL)
$= 20 \times$ pleural separation (mm)

It is important to measure the pleural separation size at the lung base with a transverse scan in the posterior axillary line. A longitudinal scan angled posteriorly may overestimate the size of an effusion.

Another simple way of estimating effusion size has been described and requires measuring the depth of the effusion in expiration at the most posterolateral alveolar/pleural syndrome (PLAPS) point (see Table 15.1).

Large effusions cause a significant increase in intrapleural pressure that may result in inversion of the

Table 15.1 Estimating the volume of a pleural effusion using measured depth at the postero-lateral ('PLAPS') point

Depth of effusion at PLAPS point in expiration	Approximate size (mL)
1–3 mm	15–30
1 cm	75–150
2 cm	300–600
3.5 cm	1500–2500

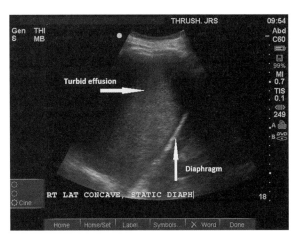

Figure 15.9 Massive purulent effusion. The fluid has a similar echogenicity to the liver or spleen but can be seen swirling around in the pleural cavity.

diaphragm and paradoxical movement with respiration (Figure 15.8 and Video 1.11.7 ▣).

Appearance of transudate, exudate, and loculated effusions

A transudate, which is caused by an imbalance of the normal forces resulting in the production and re-absorption of pleural fluid, appears anechoic on US. Common conditions associated with transudative effusions include heart failure, fluid overload, reduced serum protein, cirrhosis, and nephrotic syndrome.

An exudate can vary from anechoic to particulate and is secondary to an inflammatory process (infection, malignancy, pancreatitis). It can contain multiple particles seen swirling within the fluid or septations that float within the effusion and sometimes seem to tether the lung to the diaphragm or parietal pleura.

The US appearance of a haemothorax will vary, depending on its age. Acutely, blood within the thoracic cavity will appear anechoic, but this will become more echoic over time, often accompanied by the formation of septations.

Frankly purulent pleural fluid can sometimes have a similar echogenicity to the liver or spleen (Figure 15.9). The turbid fluid can normally be seen swirling within the pleural cavity, and this can be confirmed using colour Doppler. The fluid can be seen to move and swirl freely within the pleural cavity and is not pulsatile (Video 1.11.8 ▣).

Loculated pleural effusions are clearly visualized using US. Each pocket of fluid is seen within septated margins. Given the nature of a loculated effusion, they can occur anywhere within the chest cavity and their position is independent of gravity and the position of the patient (Figure 15.10).

Pitfalls in interpretation

Pleural thickening or pleural effusion

A thickened pleura, secondary to plaque formation or malignant infiltration, can look very similar to a small pleural effusion. The use of M-mode scanning to demonstrate the sinusoid sign is useful to differentiate fluid from other pleural pathology. Pleural thickening is uniform and does not vary in size with respiration.

Pleural fluid or ascitic fluid

In the critically ill patient, pleural fluid is often accompanied by ascitic fluid. Ascites can often be seen above

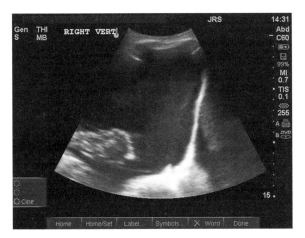

Figure 15.8 Large pleural effusion. Note the inverted hemidiaphragm and paradoxical movement reflecting raised intra-pleural pressure (seen on Video 1.11.7 ▣).

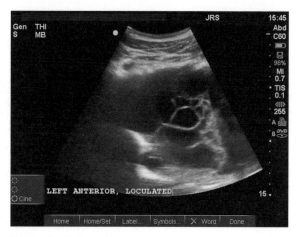

Figure 15.10 Loculated anterior pleural effusion. The locules of fluid are clearly visible and remain in the anterior position when the patient is upright.

the abdominal viscera in the semi-recumbent patient. It is vital to be confident with the US appearance of the sub-diaphragmatic anatomy to accurately determine the position of free fluid. It is essential to clearly identify all sub- and supra-diaphragmatic anatomy in order to accurately determine the position of any fluid, prior to attempting thoracocentesis.

Complex exudative/purulent effusion or consolidated lung

The differentiation of a turbid pleural exudate and consolidated lung can be challenging. There are a few US characteristics that can help this differentiation. Turbid/particulate pleural fluid should move freely and non-uniformly within the pleural cavity throughout the respiratory cycle. If this free, swirling movement is not

clear using the 2D mode, colour Doppler can be used. The use of colour Doppler will also identify the pulsatile nature of consolidated lung or abdominal viscera, which is not seen with pleural fluid. If there is any doubt, it is essential to undertake further imaging with lung CT scan to exclude the presence of consolidated lung, before considering pleural drainage.

> **Pitfall**
>
> Pleural thickening, sub-diaphragmatic fluid, or consolidated lung can be misdiagnosed as pleural fluid.

✅ Multiple choice questions

Interactive multiple choice questions to test your knowledge can be found in the Online appendix at www.oxfordmedicine.com/focusedicu. Please refer to your access card for further details.

Further reading

Husain LF, Hagopian L, Baker WE, Carmody KA. Sonographic diagnosis of pneumothorax. *Journal of Emergencies, Trauma, and Shock* 2012;**5**:76–81.

Lichtenstein D. Pleural effusion and introduction to the lung ultrasound technique. In: Lichtenstein D. *General Ultrasound in the Critically Ill*. Berlin: Springer-Verlag; 2007. pp. 96–104.

Lichtenstein D. Pneumothorax and introduction to ultrasound signs in the lung. In: Lichtenstein D. *General Ultrasound in the Critically Ill*. Berlin: Springer-Verlag; 2007. pp. 105–15.

Lichtenstein D, Mezière G, Biderman P, Gepner A. The 'lung point': an ultrasound sign specific to pneumothorax. *Intensive Care Medicine* 2000;**26**:1434–40.

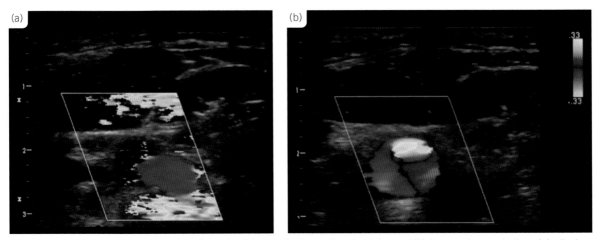

Figure 3.6 A PW Doppler image, taken from the left ventricular outflow tract in an A5C image, demonstrating: (a) aliasing; (b) aliasing resolved by setting the correct baseline.

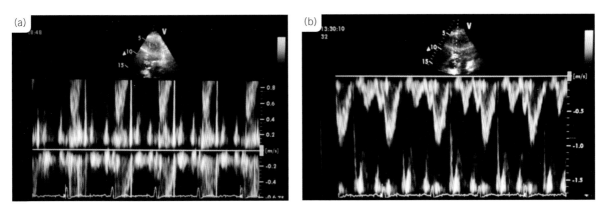

Figure 3.7 An image of the internal carotid artery with colour Doppler, demonstrating: (a) excessive gain causing speckling outside the blood vessel; (b) adequate gain setting with the colour signal limited to the contours of the artery.

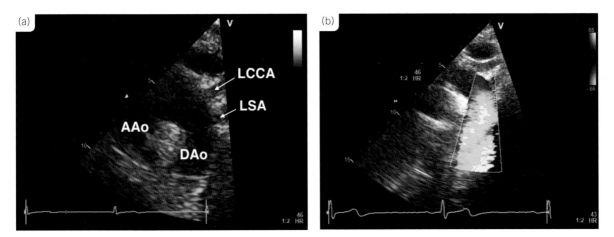

Figure 5.9. Suprasternal view: (a) 2D sonoanatomy; (b) with colour flow Doppler. AAo, ascending aorta; DAo, descending aorta; LCCA, left common carotid artery; LSA, left subclavian artery.

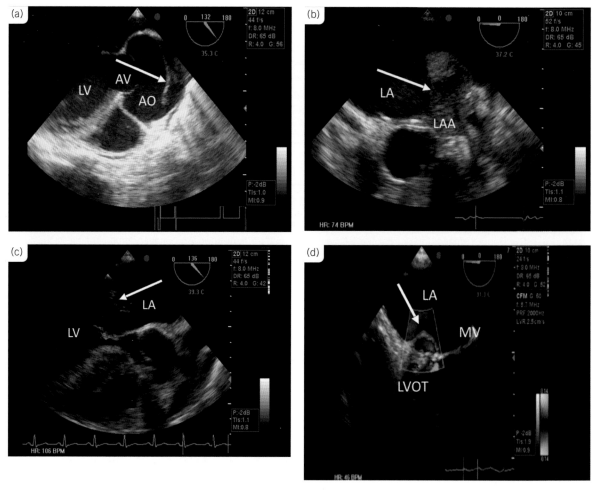

Figure 6.4 Various TOE images. (a) Aortic dissection showing a prominent intimal flap and dilated aortic valve. (b) A large atrial appendage thrombus encroaching on the left atrium. (c) Flail posterior leaflet of the mitral valve. (d) Aortic root abscess with colour Doppler to show its pulsatility. Ao, aorta; AV, aortic valve; LA, left atrium; LAA, left atrial appendage; LV, left ventricle; LVOT, left ventricular outflow tract; MV, mitral valve.

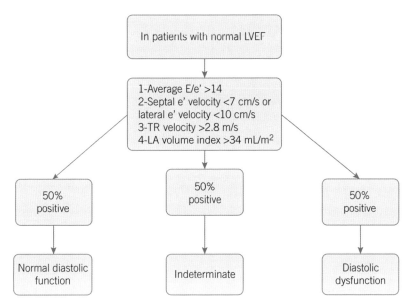

Figure 7.8 Updated guidelines on assessing left ventricular diastolic function in patients with normal LVEF.

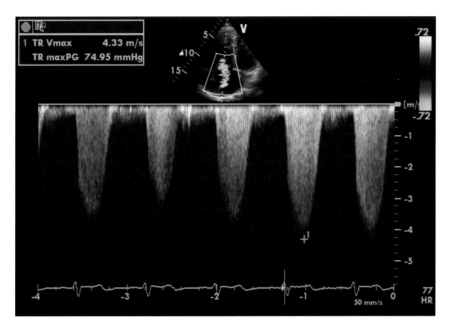

Figure 8.9 CW Doppler trace of TR. The extremely high-velocity TR jet indicates severe pulmonary hypertension that is likely to be chronic.

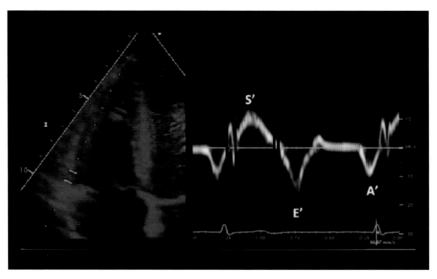

Figure 8.10 TDI calculation of S′. The RV has the same TDI properties as the LV, with an E′ and A′ wave, and S′ wave in the opposite (positive) direction.

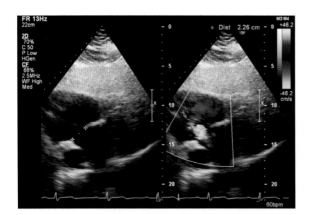

Figure 9.7 Subcostal view (two-dimensional and colour Doppler) demonstrating a large secundum atrial septal defect with a left-to-right shunt. Note: orange flow towards the transducer (see also Video 1.5.5).

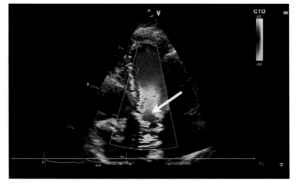

Figure 11.5 An A5C view demonstrating proximal flow acceleration, with aliasing of the colour Doppler jet seen proximal to the aortic stenosis. Note: the red mosaic jet (arrowed) represents abnormally high-velocity blood in the LVOT.

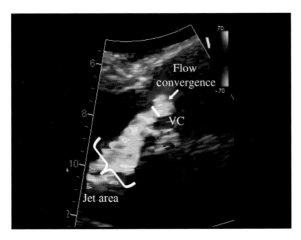

Figure 11.6 PLAX view demonstrating the vena contracta and proximal flow convergence caused by AR.

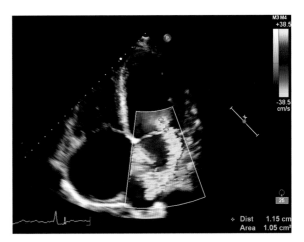

Figure 12.5 An A4C still image of severe MR, with a large hemisphere of proximal flow recruitment. Here you can see an eccentric jet of swirl down the side of the left atrium, reaching all the way to the back of the chamber, before washing forward again. These are red flags of severe MR.

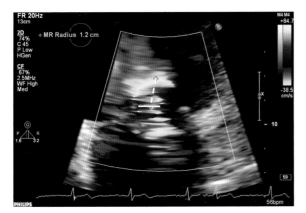

Figure 12.4 A zoomed A4C view of MR with proximal flow recruitment. The vena contracta (solid white line) of the MR jet is wide, with extensive (>1 cm) proximal flow recruitment (dashed white line). These are both markers of severe MR.

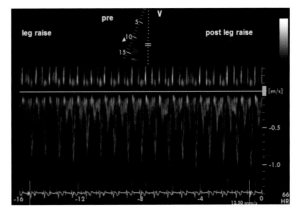

Figure 13.4 An LVOT VTI trace with low sweep speed, using PW Doppler from an A5C view. Pre-leg raise VTI measurements are shown on the left of the image, and post-leg raise measurements on the right. In this case, LVOT VTI variation was <12%, indicating that the patient was not fluid-responsive.

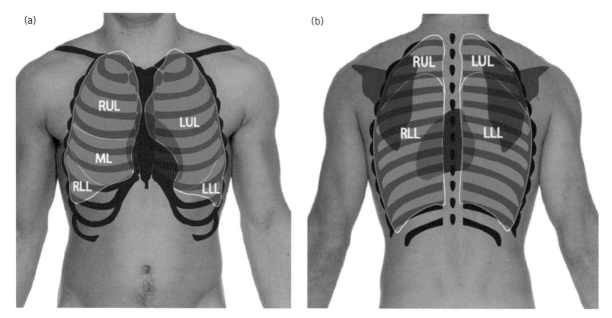

Figure 14.1 Surface anatomy of the lung.

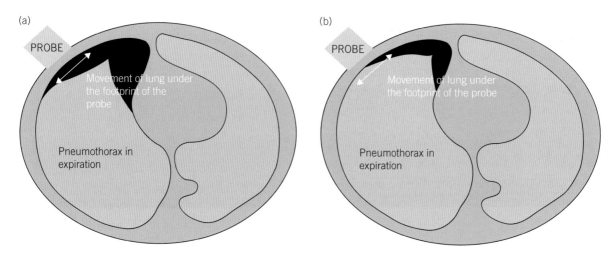

Figure 15.4 The lung point. When the probe is placed over the lung point, the aerated lung will move under the probe on inspiration and back on expiration. This can be seen as intermittent pleural sliding in 2D mode or as a transition between the seashore and stratosphere sign in M-mode.

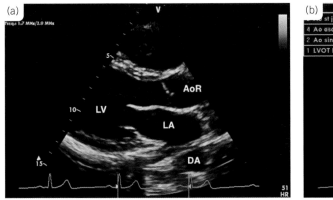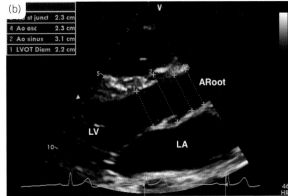

Figure 17.2 Parasternal long-axis view (PLAX). (a) See that the descending thoracic aorta (DA) sits beneath the left atrium (LA), while the left ventricular outflow tract (LVOT) and aortic root (AoR) sit above. To the left of the DA, directly beneath the insertion point of the posterior mitral valve leaflet, you can sometimes see another vessel—the coronary sinus (not clearly seen in this example). (b) Left ventricular outflow tract (1); sinuses of Valsalva (2); sinotubular junction (3); ascending aorta (4). ARoot, aortic root; LA, left atrium; LV, left ventricle.

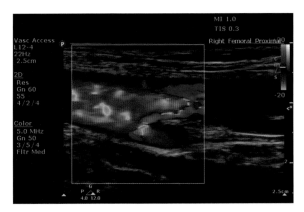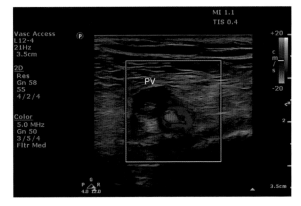

Figure 18.1 Highlighting best practices in image optimization with correct setting of the frequency, depth, focus, and gain. Colour flow Doppler imaging is used to assess blood flow towards or away from the probe. Blue is Away and Red is Towards the probe (BART).

Figure 18.12 Thrombus in the popliteal vein. There is reduced compressibility (Video 1.14.5 📷). There does not appear to be any colour flow around the thrombus. This is NOT diagnostic of an occlusive thrombus, and further tests are required to help ascertain this. PV, popliteal vein.

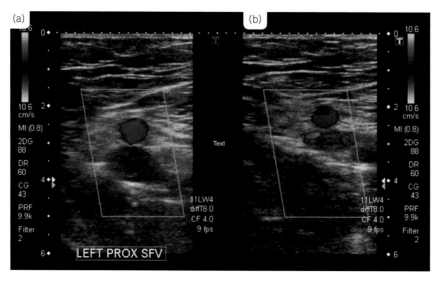

Figure 18.13 (a) Proximal superficial femoral vein (SFV) with a filling defect demonstrated with colour flow Doppler.
(b) Demonstration of reduced compressibility. Colour flow can also be seen around the edges of the thrombus, indicative of a non-occlusive thrombus.

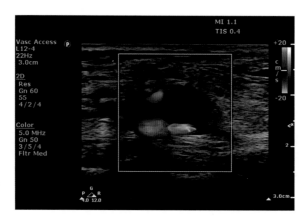

Figure 18.14 Squeeze of the distal limb will increase flow through the venous structure. In this example, there is a filling defect, with flow augmentation after squeezing. If no thrombosis were present, the whole of the vessel would show augmented flow.

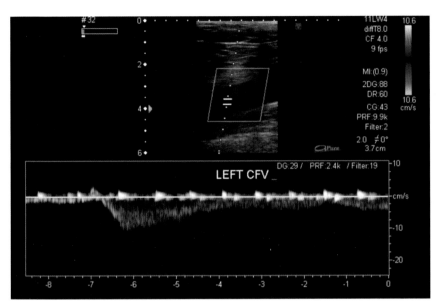

Figure 18.15 Pulsed wave Doppler focused on the femoral vein is used to show clear augmentation of flow on deep inspiration, suggesting that there is communication of flow between the thorax and this femoral vessel.

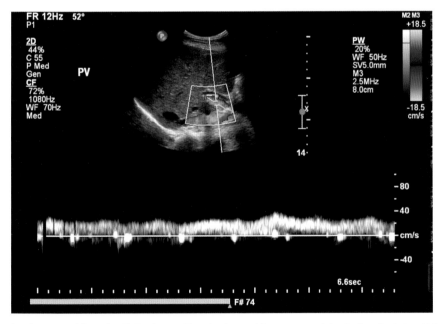

Figure 19.3 Portal vein spectral Doppler. Pulsed wave Doppler is used to assess portal vein flow that should be a continuous forward flow of low velocity (20–25 cm/s) with some respiratory variation.

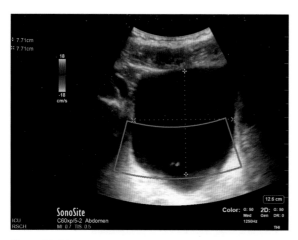

Figure 19.10 Bladder in the transverse section showing measurements and a ureteric jet (colour and black and white).

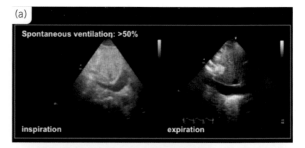

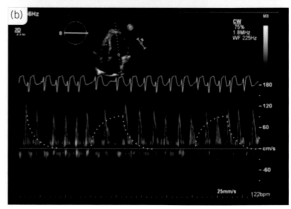

Figure 25.1 Echo parameters used to demonstrate potential responsiveness to volume loading in (a) spontaneous breathing and (b) positive pressure ventilation. (a) During inspiration, the IVC (subcostal view) collapses. Where this exceeds 50%, it may indicate that the patient will respond to volume loading by increasing cardiac output. (b) Trans-mitral PW Doppler (A4C view) in a patient with hypovolaemia. Note the increase in trans-mitral velocities shortly during inspiration (with a short delay for pulmonary transit time) shown in the green broken line. This is the opposite effect of that seen in spontaneous ventilation where left-sided Doppler velocities decrease with inspiration.

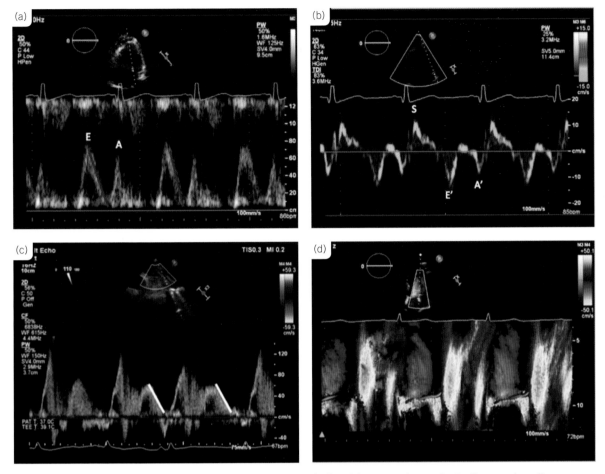

Figure 25.2 Echocardiographic modalities used for estimation of left atrial pressure in a patient with normal cardiac function. (a) Normal trans-mitral PW Doppler in a young patient, showing dominant early trans-mitral filling (E), compared with the peak late diastolic filling resulting from atrial contraction (A). The E deceleration time (red line) is normal (120–200 ms). (b) Tissue Doppler imaging of the lateral mitral annulus, showing the systolic velocity (S) and early (E′) and late (A′) annular diastolic velocities. The E′/A′ is >1 and E/E′ <8, consistent with non-elevated left atrial pressure. (c) Transoesophageal echo showing PW Doppler of the right upper pulmonary vein, with the deceleration slope of diastolic flow (solid white line) of >150 cm/s. (d) Trans-mitral M-mode colour velocity propagation time (transthoracic echo, A4C view), with the first aliasing velocity of >50 cm/s. These parameters are used in combination to support non-elevated versus elevated left atrial pressure estimation.

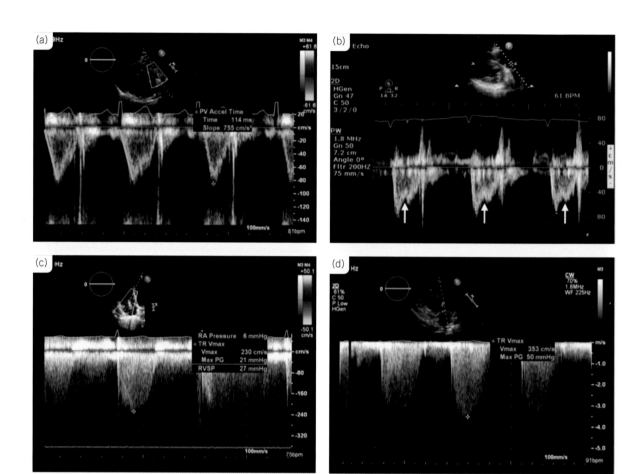

Figure 25.3 Doppler features of normal and elevated pulmonary vascular resistance and pulmonary hypertension.
(a) PAT: the time from the onset of pulmonary flow to its peak is measured using PW Doppler (solid green line). An average of at least three beats (sinus rhythm) should be taken, with care not to overestimate the peak, in particular where the gain is too high. Here, the PAT is 114 ms, indicating normal pulmonary vascular resistance. (b) PAT in a patient with significantly elevated pulmonary vascular resistance. Note the very short PAT (<80 ms, broken green lines) and the mid-systolic notch (solid white arrow). (c) PASP estimated in a patient with normal pulmonary artery pressure undergoing positive pressure ventilation, measured by using CW Doppler across the tricuspid valve (A4C view). In the miniaturized 2D image, colour Doppler is used to align the CW Doppler to the regurgitant jet. Using the echo machine software, the peak velocity between the RV and RA is measured as 21 mmHg, and with an RAP of 6 mmHg, the PASP is estimated at 27 mmHg. (d) CW Doppler across the tricuspid valve of a patient with acute pulmonary hypertension. The pressure difference between the RV and RA is estimated at 50 mmHg, and with a measured RAP of 10 mmHg, the PASP is estimated at 60 mmHg.

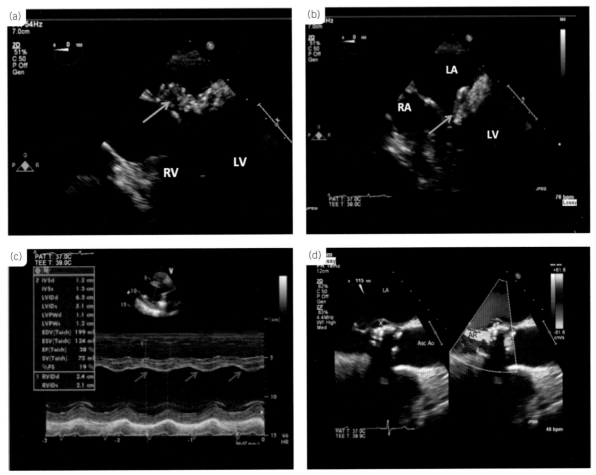

Figure 25.4 Some of the echocardiographic features of infective endocarditis. (a) and (b) TOE in a patient with mitral valve endocarditis, with a large vegetation (arrow) seen prolapsing into the LA during systole (a) and into the LV during diastole (b). (c) TTE parasternal long-axis view showing M-mode across the IVS and LV in a patient presenting with clinical features suggestive of pneumonia (bilateral pulmonary infiltrates on chest radiograph, hypoxia, elevated inflammatory markers). The patient had undergone mitral valve surgery 10 years previously. The septum shows normalization of movement (arrows), and in this clinical context, mitral valve dysfunction should be suspected and TOE performed to exclude endocarditis. (d) TOE (LVOT view, zoomed on the aortic valve) in a patient with aortic valve endocarditis and an associated root abscess (X). The valve is thickened and abnormal, and there is aortic regurgitation. Asc Ao, ascending aorta; LA, left atrium.

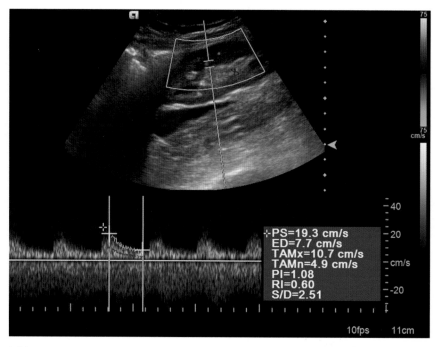

Figure 26.7 Renal RI measurement and the waveform produced.

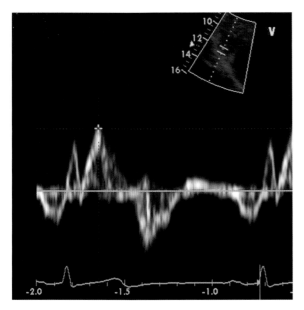

Figure 27.7 Tissue Doppler imaging of the right ventricle from an A4C view, with measurement of the peak systolic wave (RV TDI S′).

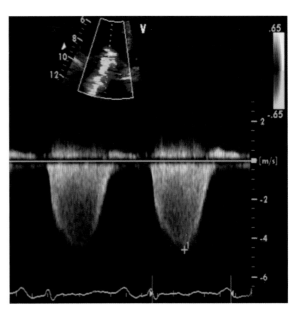

Figure 27.8 Continuous wave Doppler of tricuspid regurgitation from an A4C view, with measurement of the peak velocity.

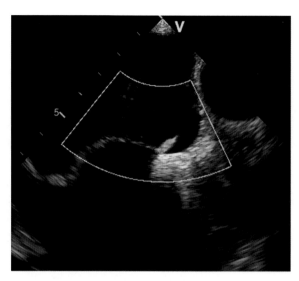

Figure 27.9 Mid-oesophageal-level TOE image focusing on the IAS. The image demonstrates right-to-left shunting across a PFO and an IAS that bows to the left, consistent with raised right atrial pressures.

16

Lung assessment

Andrew Walden

Introduction

This chapter describes the US appearances of common pathology involving the lung parenchyma. The features of consolidation and atelectasis are described and differentiated. The alveolar-interstitial syndrome is outlined, and the US characteristics that allow ARDS and cardiogenic pulmonary oedema (CPO) to be differentiated are listed. The advanced section describes the use of US to assess diaphragmatic function.

Limitations of clinical assessment of the lung

Clinical assessment of the lung parenchyma in critically ill patients is notoriously difficult. Patients are typically managed semi-recumbent and cannot be sat forward or make large inspiratory efforts to command, rendering the standard system of respiratory examination near impossible. Similarly, chest X-ray has been shown to be insensitive when trying to determine the causes of acute respiratory failure and even worse than clinical examination alone. This is problematic, given the incidence of respiratory problems in the critically ill. Undoubtedly, the reference imaging standard is CT. However, this requires the transfer of unwell patients and is associated with significant costs and morbidity and cannot be repeated too frequently due to significant exposure to ionizing radiation.

Historically, it was felt US was of no value in the assessment of lung parenchyma due to the low acoustic impedance of air. However, as the lung becomes diseased, the changes in acoustics lead to characteristic appearances. Indeed US has demonstrated excellent diagnostic accuracy in determining the causes of respiratory failure both in patients within the emergency department as well as those within ICU on mechanical ventilation. With the increasing availability of smaller and more powerful machines, LUS is becoming the primary tool in the assessment of respiratory failure in this patient group. LUS has distinct advantages over other imaging modalities in that it can be performed rapidly at the bedside and be repeated frequently without any risk of ionizing radiation exposure.

Ultrasound of the lung parenchyma

While US cannot replace CT (and, in rare cases, histology), it has high sensitivity and specificity at recognizing common causes of acute respiratory failure. These can be categorized according to their ultrasonographic appearances into alveolar conditions (lung consolidation and atelectasis) and alveolar-interstitial conditions such as ARDS, pulmonary oedema, and interstitial pneumonia (Table 16.1).

Healthy lung has high air content and very low acoustic impedance, which results in 99% of US waves being reflected, preventing any useful US imaging below the pleural line. In disease, elements of the lung parenchyma may change their fluid and air content, allowing either direct visualization of structures with high water content or the creation of characteristic artefacts such as B-lines and lung rockets due to increases in the fluid content of subpleural structures. These changes are now well described and have been validated against CT scanning, demonstrating excellent diagnostic accuracy. This can help both in

Table 16.1 Ultrasound classification of pulmonary pathology

Condition	Examples
Alveolar	Pneumonic consolidation
	Atelectasis
Alveolar-interstitial	Acute respiratory distress syndrome
	Cardiogenic pulmonary oedema
	Atypical pneumonia
Predominantly interstitial	Inflammatory pneumonia
	Lymphangitis carcinomatosis

terms of understanding the underlying diagnosis as well as identifying new problems that develop as part of the patient's stay on ICU.

Alveolar conditions

Alveolar conditions are those where the content of air within the lungs changes, such that it is possible to directly visualize parts of the lung with US. The main two clinical entities responsible for this pattern are pneumonic consolidation and atelectasis. The differentiation of these two conditions can be difficult. This section will try to explain the common findings in each condition and then will consider how best to differentiate the two conditions.

Consolidation

LUS is very useful at identifying consolidation. Ninety-eight per cent of lung consolidation abuts the pleura, and the pathological changes in the air/fluid content of the lung result in characteristic features. Where the consolidation is translobar, the lung develops a solid tissue-like pattern whereby it takes on the appearance of the liver. This is also called 'hepatization' as a pure descriptive term (Figure 16.1).

Where consolidation is not translobar, the lung develops the 'shred' sign. This is another descriptive term characterizing the loss of normal lung pattern at the pleural line. There is an irregular border of normally aerated lung and consolidated lung which has a higher fluid content. There are often comet tail artefacts emanating from the irregular border of the consolidated lung (Figure 16.2).

In both translobar and non-translobar consolidation, air/fluid bronchograms may be identified (Figure 16.3). However, these are also features that may be found in atelectatic lung. Indeed, distinguishing translobar

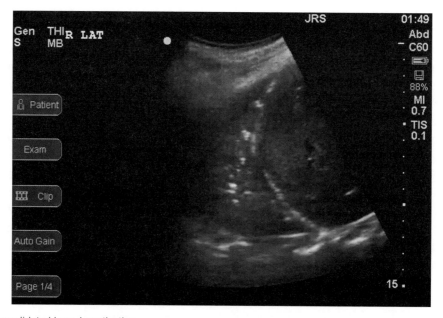

Figure 16.1 Consolidated lung: hepatization.

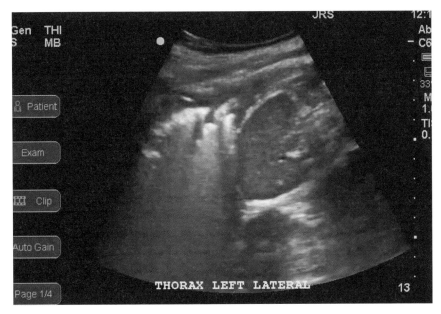

Figure 16.2 Shred sign of consolidated lung.

consolidation from atelectasis may be one of the limitations of LUS.

Atelectasis

Lung collapse in critically ill patients is often multifactorial. Patients on positive pressure ventilation can suffer from derecruitment as a consequence of inadequate doses of PEEP or following disconnection from the mechanical ventilator. In addition, inspissation of secretions can lead to airway blockage, leading to atelectasis, as can inadvertent one-lung intubation and ventilation. Another consideration in longer-term critically ill patients is the development of large-volume pleural effusions, which is common (Chapter 15).

The predominant aetiology may often lead to more characteristic patterns of lung collapse. In the situation

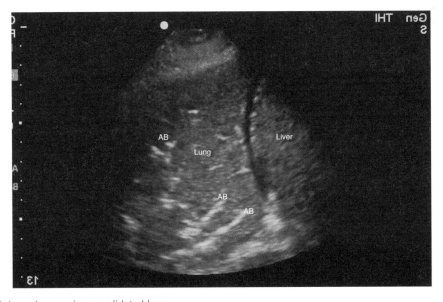

Figure 16.3 Air bronchogram in consolidated lung.

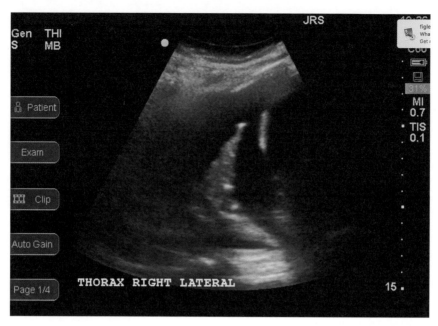

Figure 16.4 'Jellyfish sign': atelectatic lung in pleural effusion.

where pleural effusion is the main reason for collapse, the lung collapses to a point with smooth edges and becomes a sylph-like structure (Figure 16.4 and Video 1.12.1). This has previously been described as the 'jellyfish' sign.

Where collapse occurs mainly due to derecruitment or secretion retention, the lung can often take on a picture similar to consolidation with the presence of air bronchograms and a lung which becomes similar in homogeneity to the underlying liver or spleen. There can still be pleural effusion present, but often not to the same degree. The differentiation can be difficult.

A fairly unique situation occurs following endo-tracheal intubation when the endotracheal tube is in-serted in the right main bronchus. Due to the sudden lack of ventilation in the left lung, there are none of the features of volume loss or altered homogeneity described previously. However, there will be absence of pleural sliding due to a lack of ventilation, with the presence of the lung pulse to the pleural line as car-diac pulsations are transmitted through the motionless lung (Video 1.12.2).

Differentiating atelectasis from consolidation

Table 16.2 summarizes the features that distinguish consolidation from atelectasis. One pathognomonic

sign of consolidation is the dynamic air/fluid bronchogram (Video 1.12.3). In a portion of con-solidated lung when there is free movement of air and fluid, it is possible to see a shifting pattern of air and fluid moving during the respiratory cycle. In atelectatic lung which is obstructed or derecruited, this movement of air and fluid does not occur. The dynamic air bronchogram has a very high positive predictive value for consolidation, but a poor nega-tive predictive value.

In contrast, atelectatic lung will increase in size during a recruitment manoeuvre and will lose its tissular pattern as aeration increases, often taking on the appearance of normal lung, but with multiple lung rockets or B-lines.

Alveolar-interstitial conditions

The alveolar-interstitial syndrome describes a group of conditions where both the alveolar tissues and the interstitium are involved and may be broadly categor-ized into those conditions that mainly affect the alveoli, such as ARDS or CPO, and those that predominantly affect the interstitium such as interstitial pneumonia or lymphangitis carcinomatosis. The common US finding that links all these conditions is the presence of B-lines (Figure 16.5).

Table 16.2 Ultrasound features of consolidation and atelectasis

	Consolidation	Atelectasis
Tissular pattern	Yes	Yes
Shred sign	Yes	No
Air bronchograms	Yes	Yes
Fluid bronchograms	Yes	Rare
Dynamic bronchograms	Yes	No
Pleural sliding	Diminished	Greatly diminished
Lung pulse	Present but diminished	With absent pleural sliding highly likely
Pleural effusion	Evidence of septation	Free-flowing effusion
Other—dynamic effect of recruitment	Little change with recruitment	Increased size and aeration with recruitment

The mechanism of B-line artefacts is key to understanding the pathophysiology of alveolar-interstitial conditions. The usual US pattern of the lung in health is regularly spaced A-lines, a normal reverberation artefact (Figure 16.6). When the US beam reaches the normal pleura/air interface, the marked change in acoustic impedance results in most of the US waves being reflected to the probe, which is processed to show the presence of the pleural line. However, some of the returning beam is reflected back from the probe to the pleural line where the same change in acoustic impedance leads to further reflection back to the probe, resulting in the generation of a second deeper, but artefactual, pleural line. This process of reverberation between the US probe and the pleural line may be repeated a number of times, resulting in the generation of multiple regularly spaced A-lines (Figure 16.7).

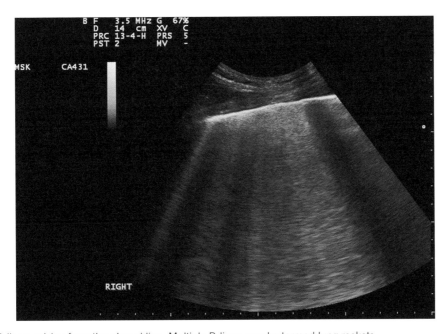

Figure 16.5 B-lines: arising from the pleural line. Multiple B-lines may be termed lung rockets.

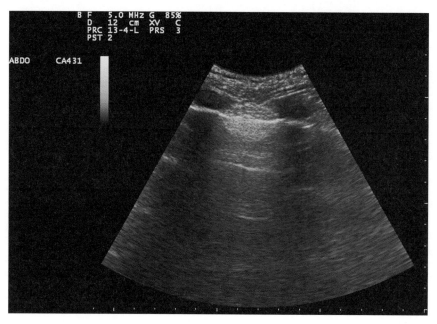

Figure 16.6 A-lines: repeating horizontal lines that are the same distance apart and are reverberations of the pleural line.

In alveolar-interstitial disorders, subpleural structures become thickened and engorged. This leads to a change in the acoustic impedance of these structures, such that the US beam is repeatedly reflected within them, and each time a signal is sent back to the probe, a small line is generated. This leads to multiple small lines concertinaed on top of each other, which gives the sense of a line emanating from the pleural line to the edge of the screen (Figure 16.7).

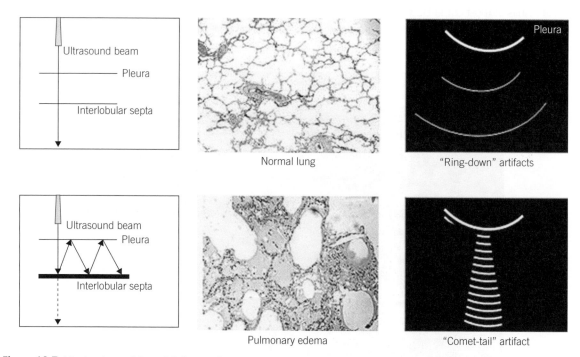

Figure 16.7 Mechanisms of A- and B-line artefacts.

Reprinted from *The American Journal of Cardiology*, **93**, 10, Jamrik *et al.*, 'Usefulness of ultrasound lung comets as a non radiological sign of extravascular lung water', pp. 1265–1270. Figure 7. Copyright © 2004 Excerpta Medica Inc. All rights reserved., with permission from Elsevier.

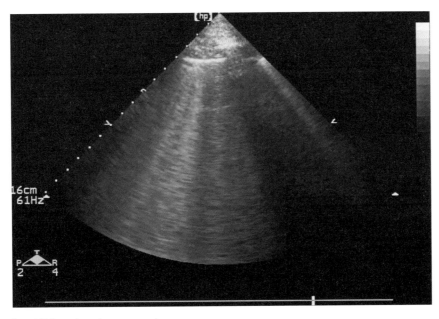

Figure 16.8 Confluent B-lines in pulmonary oedema.

The distance between each B-line may represent the underlying pathophysiology. Ultrastructurally, subpleural lymphatics are much more closely aligned, such that conditions that tend to cause predominantly lymphatic engorgement, such as pulmonary oedema, lead to a spacing much closer together than in conditions such as pulmonary fibrosis which predominantly affects the septa. Indeed case series have shown that where the spacing of B-lines is <3 mm, the aetiology is likely to be due to high levels of extravascular lung water, such as ARDS or pulmonary oedema (Figure 16.8 and Video 1.12.4 ⬤), whereas a spacing of >7 mm would favour pulmonary fibrosis or an inflammatory pneumonia (Figure 16.9 and Video 1.12.5 ⬤).

B-lines are frequently observed in ICU patients, usually as a consequence of pulmonary oedema, with the

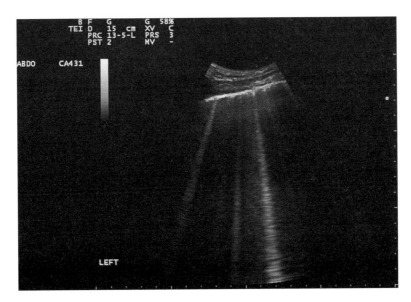

Figure 16.9 Interstitial pattern B-lines.

Table 16.3 Ultrasound features of acute respiratory distress syndrome (ARDS) and cardiogenic pulmonary oedema (CPO)

	ARDS	CPO
Bilateral B-lines	Yes	Yes
Homogenous B-lines	No	Yes
Subpleural irregularities	Yes	No
Reduced B-line in response to diuresis	No	Yes
Higher density posteriorly	Variable	Always
Pleural sliding	Diminished	Greatly diminished
Lung pulse	Present but diminished	With absent pleural sliding highly likely
Pleural effusion	Evidence of septation	Free-flowing effusion
Other—dynamic effect of recruitment	Little change with recruitment	Increased size and aeration with recruitment

number seen in each rib space examined correlating with measurements of extravascular lung water. US assessment has been shown to be more sensitive than chest radiography in identifying pulmonary oedema. Furthermore, B-lines will appear and disappear in a time frame that closely matches the course of pulmonary oedema and can be used to monitor therapy. It has been proposed that LUS can be used to monitor fluid resuscitation, with the appearance of B-lines during resuscitation as a sign of adequate fluid filling.

Not all B-lines are pathological. A few B-lines may be visible in the dependent regions of normal lungs, while B-lines in the non-dependent anterior regions are nearly always significant.

Differentiating acute respiratory distress syndrome from cardiogenic pulmonary oedema

ARDS and CPO are two of the more common conditions encountered in critically ill patients. They are both characterized by generalized increases in extravascular lung water. Both therefore lead to bilateral B-line patterns on US examination. Table 16.3 summarizes the differences that may help to distinguish ARDS and CPO.

Advanced ultrasonography

Ultrasound assessment of diaphragmatic function

The diaphragm is the most important muscle for respiration, and its function can be impaired during critical illness. Trauma, post-operative damage, specific neuromuscular conditions, and atrophy from prolonged periods of misuse can all impair diaphragmatic function and result in prolonged weaning from mechanical ventilation and increased ICU length of stay. Fluoroscopy, CT scanning, MRI, transdiaphragmatic pressure measurements, and electromyography (EMG) have all been used to determine diaphragmatic function. However, in the critically ill population, these are either impractical or unnecessarily invasive. There is accumulating evidence that US of the diaphragm provides both a good assessment of function but also may help to predict those patients who may struggle to breathe spontaneously. This information may help to guide weaning strategies and the decisions on tracheostomy tube placement.

Standard scanning technique and measurements

There are two main views of the diaphragm that are used. Using a curvilinear 3.5–5 MHz probe placed cranio-caudally in the subcostal area in the mid-clavicular line, with the probe angled 30–45°, allows visualization of the diaphragm, using the liver as a window (Figure 16.10a and b). With 2D mode, it is possible to look at the overall function and movement of the hemidiaphragm. However, more accurate and reproducible information can be gleaned by placing an

M-mode line through the diaphragm (Figure 16.10c). It is essential that the line of M-mode is kept perpendicular to the line of the diaphragm, either by adjusting the probe position or, where this is not possible, by using compass M-mode. It is then possible to measure the excursion of the diaphragm during quiet breathing and following a deep inspiration (Figure 16.11). The following parameters can be measured to assess diaphragmatic function: the peak excursion distance *a* in centimetres, the time to peak excursion *b* in seconds, and the velocity of diaphragm movement (*a*/*b*) in centimetres per second.

The second point of measurement is the zone of apposition where the diaphragm inserts into the lower chest wall. By using a curvilinear or linear probe in the mid-axillary line between rib spaces 8 and 10, it is possible to see the three layers of the muscular portion of the hemidiaphragm. Using M-mode, it is possible to measure the thickness of the hemidiaphragm (tdi) as well as fractional thickening during inspiration. This is calculated by subtracting the thickness at the end of expiration from the thickness at the end of inspiration and dividing the product by the thickness at the end of expiration.

Assessment of diaphragmatic weakness or paralysis needs to be undertaken during spontaneous breathing, as there will be passive normal movement during controlled mechanical ventilation, independent of diaphragmatic function. US evaluation needs to be undertaken during a brief period of unsupported spontaneous breathing.

Diaphragmatic paralysis or weakness

There are several situations in which diaphragmatic paralysis or weakness may be present in critically ill patients. Damage to the phrenic nerve can follow thoracic trauma or can be a post-operative complication following cardiothoracic or upper gastrointestinal surgery. Trauma to the higher cervical spine can lead to bilateral diaphragmatic weakness. Medical causes include acute polyneuropathies such as Guillain–Barré syndrome, degenerative conditions such as motor neurone disease, or primary myopathic problems such as myasthenia gravis.

The hallmark of complete paralysis of a hemidiaphragm is paradoxical movement in inspiration as a result of the other respiratory muscles

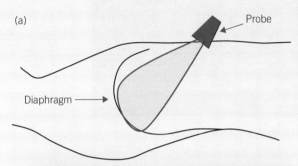

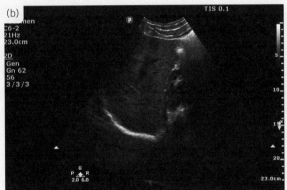

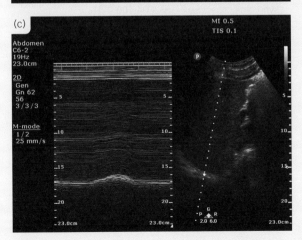

Figure 16.10 2D and M-mode assessment of diaphragm movement.

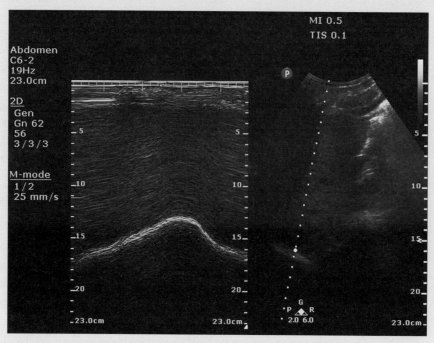

Figure 16.11 M-mode assessment of diaphragm movement during maximal inspiration.

generating a negative pressure and pulling the flaccid hemidiaphragm cephalad. This paradoxical movement is best demonstrated from M-mode in the subcostal view. Where there is weakness, rather than paralysis, the features may be more subtle. A reduction in the tdi at the zone of apposition is a feature of atrophy of the diaphragm. A thickness of <2 mm is seen in patients with motor neurone disease. However, this measurement varies with height and weight and so is not as useful as fractional thickening.

✔ Multiple choice questions

Interactive multiple choice questions to test your knowledge can be found in the Online appendix at www.oxfordmedicine.com/focusedicu. Please refer to your access card for further details.

Further reading

Lichtenstein D, Goldstein I, Mourgeon E, *et al.* Comparative diagnostic performances of auscultation, chest radiography, and lung ultrasonography in acute respiratory distress syndrome. *Anesthesiology* 2004;**100**:9–15.

Lichtenstein D, Mezière G. Relevance of lung ultrasound in the diagnosis of acute respiratory failure: the Blue Protocol. *Chest* 2008;**134**:117–25.

Matamis D, Soilemezi E, Tsagourias M, *et al.* Sonographic assessment of the diaphragm in critically ill patients. Technique and clinical applications. *Intensive Care Medicine* 2013;**39**:801–10.

Mayo PH, Doelken P. Pleural ultrasonography. *Clinics in Chest Medicine* 2006;**27**:215–27.

17

Aortic assessment

Thomas Clark and Peter Macnaughton

Introduction

Assessment of the thoracic and abdominal aorta is an advanced skill that includes TTE, TOE, abdominal US, CT scanning, and MRI. However, the critical care sonographer may identify important pathology simply using focused TTE and basic abdominal US. This chapter outlines the approach to imaging the aorta and the common pathology that may be identified. It must be noted that imaging of the aorta, even at its most basic, is an advanced-level skill and referral for evaluation by an expert sonographer will be required should aortic disease be suspected or require absolute exclusion.

Benefits of ultrasound

Focused TTE provides a rapid 'rule-in' method of diagnosing a number of acute aortic pathologies that can be responsible for acute haemodynamic collapse. It is therefore a good investigation to deploy when faced with the shocked patient—it may provide rapid diagnosis and help outcome. The accuracy of this test is user-dependent, and any concern (either from clinical features or focused TTE findings) requires further investigation. The most appropriate modality will be determined by the clinical situation and available services. These include a diagnostic TTE, TOE, CT, or MRI. It is worth remembering that TTE predominantly provides views of the aortic root and limited views of the aortic arch. TOE can give definitive views of the proximal ascending aorta (PAA), the arch, and the descending aorta. Unfortunately, parts of the aortic arch remain hidden from TOE due to its proximity to the trachea.

An understanding of aortic sonographic anatomy is important when completing a basic focused TTE examination. The descending aorta provides an important landmark to allow the differentiation between a pleural and a pericardial effusion. Abnormalities of the PAA are commonly associated with AV pathology, so imaging both it and the aortic arch are mandatory in patients with significant AV disease. Aortic examination therefore complements AV examination.

Aortic dissection may cause acute AR, acute pericardial effusion, and coronary artery regional wall abnormalities and must be considered in all patients with acute haemodynamic compromise associated with these echocardiographic abnormalities.

A ruptured abdominal aortic aneurysm is an important cause of shock with high mortality that needs to be diagnosed promptly to improve outcome. Basic abdominal US examination can provide a rapid and sensitive test to identify the presence of an abdominal aortic aneurysm. Confirming rupture using US is much more challenging, such that US is largely used to rule out a ruptured aneurysm; if the aorta is normal in dimension, rupture is unlikely. US images of the aorta may be obscured by bowel gas, so that CT and MRI are the best and most accurate imaging modalities to fully evaluate the abdominal aorta (as for the thoracic aorta).

Pitfall

Focused TTE assessment of the aorta may 'rule in' certain aortic pathology but cannot exclude a diagnosis if clinical suspicion remains.

Focused abdominal assessment of the aorta may 'rule out' an aneurysm but cannot be used to confirm rupture.

Section 1: thoracic aorta

Anatomy of thoracic aorta

The thoracic aorta itself can be divided into a number of segments: aortic root, Asc Ao, aortic arch, and descending aorta (Figure 17.1 and Table 17.1). All must be seen to exclude pathology. The PAA comprises: (1) the AV annulus (where the hinge points of the AV cusps meet the wall), (2) the aortic root (that includes the sinuses of Valsalva where the coronary arteries arise), (3) the STj, and (4) the ascending tubular aorta.

Sonoanatomy: focused echocardiographic assessment

The thoracic aorta cannot be seen in its entirety from any one single view. You must be satisfied in imaging different sections of the aorta, using a range of approaches. TTE can provide good views of the aortic root, PAA, and aortic arch.

Parasternal long-axis view (PLAX)

In this view, you may see both the long axis of the PAA and a cross-sectional view of the descending aorta (Figure 17.2a and b). The PAA is very accessible to imaging, as it lies close to your probe and perpendicular to the US beam. This provides good 'axial resolution', meaning a clear image for accurate measurement.

The PLAX view provides the best image of the aorta for focused assessment. Take time to optimize your picture; adjust the depth and gain and your focus point. Two views may need to be captured—the first of the AV and aortic root, and the second of the Asc Ao (this often requires the probe to be tilted towards the head or by sliding up one space). This one view may

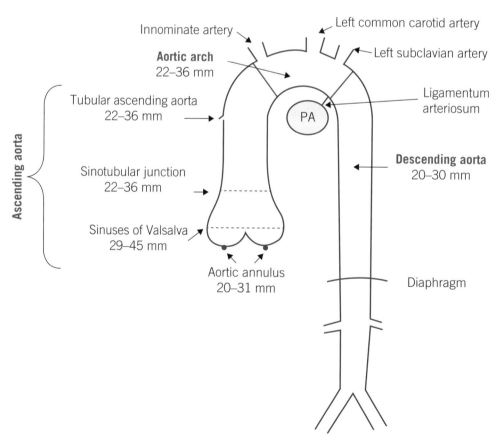

Figure 17.1 Nomenclature and dimensions of the thoracic aorta.

Adapted from Feigenbaum H, Armstrong WF, Ryan T, eds. *Feigenbaum's Echocardiography.* 6th ed. Philadelphia, PA: Lippincott Williams & Wilkins; 2005.

Table 17.1 Aortic nomenclature

Proximal ascending aorta	Aortic annulus, aortic root, sinotubular junction, and tubular proximal ascending aorta
Aortic root	Sinuses of Valsalva—widest section of the ascending aorta and origin of the coronary arteries
Aortic annulus	Point of the aorta where the coronary cusps hinge
Sinotubular junction	Narrowing where the aortic root joins the tubular ascending aorta
Left ventricular outflow tract	Exit tunnel of the left ventricle, sits in continuation with the aortic annulus and aorta

identify the following major pathologies: severe root dilatation, aortic dissection, severe AS, and severe AR.

The AV appears as two cusps opening and closing during the cardiac cycle. You will only see two of the three AV cusps, and these can be difficult to name. They are usually the right coronary cusp (uppermost, next to the RVOT at the top of your sector) and either the left coronary cusp or the non-coronary cusp (just above the LA). This view is very important in looking for abnormalities of the AV itself that can be related to aortic pathology.

The sinuses of Valsalva appear as outpouchings just distal to the AV and are where the coronary arteries originate. They comprise the aortic root and are the widest section of the PAA. Type A aortic dissections of the aortic root may involve the coronary arteries at this point. The STj is a slight narrowing after the root where the tubular Asc Ao connects. This detail may be lost with aortic dilatation. When imaging the root, it is important to get a view that is not foreshortened, especially when making measurements—the AV cusps should coapt in the centre of the root, with the sinuses of Valsalva correctly orientated on either side.

The PLAX view also provides a cross-sectional image of the descending aorta. This vessel sits behind the LA in the atrioventricular groove and OUTSIDE the pericardium. Identification of the aorta in this position is key, as it allows a pleural effusion (which sits posterior to the aorta) to be differentiated from a pericardial effusion (which will sit anterior to this vessel).

Parasternal short-axis view (PSAX)

The PSAX view provides a short-axis image of the PAA and, on occasion, the descending aorta (in long axis)

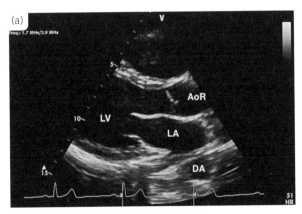 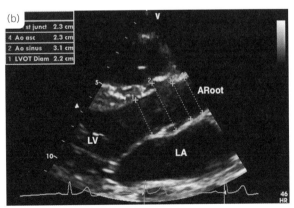

Figure 17.2 Parasternal long-axis view (PLAX). (a) See that the descending thoracic aorta (DA) sits beneath the left atrium (LA), while the left ventricular outflow tract (LVOT) and aortic root (AoR) sit above. To the left of the DA, directly beneath the insertion point of the posterior mitral valve leaflet, you can sometimes see another vessel—the coronary sinus (not clearly seen in this example). (b) Left ventricular outflow tract (1); sinuses of Valsalva (2); sinotubular junction (3); ascending aorta (4). ARoot, aortic root; LA, left atrium; LV, left ventricle. For a colour version of this figure, please see colour plate section.

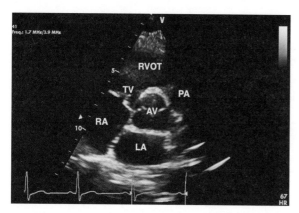

Figure 17.3 Parasternal short-axis view (PSAX) at high aortic level. AV, aortic valve; LA, left atrium; PA, pulmonary artery; RA, right atrium; RVOT, right ventricular outflow tract; TV, tricuspid valve. Tilt the probe higher to visualize the aortic root, including the coronary arteries (the left main stem exits around 2 o'clock).

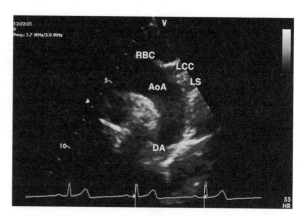

Figure 17.4 Aortic arch imaged with the suprasternal view. AoA, aortic arch; RBC, origin of the right brachiocephalic artery; DA, start of the descending aorta; LCC, left common carotid artery; LS, left subclavian artery.

(Figure 17.3). Scanning in a plane above the level of the AV cusps provides images of the sinuses of Valsalva, STj, and Asc Ao. Occasionally, the coronary vessels, usually the left, can be seen. The descending thoracic aorta is sometimes visible behind the LV (PM level) at the bottom of the image sector, although a good picture is rare.

Apical 4-chamber view (A4C)

This view gives little information on the aorta itself. By tilting 'up' from the A4C view, the AV will appear (A5C view). This view provides little information regarding the aortic root but is used to detect AR with colour Doppler (an important consequence of aortic pathology) and AS (an important cause of aortic dilatation).

In the A4C view, the descending aorta may be seen behind the LA and may appear to slightly compress the LA in this view. The aorta is too far from the probe to allow accurate measurement, but gross dilatation of the descending thoracic aorta may be appreciated.

Suprasternal (SPT)—(advanced view)

To obtain this view, place the probe into the suprasternal notch, with the marker pointed slightly towards the left ear. You then tilt to look 'down' at the aortic arch to produce your image. To get a good picture requires small modifications and a little patience. You will usually produce an image that shows the mid point of the arch onwards and includes the left CCA and left subclavian

artery root (Figure 17.4). As for the PLAX, the fact that you are perpendicular to your structure of interest gives you good 'axial resolution' and both views can show aortic dissection flaps rather well.

> **Pitfall**
>
> Only very limited sections of the descending thoracic aorta can be seen with TTE, so pathology of this segment is easily missed.

Common pathology of the thoracic aorta

Thoracic aortic dilatation

Focused TTE provides a good opportunity to diagnose aortic root dilatation from widening of the aortic structure and may identify dilatation in other areas (Figure 17.5). However, more advanced imaging is required to fully assess the Asc Ao, aortic arch, and descending thoracic aorta.

Thoracic aneurysms make up around one-third of all aortic aneurysms, and their incidence is on the rise (Box 17.1). They often remain asymptomatic until very large, when they are at high risk of rupture.

The widest section of the aorta is the root. The sinuses may measure up to 3.9 cm, depending on age, height, weight, and sex. Anything over 4 cm is more likely to be enlarged, over 5 cm worryingly so. The Asc Ao and mid-descending aorta will typically be <3 cm.

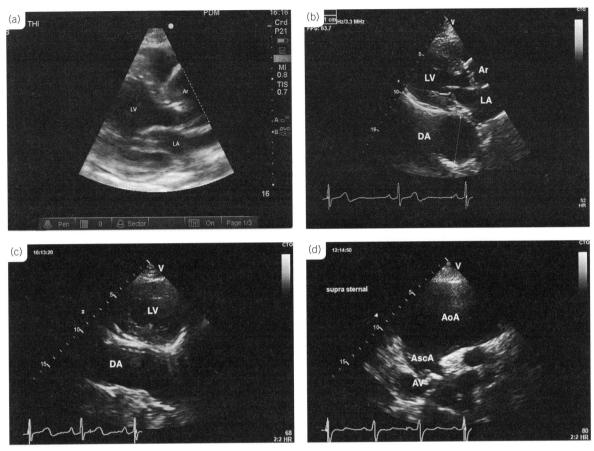

Figure 17.5 (a) Aortic root dilatation (parasternal long-axis view). Patient with mixed aortic valve disease secondary to bicuspid aortic valve. Ar, aortic root; LA, left atrium; LV, left ventricle. The aortic root is highlighted and measures >6 cm. (b) Parasternal long-axis view of a dilated thoracic aorta. The descending aorta (DA) is grossly dilated, measuring 5.1 cm. Ar, aortic root; LA, left atrium; LV, left ventricle. (c) Parasternal short-axis view of a dilated thoracic aorta. The DA is seen in long axis, sitting deep to the LV. (d) Suprasternal view of a grossly dilated aorta. AoA, aortic arch; AscA, ascending aorta; AV, aortic valve.

> **Box 17.1** Causes of thoracic aneurysm
>
> - Hypertension
> - Atherosclerotic disease
> - Aortic stenosis (post-stenotic dilatation)
> - Bicuspid aortic valve (may get dilatation without significant stenosis)
> - Connective tissue diseases (e.g. Marfan's syndrome)
> - Aortic regurgitation
> - Inflammatory diseases (e.g. arteritis)
> - Infection (e.g. syphilis)
> - Congenital (e.g. Turner's syndrome)

The most common sites for thoracic aortic aneurysms are the Asc Ao (up to the innominate artery) and the descending aorta (left subclavian artery down).

TTE measurements correlate well with CT measurements; however, any suggestion of dilatation on TTE requires further imaging with either CT or MRI. TTE measurements are always taken from 'internal edge to internal edge' and perpendicular to direction of blood flow.

Complications of a large aneurysm include leakage, rupture, dissection, and AR (acute and chronic). The most important determinant of rupture risk is aneurysm size (Box 17.2).

Box 17.2 How to measure the aortic root size

- Get a good view of the aortic root using PLAX.
- Optimize your picture—focus point, gain, and depth.
- Reduce the depth, so the aortic root fills the picture.
- Freeze and scroll, so that you have a picture captured in systole when the aorta is at its maximum diameter and seen most clearly.
- Measure internal edge to internal edge in each of the four positions (perpendicular to the direction of blood flow)—aortic valve annulus, sinuses of Valsalva, sinotubular junction, and ascending aorta.

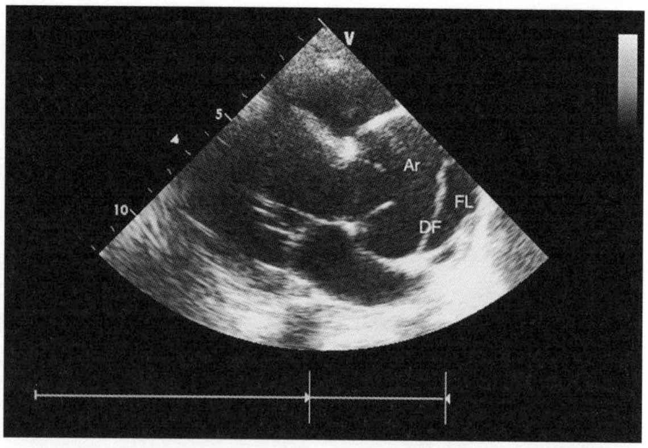

Figure 17.6 Thoracic aortic dissection (PLAX view). Very poor left ventricular function (Video 1.14.1), indicating coronary artery involvement. Ar, aortic root; FL, false lumen; DF, dissection flap.

Aortic dissection

Dissection involving the Asc Ao (type A) is a surgical emergency. The best imaging modality depends on the clinical circumstance and local capabilities. The most common modalities used are CT and TOE. However, type A aortic dissection may be identified on TTE, although views are limited and dissection can be missed easily. A dissection limited to the descending aorta (type B) is much less likely to be visualized by TTE. TTE cannot be used to investigate the extent of any dissection, although it is useful to identify the cardiac complications of a dissection, which, if seen in a patient with shock, then must be considered (Box 17.3).

The diagnostic features of aortic dissection are a dissection or an intimal flap and evidence of a false lumen (Figure 17.6 and Video 1.13.1). In focused TTE, a dissection flap MAY be seen in the PLAX or aortic arch views. TOE is usually required to identify a dissection flap (Video 1.13.2). A flap appears as a chaotic, undulating structure moving independently from surrounding structures. The flap will separate the true from the false lumen. The false lumen may exhibit sluggish blood flow that can appear grey/white, rather than black. and may also appear to 'swirl'. Colour Doppler may be used to identify the false lumen.

You must take care that you do not diagnose an artefact as a dissection flap. Because the aorta is perpendicular to the echo probe in the PLAX and suprasternal views, and because the aortic wall can behave as a 'strong reflector', then linear artefact lines can be seen in the aortic lumen. These lines mirror the shape of the aortic wall and move with their surrounding structures, not in the chaotic manner of a dissection flap.

You must always consider acute aortic dissection in all patients who present with acute AR or a pericardial tamponade (Figure 17.7 and Video 1.13.3).

Box 17.3 Cardiac complications of aortic dissection

- Thrombus in the aorta/a false lumen
- Acute aortic valve regurgitation
- Coronary artery involvement illustrated by regional wall abnormalities
- Pericardial effusion (note fresh blood on TTE looks more 'tissue-like', rather than dark black as for 'simple' fluid)

Pitfalls in interpretation of the thoracic aorta

The thoracic aorta can only be imaged in very restricted TTE views. Any echo exam is incomplete and can miss pathology related to certain segments.

Dissection flaps can be hard to identify, even when present, and can be confused for artefact.

In acute AR, consider dissection—especially if associated with regional wall abnormalities or pericardial effusion.

When measuring aortic size, do so in views where the aorta is close to the transducer and lies perpendicular

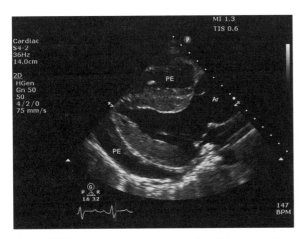

Figure 17.7 Dilated aortic root and pericardial effusion in an 18-year-old male patient with aortic dissection secondary to Marfan's disease. Aortic dissection flap not visualized but seen on CT scan (Video 1.13.3 ◉). Ar, aortic root; PE, pericardial effusion.

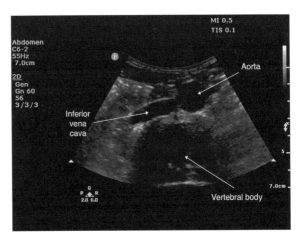

Figure 17.8 2D transverse image of the abdominal aorta and inferior vena cava. Note the vertebral body is an immediate size comparator, and the inferior vena cava is flatter than the circular aorta. There is a branch vessel coming off laterally from the aorta.

to it. Measure from inner edge to inner edge after optimizing your image. Be careful in cases where the aorta is calcified (walls appear thickened and bright)—identifying the true wall inner edge in this instance can be difficult.

Section 2: Abdominal aorta

Normal anatomy

The abdominal aorta begins at the level of the diaphragm (T12) and terminates when it divides into the iliac vessels at the level of the fourth lumbar vertebra. It lies anterior to the vertebral body to the left of the IVC, which runs parallel. It gives rise to three anterior branches that supply the gut and related viscera: the coeliac (T12), superior mesenteric (L1), and inferior mesenteric arteries (L3). The renal arteries arise at L2.

Probe selection and scanning technique

The abdominal aorta is best scanned using the curvilinear probe, although in thin patients, satisfactory images will be obtained with the phased array probe.

The probe is placed immediately below the xiphisternum in the transverse plane (90° to the aorta), with the marker facing the patient's right. The aorta lies on top of the vertebral body, with the IVC adjacent

on the right side (Figure 17.8). The entire length of the abdominal aorta is visualized by sliding the transducer distally towards the umbilicus until the aortic bifurcation is identified. Once a transverse image has been obtained, the probe can be rotated 90° to obtain a longitudinal view (Figure 17.9). Sliding the probe slowly to the right-hand side of the patient will lose the aortic view and bring the IVC into view. The IVC may be mistaken for the aorta by the novice and the US appearances which differentiate these vessels are summarized in Box 17.4.

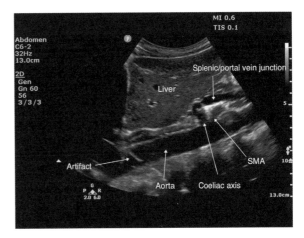

Figure 17.9 Longitudinal view of the abdominal aorta. Note the artefact crossing the anatomical boundaries. SMA, superior mesenteric artery.

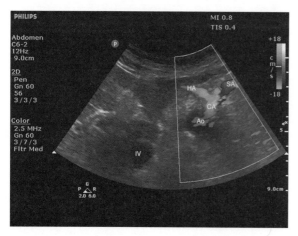

Figure 17.10 Aorta transverse view at the level of the coeliac axis highlighted with colour dopper. 'Seagull sign': division of the coeliac axis into the hepatic artery (HA) and splenic artery (SA).

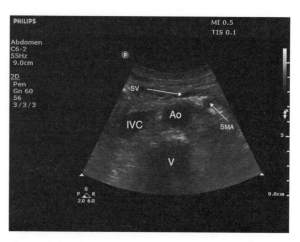

Figure 17.11 Aorta transverse view at the level of the superior mesenteric artery (SMA). The SMA and splenic vein (SV) are highlighted. Ao, aorta; IVC, inferior vena cava; V, vertebral body.

Stomach and bowel gas may obscure the view of the abdominal aorta. Typically, it is the transverse colon and the image may reappear, as the probe is moved caudad. Firm pressure may be required to displace bowel gas. Other approaches to obtaining a view include moving the probe laterally slightly or if the patient can roll onto the left-hand side, then imaging through the liver.

Normal sonoanatomy

In the transverse view, the coeliac axis will be seen to arise from the anterior wall of the aorta and divide into the hepatic and splenic arteries (Figure 17.9). The left gastric artery is not usually seen. Inferior to the origin of the coeliac axis, the superior mesenteric artery will be visualized (Figure 17.11). This is an important landmark, as it identifies the level of the renal vessels, with most abdominal aneurysms arising infra-renally. Scanning down to the umbilicus should allow the aorta to be imaged to its bifurcation into the common iliac arteries (Figure 17.12). The abdominal aorta is usually <3 cm in diameter and narrows slightly from proximal to distal. The iliac vessels are usually <1.5 cm in diameter.

It is important that any measurements are made from outer wall to outer wall and on a 90° transverse cut through the vessel. Inaccuracies can result from abnormal slicing through the vessel, resulting in elongated lumens. Longitudinal imaging can be performed as described previously, although care must be taken to stay in the centre of the vessel if any

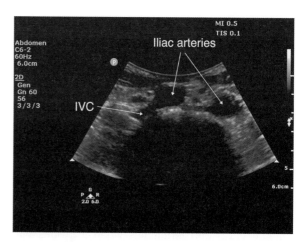

Figure 17.12 Abdominal scanning below the level of the umbilicus. The iliac arteries are apparent, with a collapsed inferior vena cava (IVC).

Box 17.4 Differentiating the abdominal aorta and inferior vena cava

- The aorta cannot be compressed with the transducer.
- The aorta has clear pulsation.
- The inferior vena cava has softer double pulsation, reflecting a central venous waveform.
- The inferior vena cava will collapse during inspiration (spontaneous breathing).

measurements are to be made, as inaccuracies can again arise from incorrect cuts through the vessel.

Abdominal aorta pathology

Abnormalities identified during abdominal aorta scanning include:

- Dilatation of the aortic or iliac vessels
- Alteration in the usual tapering of the proximal to distal aorta
- Atheroma
- Thrombus.

The normal abdominal aorta is <3 cm in diameter, and if it is >4–5 cm, then the risk of rupture is 3–12% per year, while if >5 cm, the risk increases exponentially (25–40%).

Most aneurysms arise from below the renal arteries and are fusiform in shape. More rarely, a localized or saccular aneurysm may occur.

It is essential to ensure that the measurement is made from outer wall to outer wall. Aneurysms may contain thrombus that could make the aneurysm appear smaller than it is, if the measurement only includes the lumen but excludes the thrombus. Measurements are best taken using the transverse view (Figure 17.13).

While US is a sensitive method for identifying an aortic aneurysm, it cannot reliably diagnose rupture. This is based on clinical presentation or further evaluation with CT scan. In addition to identifying evidence of a leak or rupture, CT allows greater visualization of the extent of the aneurysm and branch vessel involvement. The surgeon therefore has a greater ability to plan the required surgery.

Pitfalls in imaging the abdominal aorta

- Need to image the entire aorta to exclude an abdominal aortic aneurysm

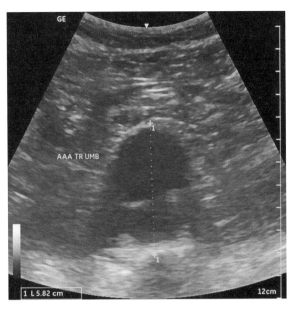

Figure 17.13 Dilated abdominal aorta with thrombus within the aneurysm. Measure outer wall to outer wall. Posterior to the aorta, the vertebral body can just be seen as a visual comparator for size.

- Spine mistaken as an abdominal aortic aneurysm
- The IVC mistaken for the aorta
- Bowel gas and obesity may make imaging the aorta challenging

✅ Multiple choice questions

Interactive multiple choice questions to test your knowledge can be found in the Online appendix at www.oxfordmedicine.com/focusedicu. Please refer to your access card for further details.

18

Vascular assessment

Colin Bigham

Introduction

US-guided vascular access requires knowledge of the anatomy and the US appearances of normal and abnormal vessels in all regions where vascular access may be undertaken. This chapter describes the optimal US technique for imaging vessels, how to differentiate arteries and veins, and the normal appearances of the jugular, axillary, femoral, and upper and lower limb vessels. The technique for undertaking a lower limb scan to assess for venous thrombosis is outlined.

Limitations of clinical assessment

Almost all patients in intensive care will require invasive vascular access such as an arterial line, a multi-lumen central line, or a peripherally placed long line. The use of US to identify vessels and guide cannulation in real time greatly improves success and reduces complications, compared to traditional landmark techniques.

Critically ill patients develop swollen limbs frequently and from a number of causes, including fluid overload, immobility, and deep venous thrombosis (DVT), which are not always easy to distinguish clinically. The ability to confirm or exclude thrombosis with US is a useful, rapid, non-invasive test that can be performed at the bedside and is relatively easy to learn.

Probe selection and image optimization

The vasculature of the limbs and junctional areas (groin, neck, axilla) are visualized using a linear high-frequency probe (6–18 MHz), which provides the best resolution but has limited ability to visualize deeper structures, with a maximal working depth of about 6 cm. A mid-frequency (5–8 MHz) curvilinear probe may be required when assessing lower limb vessels in obese patients.

Place the object of interest in the centre of the screen, at one-half to two-thirds of the depth of the US field. If adjustable, ensure that the focus is set at the depth of interest. In thinner patients, the frequency of the probe can be set at maximum (or R for Resolution) to improve image quality. In obese patients, a lower frequency will need to be used (or P for Penetrating) to allow greater tissue penetration, at the expense of resolution. The gain should be adjusted to optimize the image appearance for your needs.

Figure 18.1 highlights many of the best practices in image optimization. Colour flow Doppler imaging assesses the movement of high-velocity structures towards or away from the probe. The direction of flow is defined by the acronym 'BART': Blue is Away from the probe, Red is Towards. In this setting, the Nyquist limit is 20 cm/s, indicating when aliasing of the colour will occur (as seen in the regions of femoral artery flow).

Differentiating arteries and veins using ultrasound

Arteries are pulsatile and relatively non-compressible. If there is any doubt, then colour flow Doppler can be used to demonstrate pulsatile flow, or spectral Doppler to reveal the characteristic pulsatile arterial velocity profile.

Veins are easily compressed by applying gentle pressure with the probe. Colour flow Doppler or spectral Doppler will reveal phasic flow that varies with the respiratory cycle.

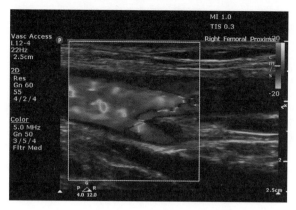

Figure 18.1 Highlighting best practices in image optimization with correct setting of the frequency, depth, focus, and gain. Colour flow Doppler imaging is used to assess blood flow towards or away from the probe. Blue is Away and Red is Towards the probe (BART). For a colour version of this figure, please see colour plate section.

Sonoanatomy

Internal jugular vein

The internal jugular veins (IJVs) lie lateral to the trachea, thyroid, and larynx. Depending on individual variation and position of scanning in the neck, the IJV can lie medial, deep, or lateral to the sternocleidomastoid muscle. The carotid artery is most commonly medial and deep to the IJV, although variations are not unusual. Figure 18.2 shows the frequency of different anatomical relationships between the carotid artery and jugular vein. Lying posterior and lateral to the

vessels are the roots and cords of the brachial plexus. The thoracic duct joins at the junction between the left internal jugular and subclavian veins (SCVs).

Figure 18.3 demonstrates the right IJV and its immediate anatomical relations on US in the transverse plane.

Subclavian/axillary vessels

The axillary artery and vein become the subclavian artery and vein, respectively, at the inferior border of the clavicle. Therefore, technically, infraclavicular US scanning visualizes the proximal axillary veins. This approach is useful for vascular access and detecting venous (and arterial) thrombosis.

With the probe angled at 90° to the vessels (with the probe pointing towards the acromioclavicular joint), the artery and vein can be seen in close proximity (Figure 18.4). The vessels also lie very close to the pleura, especially in thin people. The traditional landmark technique for cannulating the SCV is difficult to undertake using US guidance, as the clavicle creates an acoustic shadow, and an axillary approach is usually required.

Upper arm vessels

The venous system of the upper arm is divided into the deep and superficial veins. The deep brachial veins lie around the brachial artery and vary in size and number but coalesce to form the axillary vein (Figure 18.5). The main superficial veins are the basilic and cephalic veins, which extend medially and laterally down the proximal arm, respectively. They penetrate the deep fascia in the

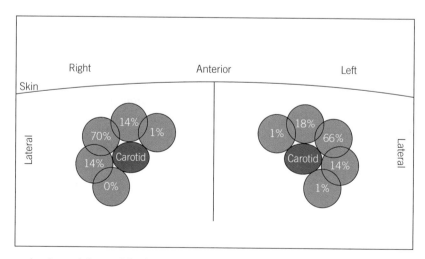

Figure 18.2 Diagram showing variation and the frequency of the different carotid artery and internal jugular vein relationships.
Courtesy of Sinoe Medical Association (reproduced with permission from: http://sinoemedicalassociation.org/usmle2/anatomyreview1.htm).

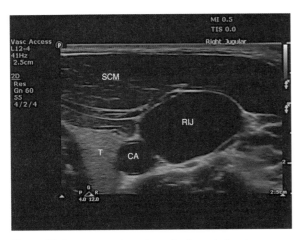

Figure 18.3 Right jugular vein and adjacent structures. CA, carotid artery; RIJ, right internal jugular vein; SCM, sternocleidomastoid muscle; T, thyroid gland.

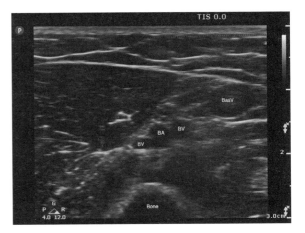

Figure 18.5 Upper arm vasculature. BA, brachial artery; BasV, basilic vein; BV, brachial vein.

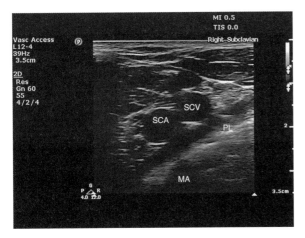

Figure 18.4 Right subclavian artery and vein, seen in short axis. These vessels can be seen to lie immediately anterior to the pleura, highlighting the risk of pneumothorax. The artery should be distinguished from the vein by its pulsatile nature and the use of colour flow and spectral Doppler. MA, mirror artefact from reflection of the subclavian artery; PL, pleural line; SCA, subclavian artery; SCV, subclavian vein.

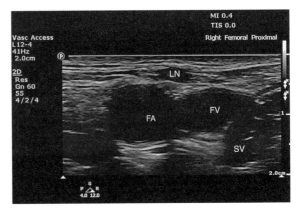

Figure 18.6 Normal femoral vessels in the groin. In single-plane 2D images, a lymph node can look very similar to a vessel or DVT (it is non-compressible). Scanning up and down to determine the spherical structure and using colour flow Doppler should identify this as a node. The saphenous vein is also visible as it enters the femoral vein. FA, femoral artery; FV, femoral vein; LN, lymph node; SV, saphenous vein.

upper arm to join the axillary vein. The basilic vein is the favoured access point for long-term peripheral line access [midlines and peripherally inserted central catheter (PICC) lines], as it follows a relatively straight course into the axillary vein that facilitates catheter advancement.

US assessment of the brachial artery may be undertaken during arterial line access or for the investigation of an acutely ischaemic arm. Arterial lines in the brachial artery should be avoided as it is an end-artery and several cases of associated limb ischaemia have been reported.

Femoral and lower limb vessels

The femoral vessels can be easily visualized by US, used either as a guide for venous or arterial cannulation or for assessing for the presence of DVT. The femoral vein lies medial to the artery, with the femoral nerve lying lateral (from medial to lateral: Vein, Artery, Nerve). At the inferior border of the iliac ligament, the femoral vessels become the external iliac vein. The saphenous vein is a superficial vein that runs along the length of the medial aspect of the leg and joins the femoral vein in the femoral triangle (Figure 18.6).

Lymph nodes reside in the groin and can be easily mistaken for a vessel or thrombosis. Scanning up and down the leg to determine the spherical nature of the structure should be enough to prevent misdiagnosis.

The superficial femoral vein can be visualized to mid thigh by tracing down from the common femoral vein (Figure 18.7). The popliteal vein is visualized, with the

probe applied to the posterior side of the knee (Figure 18.8). In a cooperative patient, this is often easy; in the critically ill, help from an assistant is usually required.

Assessment for venous thrombosis

It is important to identify venous thrombosis both to prevent an inappropriate attempt at cannulation and to

(a)

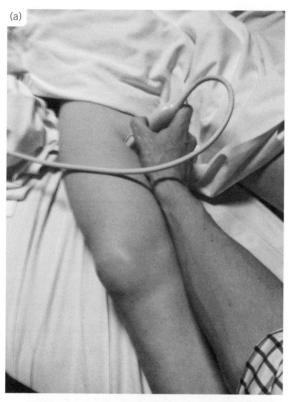

(b)

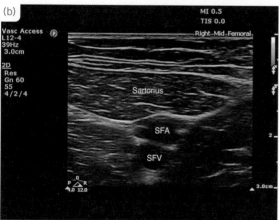

Figure 18.7 (a) Scanning position to image femoral vessels in the mid thigh. (b) Ultrasound appearances of mid-thigh femoral vessels. SFA, superficial femoral artery; SFV, superficial femoral vein.

(a)

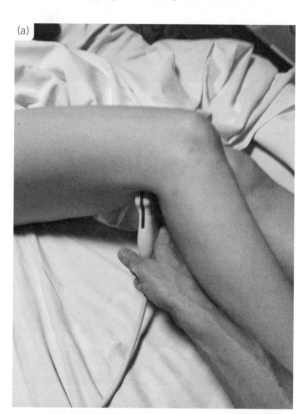

(b)

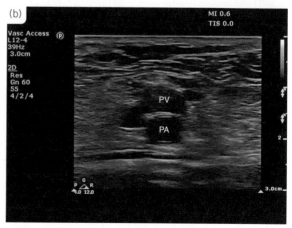

Figure 18.8 (a) Scanning position to image popliteal vessels. (b) Ultrasound appearances of popliteal vessels. The vein lies superficial to the artery in the popliteal crease. PA, popliteal artery; PV, popliteal vein.

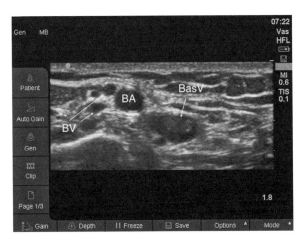

Figure 18.9 Upper arm vessels with a non-occlusive thrombus visible within the basilic vein. Use of colour flow Doppler makes the clot more obvious (Video 1.14.4 ⊙). BA, brachial artery; BasV, basilic vein; BV, brachial vein.

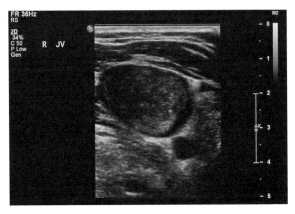

Figure 18.10 Thrombus in the internal jugular. Even on 2D imaging, this is close to occlusive.

identify when therapeutic anticoagulation is indicated. In the lower limb, popliteal, superficial femoral, and femoral vein thromboses have the potential to embolize, while below-knee thromboses have a very low risk of embolization (Videos 1.14.1 to 1.14.5 ⊙). Pelvic thrombosis cannot be detected directly on US but can be inferred from assessing venous flow patterns (see later text).

The significance of upper limb thrombosis is less clear, although the risk of embolization is significantly less than that with lower limb thrombosis, while post-thrombotic syndromes are not uncommon.

When assessing a vein for the presence of thrombus, the following approach should be followed:

1. Check for a visible clot in the lumen. A visible clot may be seen within the lumen of the vessel. This can represent a well-organized, layered clot that has been present for some days, although there are many exceptions to this supposition. An acute clot can be almost invisible on 2D scanning and go unrecognized without further assessment with compression and colour flow imaging (Figures 18.9 and 18.10).

2. Assess compressibility of the vein. If the vein is compressible, there is no thrombus preventing collapse (Video 1.14.1 ⊙). Vessels that cannot be compressed will almost inevitably have a thrombus within their lumen (Figure 18.11, and Videos 1.14.2 and 1.14.5 ⊙).

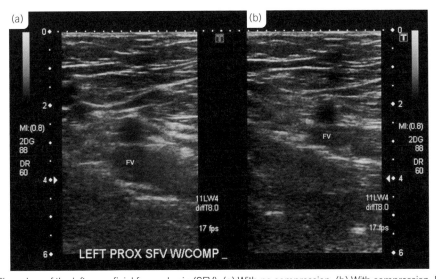

Figure 18.11 Thrombus of the left superficial femoral vein (SFV). (a) With no compression. (b) With compression. FV, femoral vein.

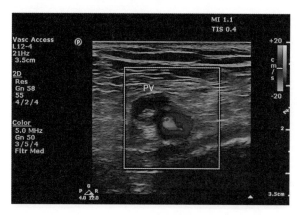

Figure 18.12 Thrombus in the popliteal vein. There is reduced compressibility (Video 1.14.5 🔘). There does not appear to be any colour flow around the thrombus. This is NOT diagnostic of an occlusive thrombus, and further tests are required to help ascertain this. PV, popliteal vein. For a colour version of this figure, please see colour plate section.

3. Apply colour flow Doppler to detect any flow around the margins of a clot. Colour flow mapping can help reaffirm no flow within the venous structures (Video 1.14.2 🔘). The flow in the blood vessels is at 90° to the transducer and so may not be detectable by the US machine. Therefore, this element of the test is best interpreted in conjunction with further compression and the squeeze tests. However, when a colour flow signal is clearly seen around a

thrombus, or there are clear areas of augmented blood flow with clear areas of no augmentation, then this suggests venous thrombus (Figures 18.12 and 18.13, and Video 1.14.3 🔘).

4. Check for augmented flow by performing a gentle distal squeeze of the affected limb, while the colour flow is still on the region of interest (Figure 18.14 and Video 1.14.3 🔘). Gentle compression of the distal part of the limb can augment the flow proximally to the region that is being scanned. This should not be too vigorous, as there is a theoretical risk of inducing an embolus. Augmentation of blood flow can rule out a thrombus if flow is visible filling the whole vein, and it can be assumed there is no occlusion between the lower limb vessels and the area being scanned. Sometimes, clear augmentation of flow can be seen around a thrombus (Video 1.14.4 🔘).

5. Check for proximal clot (in the pelvis) by assessing for respiratory variation in the femoral vein flow using PW Doppler (Figure 18.15). This is best performed in spontaneously breathing patients who can assist. Mechanical ventilation will significantly impair the reliability of this test.

By asking the patient to take a big breath in and out, increased flow in the femoral vessels can be observed if there is no thrombus or obstruction in the

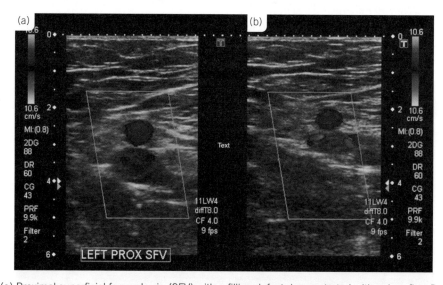

Figure 18.13 (a) Proximal superficial femoral vein (SFV) with a filling defect demonstrated with colour flow Doppler. (b) Demonstration of reduced compressibility. Colour flow can also be seen around the edges of the thrombus, indicative of a non-occlusive thrombus. For a colour version of this figure, please see colour plate section.

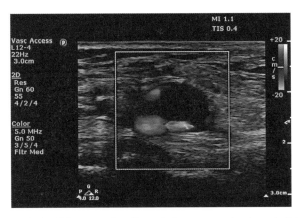

Figure 18.14 Squeeze of the distal limb will increase flow through the venous structure. In this example, there is a filling defect, with flow augmentation after squeezing. If no thrombosis were present, the whole of the vessel would show augmented flow. For a colour version of this figure, please see colour plate section.

proximal veins. This is a subtle change in flow, best observed using PW Doppler, with the sampling volume positioned in the vessel and angulated to be as in line with the vessel as possible.

Procedure for scanning the upper limb to assess for thrombosis

Start with a transverse scan at the anterolateral base of the neck, and identify the origin of the SCV where it joins the IJV. The vein should be followed laterally, looking for compressibility and the presence of non-occlusive filling defects. The axillary vein is scanned lateral to the clavicle and in the axilla, with the arm abducted and elbow flexed. In the proximal upper arm, the axillary vein divides into the brachial and basilic veins, which can be traced to the antecubital fossae, with the arm supinated. At the antecubital fossae, the brachial vein divides into the radial and ulnar veins.

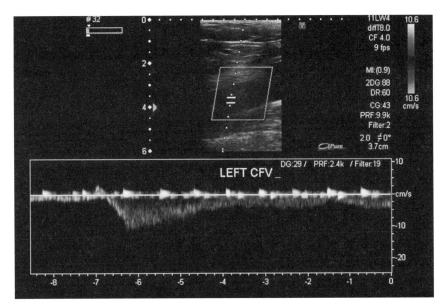

Figure 18.15 Pulsed wave Doppler focused on the femoral vein is used to show clear augmentation of flow on deep inspiration, suggesting that there is communication of flow between the thorax and this femoral vessel. For a colour version of this figure, please see colour plate section.

Procedure for scanning the lower limb to assess for thrombosis

The patient should be positioned in a 30–45° reverse Trendelenberg position to increase venous size, with the hip flexed and externally rotated to assist visualization of the deep veins of the thigh. The whole path of the femoral vein can be followed down from the groin to the popliteal vein, when assessing for a lower limb DVT. However, a number of studies have indicated that a 2-point assessment of the leg veins (at the groin and just above the popliteal fossae) has a high sensitivity and specificity for diagnosing DVT. The common femoral vein should be scanned 2 cm proximal and 2 cm distal to its junction with the saphenous vein. The distal 2 cm of the popliteal vein should be examined, together with the proximal part of its trifurcation into the anterior and posterior tibial veins and peroneal vein.

> **Pitfall**
>
> Other normal and pathological structures (e.g. lymph nodes, nerves, cysts, abscesses) can be mistaken for vessels.
>
> Obesity can significantly impair US images and reduce sensitivity of identifying thrombosis.

✅ Multiple choice questions

Interactive multiple choice questions to test your knowledge can be found in the Online appendix at www.oxfordmedicine.com/focusedicu. Please refer to your access card for further details.

19

Abdominal assessment

Justin Kirk-Bayley and James Doyle

Introduction

The role of focused abdominal scanning includes during the initial assessment of severe trauma and to guide safe drainage of ascites. Knowledge of the normal abdominal appearance is essential for the safe interpretation of focused abdominal scanning. Assessment of the sub-diaphragmatic structures is also integral to undertaking LUS. This chapter describes the technique of abdominal scanning, the ultrasonographic features of the major intra-abdominal organs, and the appearances of some common pathology.

Benefits of ultrasound

Focused abdominal US can provide a useful adjunct to the clinical assessment of critically ill patients. A variety of important clinical questions may be addressed by a directed abdominal US examination. Like all other focused assessments, simple and mostly binary questions are asked of the examination to complement and enhance clinical evaluation. The structures that may be easily identified by focused abdominal scanning are the liver, gall bladder, kidneys, spleen, and bladder. The bowel and stomach may also be visualized, depending on whether they are fluid- or gas-filled. The abdominal aorta and IVC may also be identified, to some extent, in the majority of patients.

In the context of trauma, the FAST (Focused Assessment with Sonography for Trauma) (Chapter 24) scan is used to allow rapid detection of free fluid indicating likely haemorrhage. In the ICU setting, focused abdominal scanning is much more accurate than clinical assessment for identifying the presence of, and quantifying, ascites. US-guided ascitic drainage is associated with a higher success rate and reduced complications, when compared to reliance upon clinical assessment (see Chapter 32 for details of the technique). US is the preferred method of assessment of the gall bladder and biliary tree in usual clinical practice and is used to confirm a diagnosis of acalculous cholecystitis, which is being recognized with increasing frequency in the critically ill. US examination of the renal tract is indicated in the assessment of patients with renal failure of unclear cause (Chapter 26).

Assessment of the size of the abdominal aorta allows confirmation of the presence of an aortic aneurysm, while assessment of the IVC (as the 'intra-hepatic' IVC enters the right atrium) can be used to indicate the intravascular volume status of the patient (Chapter 13).

Identifying the normal sub-diaphragmatic structures (liver, spleen, and kidneys) is also an integral and essential component of the LUS examination, while recognition and assessment of free abdominal fluid and the bladder are considered core US skills for those performing point-of-care US examination in ICU.

Probe choice

A large, curvilinear low-frequency probe is used for abdominal scanning, which typically uses a frequency range of between 2 and 7 MHz and allows scanning to depths of up to 20 cm. Although a low-frequency probe allows greater penetration into the abdominal compartment, resolution is reduced and the shallowest depth setting to obtain a view of the tissue being scanned should be used. The abdominal settings on the machine (where available) should also be used for optimal gain and dynamic range adjustment. Adjust the frequency, if required, to gain the best image.

Depth settings required depend very much on the target for acquisition and the habitus of the patient being examined. One benefit of a large probe footprint is that pressure may be applied, with reduced discomfort to the patient, especially if one seeks to displace bowel gas to improve a view.

Scanning technique and normal sonoanatomy

Liver

The liver, as a large pyramid-shaped organ, sits at the costal margin on the right side of the abdomen and is examined ultrasonographically by scanning both inter- and subcostally. Start with a subcostal transverse view, and slowly rock the probe to scan through the whole liver (Video 1.15.1 ⬤). The probe is then turned 90° and rocked from right to left in order to obtain a longitudinal view. An intercostal approach is required if views cannot be obtained subcostally. In general, focused liver US can detect the normal liver, hepatic vessels (± Doppler), portal hypertension, diffuse liver disease patterns, and focal liver masses.

The normal liver

The normal liver has a relatively homogenous texture, being darker than the spleen, but brighter than the renal cortex, and a prominent hypoechoic vasculature comprising hepatic arteries and veins. The bile duct system is also hypoechoic. The portal vein walls tend to be hyperechoic, owing to the relationship of the portal triad and connective tissue (Figure 19.1). Within the parenchyma, one can view the portal and hepatic veins, while hepatic arterioles and bile ducts are not usually visualized and, if seen, suggest abnormal dilatation. The only exception to this is around the porta hepatis (transverse fissure). It can be useful to remember that the hepatic veins are anatomical dividers (Table 19.1), while the portal veins define segments. Stored images should always contain a vessel, as this allows orientation of the findings into the eight Couinaud lobes (Figure 19.2).

If a measurement of size is taken in the mid-clavicular line from the anterior diaphragm to the lowest edge of the liver, then this should be no more than 13 cm.

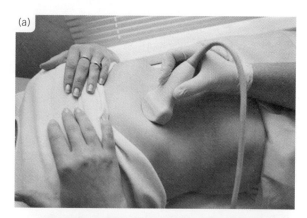

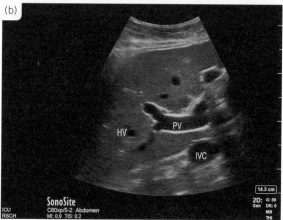

Figure 19.1 Normal transverse scan of the liver. HV, hepatic vein (branch); IVC, inferior vena cava; PV, portal vein with characteristic bright (hyperechoic) walls.

While size measurements are not of routine value, this may give a guide to gross hepatomegaly.

Hepatic vessel Doppler

The main portal vein should have a low-velocity (20–25 cm/s), continuous forward flow. An undulating pattern is seen, with increased flow on inspiration (Figure 19.3). However, a pulsatile flow is abnormal

Table 19.1 Anatomical division by hepatic veins

Vein	Division
Middle hepatic vein	Right and left lobes
Right hepatic vein	Anterior and posterior segments
Left hepatic vein	Medial and lateral segments

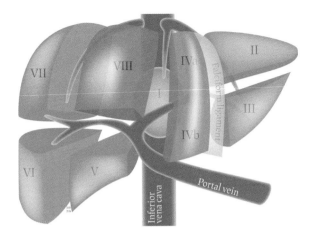

Figure 19.2 Couinaud segments of the liver. The eight segments represent independent functional units, each with a dual vascular supply and biliary and lymphatic drainage.

and may represent TR or other right heart pathology. A flattened flow is associated with hepatic fibrosis or cirrhosis.

Hepatic artery Doppler should show continuous forward flow and rapid systolic acceleration. The presence of low diastolic flow may suggest portal hypertension. Note that blood flow in the main portal vein and hepatic artery will be in the same direction, and therefore the same colour.

Portal hypertension

In addition to the Doppler signs mentioned previously, signs of portal hypertension include biphasic or reversal of flow in the portal veins, enlarged hepatic arteries, and the presence of collaterals. Look for associated ascites and splenomegaly.

Diffuse liver disease patterns

Two distinct patterns of diffuse liver disease are described: centrilobular and fatty/fibrotic. The centrilobular pattern is that of decreased echogenicity of the parenchyma and increased echogenicity and number of the hepatic vessels. Examples of diseases causing this pattern include hepatitis and right heart failure. Note this may be a normal finding in 3% of the adult population. The fatty/fibrotic pattern is that of increased echogenicity of the parenchyma, with a decreased definition of vessel walls. There may be attenuation of the posterior aspects. Examples include fatty infiltrate, cirrhosis, and acute alcoholic hepatitis. Nodularity of the liver surface may be the only sign of liver cirrhosis, with good specificity, and a loss of the clear, sharp surface of

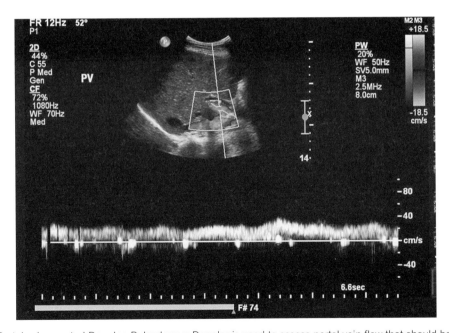

Figure 19.3 Portal vein spectral Doppler. Pulsed wave Doppler is used to assess portal vein flow that should be a continuous forward flow of low velocity (20–25 cm/s) with some respiratory variation. For a colour version of this figure, please see colour plate section.

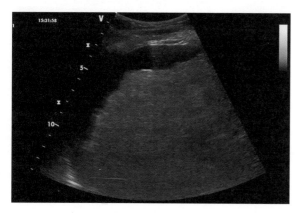

Figure 19.4 Cirrhotic liver edge.

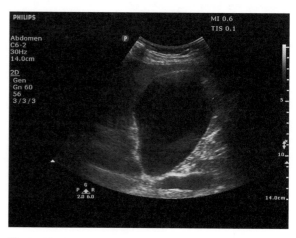

Figure 19.5 Enlarged gall bladder. The wall is normal thickness

the liver character due to the specular reflection of US that it creates (Figure 19.4). Portal hypertension is most commonly caused by cirrhosis, so this finding should prompt an assessment for it.

Focal liver masses

US is an excellent modality for detecting the presence of focal lesions, however, not in differentiating between the causes. Cysts, abscesses, old haematomas, and aneurysms may all appear similar. While not within the scope of this chapter, the use of US-guided aspiration, biopsy, and drainage is advantageous.

Other pathology

Biliary duct obstruction, gall bladder pathology (see Gall bladder, next section), and necrosis may also be seen on focused liver US.

Gall bladder

The gall bladder is best scanned with the probe aligned parasagittally in the right upper quadrant of the abdomen, with good views to be obtained when using the liver as a window. While available to be scanned in the supine position, the best views are obtained with the patient in the left lateral position. This may help eliminate overlying bowel gas, which can significantly hinder examination. Place the probe in the mid-clavicular line on an oblique line, 90° to the costal margin, angled slightly towards the right shoulder, with the marker end of the transducer on the lowest rib. Adjust the depth, so that the main portal vein is at the deepest structure. Sweep along the costal margin, looking for the gall bladder lumen. Once found, rotate

the probe to elongate the gall bladder to its longest dimension. From here, sweep through the gall bladder. Then rotate 90° and repeat the sweep. In this manner, you will view the entire gall bladder in two planes. Troubleshooting includes moving to the left lateral position, with the patient's abdominal musculature relaxed to allow the gall bladder to fall forward.

The normal gall bladder is pear-shaped, with a hypoechoic content, and has a thin (<3 mm anteriorly), clear wall. Its size varies, depending on the state of fasting and bile content, although it is considered to be enlarged when over 10 cm in length (Figure 19.5). Folds are commonly seen within the wall and are a normal finding. The gall bladder should be assessed for the presence of stones, thickness of the wall, and diameter of the common bile duct (CBD). Gall bladder US is usually considered as imaging for more experienced practitioners.

Gallstones are typically echogenic, creating acoustic shadows. They gather in the most dependent part of the gall bladder and may fill the lumen or be barely perceptible. They will move as the patient does and, if immobile, may represent stone impaction, polyps, or a mass.

Cholecystitis may be diagnosed in the presence of gallstones from the following signs: a thickened gall bladder wall (>3 mm anteriorly) (Figure 19.6), fluid around the gall bladder (a peritoneal assessment should be made to ensure that this does not represent ascites), and in an awake patient, pain on probe pressure (Murphy's sign). However, in the critically ill, acalculous cholecystitis may occur due to bile stasis.

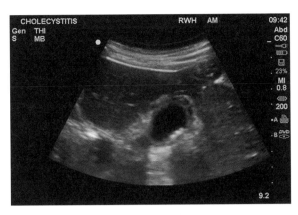

Figure 19.6 Cholecystitis with gall stones. Note the thickened gallbladder wall and echogenic stones.

Stones may be absent despite gall bladder wall thickening, although there may be 'sludge' in the distended gall bladder and the wall may be overtly oedematous and have gas within it.

Measurement of the CBD to elucidate a cause for cholestasis is highly desirable, but again, not always easy for beginners. Identifying the portal triad (containing the main portal vein, hepatic artery, and CBD) is the key to this. This is best achieved by viewing the gall bladder longitudinally, so that its neck points towards the triad. This is commonly referred to as the 'Mickey Mouse' sign (Figure 19.7). With standard probe orientation, as one looks at the screen triad, the 'ear' to the left of the screen (patient's right) is the CBD, with the other one being the hepatic artery. In this alignment, the CBD can be measured and should be <7 mm from inner wall to inner wall (there is some dilatation with

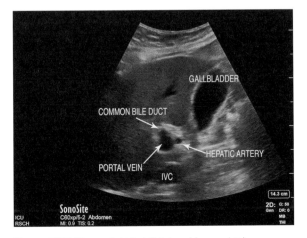

Figure 19.7 The portal triad (Mickey Mouse sign).

age, and so a diameter less than the patient's decade of life should be normal) and a measurement of over 10 mm is very likely to represent obstruction.

Kidneys

The kidneys are retroperitoneal organs, protected by the lower ribs posteriorly. As per the FAST scan (Chapter 25), the starting point for the right kidney is the mid-axillary line at the level of the eleventh to twelfth ribs in a coronal plane at an oblique lie tilted towards the retroperitoneum. This enables use of the liver as an 'acoustic window'. Additionally, the hepatorenal angle (Morrison's pouch) should be viewed for the presence of free fluid. The left kidney starting point, again as per the FAST scan, is the posterior axillary line in the intercostal space, with the probe tilted towards the retroperitoneum, so more posterior and higher compared to the right side. Importantly, inspect the splenorenal angle for free fluid. Varying degrees of inspiration may help subtly move the kidney into the best view.

The kidneys should be scanned throughout in both a longitudinal and transverse plane. In the longitudinal plane, the kidney is elliptical, measuring 9–12 cm in length and 4–5 cm in width. In the transverse view, the kidney is C-shaped. There is usually a hyperechoic area of perinephric fat, with the renal cortex appearing comparatively hypoechoic; finally, the calyces and renal pelvis are hyperechoic. The ureters are usually not well visualized unless distended, so indicating pathology. See Chapter 26 for further details of renal scanning, including examples of pathology and normal variants.

Stomach and bowel

There is some utility in visualizing the stomach and bowel with US in the acute care setting. However, as they are likely to be air-containing structures, this is inherently challenging.

The principal use of stomach scanning in the acute setting is for the determination of the presence of gastric contents and assessment of emptying. In the realms of anaesthesia and emergency care, this may be a useful tool for assessment of fasted status. Undertaking a study that will demonstrate the stomach is best initiated by scanning left and right in the sagittal plane in the epigastrium, assessing the area beneath

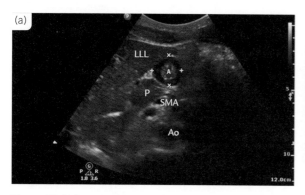
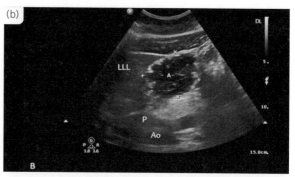

Figure 19.8 Identification of the gastric antrum a) empty stomach, b) fluid filled stomach. A, antrum; Ao, Aorta; LLL, left lobe of liver; P, pancreas; SMA, superior mesenteric artery.

the left lobe of the liver. Scanning will demonstrate the gastric antrum as a clearly defined multi-lamellated ring structure sitting between the liver and pancreas (Figure 19.8a). It is usually located relatively superficially (3–5 cm), and its relative distension (or not) reflects the total gastric volume. If there is difficulty visualizing the gastric antrum, turning the patient towards the right lateral position may aid identification. The body and fundus can be found but more often contain air, limiting its value.

With an empty stomach, the antrum is a muscular, round 'target', or slightly flattened, round structure with negligible internal content. A fluid-filled stomach will be seen as a thin-walled antrum with a hypoechoic core. Solid content will present a mixed echogenicity, and the presence of ingested air will cause acoustic shadowing, making posterior structures indistinct. Mixed solid, liquid, and air content can show as a characteristic 'starry night' content of the antrum (Figure 19.8b). Tables exist relating antral diameters to approximate gastric residual volumes.

Point-of-care US may also be useful in the diagnosis of small bowel obstruction by identifying dilated small bowel loops (Figure 19.9). Additional diagnostic accuracy is obtained by combining bowel wall thickening, increased peristalsis, and extra-luminal fluid presence.

The small bowel is imaged by passing the probe to assess the whole of the abdomen and providing gentle pressure, each few centimetres, with the probe to assess for compressibility of the bowel. Obstructed bowel will be dilated (>2.5 cm at the jejunum and >1.5 cm at

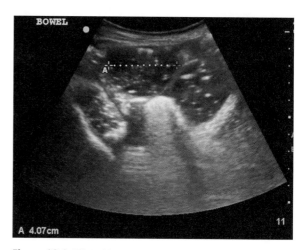

Figure 19.9 Dilated loops of the small bowel.

the ileum) and non-compressible, proximal to the obstruction. The wall of obstructed bowel may be thickened (>3 mm thick) and oedematous. The lumen size will not change with peristalsis. It may be possible to follow the obstruction to a transition point where distal bowel will be collapsed and compressible.

It is also possible to differentiate between incarcerated and strangulated bowel within hernias. The absence of peristaltic activity may suggest strangulated bowel and hence expedite management to limit the extent of bowel infarction.

Bladder

The bladder is normally a pelvic organ and, when filled with even the smallest amount of urine, becomes easy to see with US, being a thin-walled structure with a hypoechoic centre, although it may be obscured on occasion by overlying bowel gas. In critical care, the bladder volume may be assessed easily and causes for anuria sought.

The bladder may be examined in the sagittal plane with a curvilinear probe. Sweeping from side to side, you can find the maximum sagittal distance and measure it (*A*) in centimetres. Rotating the probe into a transverse orientation, the maximum bladder width (*B*) and depth (*C*) can be found (Figure 19.10). The bladder volume in millilitres approximates to $A \times B \times C \times 0.52$, which is the simplest of many formulae, none having any evidence-based superiority over another.

In both the transverse and sagittal views, imaging the bladder base, applying colour Doppler, and waiting with an immobile probe may reveal ureteric jets. Their frequency is variable and laterality random, and it may take several minutes to see one, depending on the state of hydration of the patient. However, the detection of a jet will confirm some ureteric patency for that side. Lack of detection conversely does not confirm obstruction.

Abnormalities contributing to diagnosis may be found when imaging the bladder such as large prostatic hypertrophy protruding into the bladder lumen (as a cause of obstructive uropathy) or mixed-echogenicity

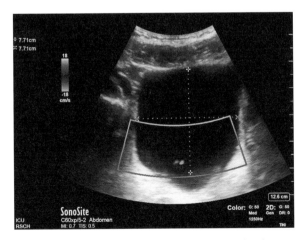

Figure 19.10 Bladder in the transverse section showing measurements and a ureteric jet (colour and black and white). For a colour version of this figure, please see colour plate section.

fluid in the bladder (suggesting pyuria in the septic patient).

The balloon of a Foley catheter should be detected easily if in the bladder. A fully decompressed bladder, with the balloon visualized within it, should be seen before absolute anuria is declared. The author has imaged a full bladder in a catheterized patient declared to be anuric in whom the balloon was not within the bladder on occasion.

Pitfalls in interpretation

Large ovarian cysts may be confused for the bladder (or indeed any source of pelvic fluid). However, the bladder is normally a symmetrically midline organ.

Renal cysts or the presence of an extrarenal pelvis can sometimes be mistaken for hydronephrosis. Also the volume-replete patient may have mild hydronephrosis with no obstruction, and vice versa, the volume-deplete patient may have no signs of hydronephrosis when, in fact, there is an obstruction.

An elongated, tongue-like projection of the right lobe of the liver may be present in approximately 15% of people (more commonly in women). This is a Riedel lobe, a normal anatomical variant, although pathology may occur in it.

When measuring the CBD in the portal triad view, remember to add colour Doppler to ensure that you are not assessing the hepatic artery.

A highly contracted, stone-containing gall bladder may sometimes generate a 'wall echo sign', creating an echogenic anterior line to the gall bladder wall and posterior acoustic shadowing. This makes the wall echo sign appear like bowel wall. When the gall bladder is not easily found, and there is good clinical suspicion for biliary colic, the wall echo sign should suspected.

Summary

Abdominal point-of-care scanning represents more advanced practice, although there is utility in simple organ identification. However, even at that level, the operator soon learns that they may identify intra-abdominal fluid collections and, with repeated tutored analyses, develop a feeling for what represents normality, such that, with time, skills may be extended to measurements and more complex diagnostics.

✓ Multiple choice questions

Interactive multiple choice questions to test your knowledge can be found in the Online appendix at www.oxfordmedicine.com/focusedicu. Please refer to your access card for further details.

Further reading

Guttman J, Stone MB, Kimberly HH, Rempell JS. Point-of-care ultrasonography for the diagnosis of small bowel obstruction in the emergency department. *Canadian Journal of Emergency Medicine* 2015;**17**:206–9.

Van de Putte P, Perlas A. Ultrasound assessment of gastric content and volume. *British Journal of Anaesthesia* 2014;**113**:12–22.

SECTION 3

Problem-based

20

Haemodynamic instability

Lewis Gray and Craig Morris

Introduction

There has been a paradigm shift in our understanding of cardiovascular physiology. Volumetric assessment (e.g. echocardiography) has moved centre stage as pressure-derived parameters, e.g. pulmonary arterial opening pressure (PAOP), have been marginalized, manifest by the decline in pulmonary artery catheterization. However, current trends risk overlooking a crucial point—volumes, pressures, and flow are all important and linked. A complete haemodynamic picture is impossible with echocardiography in isolation.

This chapter will discuss how 2D echo can be used to evaluate ventricular performance in terms of preload (volume status), systolic function (pump status), and filling pressure (pressure status). Using these parameters, it will describe an integrative approach to haemodynamic assessment that categorizes the patient into one of seven characteristic states that become immediately recognizable. This chapter will also present useful practical tips on using echo in clinical practice and avoiding its pitfalls.

Ventricular performance

The Frank–Starling relationship ensures that ventricular outputs are precisely matched on a beat-to-beat basis. Sudden changes, or extreme differences, in pressure or volume can cause abnormalities of ventricular filling, ejection, and synchrony. It is fundamental that both ventricles have identical SVs, even when pathology only affects one, or both differ significantly in size. The relationship between left ventricular fibre length and inotropic performance in the intact heart remains unvalidated and complicated by factors

such as the complexity of radial, longitudinal, and rotational contraction, and the effects of vasoactive drugs, myocardial depression (e.g. sepsis), and mechanical ventilation.

Pitfall

A dilated LV with low EF does not always indicate a low cardiac output. It may still maintain a preserved or an increased SV, particularly in the presence of tachycardia.

Diastolic function

Quantitative assessment of diastolic ventricular function is beyond the scope of 2D focused US. We expect a rapid growth in the understanding of 'diastology' in critical illness, but most current research is observational. Diastolic indices are confounded by the presence of hypovolaemia, arrhythmias, valvular disease, or ventricular hypertrophy. 2D assessment of raised left ventricular filling pressure is possible through indirect morphological measures. Increased left atrial size is a sensitive, but not specific, sign and normal size cannot exclude acute rises.

Haemodynamic assessment: pressure, volume, and flow

The term 'haemodynamic state' refers to a detailed description of the cardiovascular system with simultaneous measurement of volume, pressure, and flow; 'instability' is a disorder of one or more of these components. Consequently, while echocardiography is hugely informative, it cannot achieve this assessment alone.

Depending on the circumstances, clinical assessment, invasive pressures, cardiac output, or lactate may all be needed for the full haemodynamic picture. Many ways exist to classify 'shock', and this chapter assumes common consensus goals in managing critically ill patients.

A suggested approach to haemodynamic instability

1. Identify a clinical syndrome (e.g. an elderly man + chest pain + shock).

2. Start simple resuscitation early.

3. Refine with haemodynamic diagnosis (e.g. echo, lactate).

4. Obtain additional imaging and tests (e.g. ECG, extra-cardiac US, CT).

5. Review with definitive investigations (e.g. laparotomy or coronary angiography).

6. Instigate appropriate therapy and monitor (e.g. serial echo during fluid and vasoactive therapy).

Diagnosing the haemodynamic state

When the diagnosis is unclear (i.e. 'undifferentiated shock'), echocardiography can provide a window through which to see the cardiovascular system and identify its failing components. We believe the system developed by Royse et al. lends itself to focused assessment by integrating large amounts of information from relatively straightforward scanning. Using this scheme, echocardiography can define the presenting haemodynamic state, from which immediate management strategies and definitive management pathways can be created.

This scheme utilizes three basic parameters to determine seven haemodynamic states, six of which are associated with haemodynamic instability and can be linked to particular therapies.

Left ventricular parameters assessed are:

1. Preload—'volume status'

2. Systolic function—'pump status'

3. Filling pressure—'pressure status'.

The seven haemodynamic states are:

1. Normal

2. Vasodilatation (distributive)

3. Hypovolaemic

4. Right ventricular failure

5. Primary systolic failure

6. Primary diastolic failure

7. Combined systolic and diastolic failure.

For the purposes of focused scanning, we strongly advocate starting with short-axis (SAX) views of the ventricles, for the following reasons:

1. Simplicity in identification and measurements of structures

2. Ninety per cent of left ventricular contraction is radial

3. Ability to compare the relative size and function of the RV and LV

4. Ability to infer right ventricular pressure from interventricular septal motion

5. Ability to assess the three main coronary territories for RWMAs.

The initial management can often be guided by single SAX view alone, and a more detailed study can be undertaken while therapy is ongoing.

Assessing preload

Left ventricular preload can be assessed with echo by assuming that left ventricular end-diastolic 'size' reflects end-diastolic volume and preload. Left ventricular size may be assessed as a linear distance, such as its end-diastolic dimension [left ventricular end-diastolic diameter (LVEDD)] or area (LVEDA), accepting that neither may be reflective of the full 3D morphology. In focused scanning, we do not advocate complex volumetric measurements (e.g. Simpson's biplane method) due to the technical challenges involved. Preload should be assessed as normal, low, or high volume.

Pitfall

Be wary of purely 'eyeball' assessment of left ventricular dimensions, unless at extremes.

Assessing left ventricular systolic function

FS and/or FAC are quicker and simpler than formal volumetric assessments (e.g. EF) and can be used if no RWMAs are apparent.

The vast majority of left ventricular contraction occurs radially, with only 10% of systolic function derived from longitudinal shortening. The opposite is true for the RV, which has predominantly longitudinal contraction, and in A4C, the LV often appears 'impaired', relative to the RV. With experience, the scanner's eyes adapt to this.

Left ventricular dilatation and impairment are not uncommon in sepsis, but cardiac output may be preserved or increased due to associated tachycardia.

Pitfall

Avoid labelling patients with 'left ventricular impairment' in the early phase (minutes to hours) following cardiac arrest, DC shock, tachyarrhythmia, or myocardial ischaemia, as in these conditions, the LV is often 'stunned' and its function typically improves. Once uttered, this spreads like wildfire in handovers!

Assessing left ventricular filling pressure

In a compromised patient, left ventricular filling pressure may be difficult to assess. Estimates can be made from left atrial size, and the position and motion of the IAS. A fixed curve of the IAS from left to right correlates well with high PAOP in anaesthetized and mechanically ventilated patients. More complex techniques (e.g. pulmonary vein and MV inflow patterns) are beyond the scope of this chapter.

Pitfall

Diastolic dysfunction is complex and poorly validated in ICU patients. Generally speaking, tachycardia worsens diastolic function, a dilated LA suggests chronic disease, and LVH usually implies at least some degree of diastolic dysfunction.

A less detailed consideration of filling pressures reduces the scheme to four clinical categories (if one disregards 'normal'), capturing the most common indications for focused echocardiography (Table 20.1).

In our experience on a 'general' ICU, hypovolaemia and distributive shock form the largest groups in ICU. We treat both with early fluid challenges and serial

Table 20.1 Categories of shock and their typical haemodynamic effect on the left ventricle

Shock category	Common causes	Preload	Systolic function	Filling pressures
Hypovolaemic	Bleeding	LV low RV low	Normal/increased	Low
Cardiogenic	Acute myocardial infarction	Normal	Decreased	Normal/raised
Distributive (vasodilatation)	Anaphylaxis, sepsis, spinal cord injury	Normal/low	Normal/high	Normal/low
Obstructive	Tension pneumothorax	LV low RV high	Normal	LV low RV high
	Pulmonary embolism	LV low RV high	Normal	LV low RV high
	Cardiac tamponade	LV low RV low	Normal	LV high RV High

Table 20.2 Typical echocardiographic features of abnormal left ventricular preload, systolic function, and filling pressure

Haemodynamic indices (LV)	Assessment	Normal	Low	High
Preload	LVEDD (PLAX)	3.5–5.6 cm	<3.5 cm	>6 cm
	LVEDA (PSAX)	8–14 cm²	<8 cm²	>14 cm²
	Eyeball		Empty Kissing papillary muscles	Full—globular dilatation and stretched-looking chamber
	Right ventricular/left ventricular area	1/3 to 2/3		≥1
Systolic function	Eyeball in SAX	Brisk (contracts 1/3)	Lazy (<1/3)	Vigorous (>1/2)
	FS	25–40%	<25%	>40%
	FAC	50–65%	<50%	>65%
Filling pressure	Left atrial diameter (PLAX)	2.5–4 cm	<2.5 cm	>4 cm
	IAS movement	L ↔ R	R → L	L → R
	IVC (SV)	1.5–2.1 cm >50% collapse	<<1.5 cm >50% collapse	>2.1 cm <50% collapse
	Evidence of pulmonary oedema	No B-lines	–	Alveolar-interstitial syndrome

reassessment, and exhaustive attempts to differentiate them are rarely helpful.

TTE has a high sensitivity and specificity for detecting (or excluding) a cardiac cause for shock. The difference between systolic failure and combined (systolic and diastolic) failure is academic, as the decision is typically whether or not to start inotropes. Primary diastolic failure is a rare cause of shock, and attention should typically focus on systolic (rather than diastolic) function (Table 20.2).

Determining 'fluid responsiveness'

Volume responsiveness is a haemodynamic state whereby rapid intravenous fluid increases cardiac output by approximately 10% or more. This paradigm is increasingly challenged, and deciding between fluid administration versus increased vasoactive therapy is a common bedside dilemma.

Many monitors estimate this semi-continuously or continuously (e.g. stroke or pulse pressure variation with mechanical ventilation). US techniques used to assess volume responsiveness (e.g. Doppler) are beyond the scope of FoCUS. However, 2D associations are outlined in Table 20.3.

A more correct haemodynamic principle may be 'correct fluid at the correct time', as both hypo- and hypervolaemia are detrimental.

The best way to determine fluid responsiveness is to assess both right and left heart parameters. One point-of-care protocol assessing jugular vein variation and SVV demonstrated predictive values for fluid responsiveness exceeding 95% (Guarracino *et al.*, 2014; PMID: 25475099).

Table 20.3 Typical echocardiographic variables consistent with fluid responsiveness

Variable consistent with fluid responsiveness	Examples
Reduced left ventricular end-diastolic volume	LVEDD <3.5 cm, LVEDA <8 cm^2
Low LAP	Small LA <2.5 cm, buckling septum
Low RAP	IVC <1.5 cm, and collapsing >50% during spontaneous breathing; distensibility index >16% on IPPV
Hyperdynamic circulation	Tachycardia and increased left ventricular function
Absent markers of overload	No B-lines, dilated LV or LA, good systolic function present

Right heart, including intermittent positive pressure ventilation and spontaneous ventilation

ACP can be defined by the combination of right ventricular end-diastolic area (RVEDA)/LVEDA ratio of >0.6 and the presence of a paradoxical end-systolic ventricular septal motion.

In health, the RV operates at low pressures (mean PAP of 25 mmHg), with high flows and compliance. One feels sympathy for it, while making it work against mechanical ventilation and PEEP, causing a non-physiological state whereby intermittent positive pressure ventilation (IPPV) exerts exactly opposite effects to spontaneous ventilation.

Acute pressure and volume overload of the RV can change right ventricular dimensions, such that its contractile function and compliance are compromised. In ACP, elevated RAP inflicts back-pressure on the liver and gut, which can reopen the foramen ovale to produce right-to-left shunt in susceptible patients. Left-sided filling may also become acutely compromised by right ventricular over-distension and displaced IVS, known as 'ventricular interdependence'.

Undifferentiated hypotension and non-cardiac scanning

Undifferentiated hypotension is common in the emergency department and ICU and is independently associated with mortality. Clinicians who extend their scanning beyond the heart undoubtedly pick up more clues to the aetiology and ultimately therapeutic intervention. For instance:

- Lungs: B-lines, pneumonia, etc.
- Free fluid in the thorax, abdomen, or pelvis.
- DVT in femoral/popliteal veins.
- Abdominal aorta and vessel scanning.

Training pathways that encourage use of non-cardiac scanning are strongly encouraged, to complement echocardiography.

Additional monitoring

One counterintuitive benefit of focused echocardiography is that by not generating 'numbers' (e.g. left ventricular function is 'good', rather than 'cardiac output 7.2 L/min'), one avoids task fixation and therapeutic exclusion (when a target is pursued, regardless of its importance or associated adverse effects). 2D echocardiography's utility in predicting fluid responsiveness is somewhat limited in practice, while pulse contour or oesophageal Doppler monitors can define SVV/pulse pressure variation to within a few per cent. As emphasized previously, additional information beyond echocardiography is required to fully define the haemodynamic state. We advocate early echo assessment and ongoing monitoring of CVP and cardiac output.

Useful tips

- Use PSAX views, as they detail left ventricular size and radial contraction.

- Repeat echo before and after interventions (e.g. a fluid bolus).

- If the LV can be kept 'adequate', things are likely to improve. Do not chase the 'perfect' LV.

- Do not get too 'technical', especially in the acute setting. A vigorous LV with hypotension will probably respond to fluid loading.

- Keep in mind that echo findings may not always directly relate to the haemodynamic state (e.g. a small pericardial effusion without tamponade, when shock is actually due to hypovolaemia).

- If in doubt, refer to an expert for a second opinion.

✔ Multiple choice questions

Interactive multiple choice questions to test your knowledge can be found in the Online appendix at www.oxfordmedicine.com/focusedicu. Please refer to your access card for further details.

Further reading

Cecconi M, De Backer D, Antonelli M, *et al.* Consensus on circulatory shock and hemodynamic monitoring. Task force of the European Society of Intensive Care Medicine. *Intensive Care Medicine* 2014;**40**:1795–815.

Colebourn C, Newton J (eds). *Acute and Critical Care Echocardiography: Oxford Clinical Imaging Guides.* Oxford: Oxford University Press; 2017.

Guarracino F, Ferro B, Forfori F, Bertini P, Magliacano L, Pinsky MR. Jugular vein distensibility predicts fluid responsiveness in septic patients. *Critical Care* 2014;**18**:647.

Royse C. Assessing the basic haemodynamic state. In: Royse C, Donnan G, Royse A (eds). *Pocket Guide to Perioperative and Critical Care Echocardiography.* London: McGraw-Hill; 2006. pp. 93–109.

21

Cardiac arrest

Gajen Sunthar Kanaganayagam, Andrew Constantine, and Susanna Price

Introduction

Survival of in-hospital cardiac arrest in adults is approximately 24%, and 45% of these events occur in ICU. All resuscitation guidelines suggest that identifying and treating the underlying cause of arrest are vital. FoCUS is the only way to diagnose many of the potentially treatable causes of cardiac arrest at the bedside. When cardiovascular pathology is severe enough to cause cardiac arrest, FoCUS findings are frequently obvious, and information gained within this time can fundamentally change patient management.

FoCUS is now recommended as part of advanced life support (ALS) algorithms, provided that appropriately trained practitioners are available and that the images are acquired during the 5-s pulse/rhythm check without compromising high-quality cardiopulmonary resuscitation (CPR). Subsequently, formal echocardiography is valuable to guide ongoing management in the post-cardiac arrest setting.

This chapter will present how ALS-compliant FoCUS can help confirm the cardiac rhythm, diagnose reversible causes, and predict favourable outcomes during CPR. It will describe how to recognize severe hypovolaemia, cardiac tamponade, coronary artery thrombosis, massive PE, and tension pneumothorax, and when to intervene. It will conclude by introducing how echo can assist clinical management during post-resuscitation care.

Practicalities of FoCUS within advanced life support

Although seemingly simple, appropriate performance of FoCUS during resuscitation requires specific training and that the practitioner and team must respect the paramount importance of high-quality CPR, with regard to timing, interpretation, and communication of findings. Performing FoCUS during chest compressions is challenging, and therefore, imaging is recommended during the 5-s pulse/rhythm check. However, this imposes a strict time frame for image acquisition. Whereas some diagnoses may be readily apparent, it is likely that repeated acquisitions (and potentially different views) might be required in successive pulse/rhythm checks. Loops should be acquired prospectively and stored for review, allowing interpretation while high-quality CPR is ongoing. Echo modalities are limited to 2D (no Doppler), using qualitative estimation of cardiac function/chamber dimensions. Initially, a subcostal view is recommended, as this is the easiest, most reproducible to obtain and does not interfere with chest compressions or defibrillation pads. Where images are not achievable, the A4C and then parasternal views should be attempted. As with any imaging in the acute setting, FoCUS must be interpreted within the clinical context, taking into account resuscitative measures that have already occurred. Interpretation and communication are in line with other decision-making in ALS, with a binary rule-in/rule-out approach.

FoCUS and cardiac rhythm

In certain circumstances, FoCUS can be useful in determining the cardiac rhythm:

• Where the ECG suggests asystole, echo may demonstrate coordinated cardiac activity, thus promoting ongoing resuscitative efforts. Whether

ECG or echo is the gold standard for diagnosis of asytole in cardiac arrest remains to be determined.

- Ventricular fibrillation (VF) appears on echocardiography as diffuse, asynchronous contractile myocardial activity. Although each minute of delay to defibrillation reduces the probability of survival to hospital discharge by 10%, whether defibrillating non-ECG detectable (fine) VF is as beneficial remains unclear. Focused echocardiography has been used to identify VF in rare cases of cardiac arrest where there are barriers to effective rhythm analysis.

- Detection of output during arrest is generally performed by palpating central pulses; however, this is inaccurate in profound hypotension, and up to 45% of trained healthcare professionals are unable to perform an accurate assessment during cardiac arrest. Pulseless electrical activity (PEA) encompasses 'true PEA' (electromechanical dissociation: organized electrical activity associated with cardiac standstill) and 'pseudo-PEA' (no palpable pulse despite coordinated cardiac electrical and mechanical activity). Demonstration of pseudo-PEA can be used to support/encourage ongoing resuscitative efforts, as the outcome is likely to be better, in particular where a reversible cause is demonstrated (Figure 21.1).

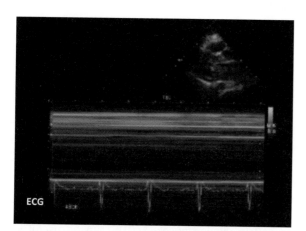

Figure 21.1 Diagnosis of pulseless electrical activity (PEA) using echocardiography. PLAX view using M-mode, demonstrating no cardiac motion despite the presence of coordinated electrical activity. The diagnosis is true PEA, or electromechanical dissociation (EMD).

- Pacing devices continue to deliver energy during cardiac arrest until deactivated and will therefore potentially produce an electrical rhythm on a monitor without leading to coordinated cardiac contraction. This can be easily misinterpreted. Differentiating true PEA from pseudo-PEA remains important and is a potential role for FoCUS.

Differential diagnoses

The major use of FoCUS in cardiac arrest is to provide diagnostic information to guide management, including potentially lifesaving procedures such as pericardiocentesis, thrombolysis, volume resuscitation, or transfer for PCI. It is then used to guide post-resuscitation care.

Hypovolaemia

Hypovolaemia causing cardiac arrest is likely to be severe, and presence of any of the following echocardiographic parameters should raise suspicion of the diagnosis:

- Hyperdynamic biventricular function
- LVEDA <5.5 cm²/m² of body surface area (BSA)
- Small IVC at end-expiration (<1 cm spontaneously ventilating, <1.5 cm positive pressure ventilation), with variable respiratory change.

In the absence of ventricular pathology, a significant reduction in preload will result in hyperdynamic biventricular function, with low EDVs. However, there are other causes for these appearances. LVH and/or right ventricular failure/PHT may also result in the appearance of an unloaded LV with a low LVEDA. Here, left ventricular size does not correlate with potential volume responsiveness. IVC dimensions are affected by changes in intrathoracic pressure, and a number of parameters have been used to estimate potential volume responsiveness by determining changes in dimension in response to ventilation. Thus, a small/collapsed IVC may represent hypovolaemia, whereas a dilated IVC may have no predictive value for RAP, in particular in the context of cardiorespiratory disease. Here, causes other than hypovolaemia should be considered,

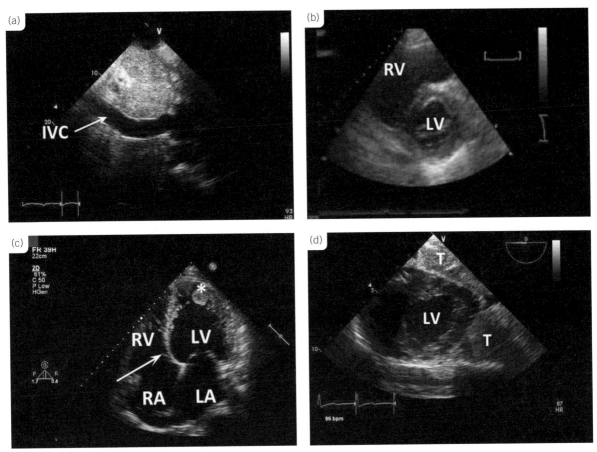

Figure 21.2 Determination of volaemic status using echo—potential pitfalls. (a) Subcostal view, TTE showing a dilated, non-collapsing IVC in a patient with tamponade. This patient may respond to volume loading acutely. (b) PSAX view in a patient with right ventricular infarction (note the dilated right heart, compared with the left heart). This patient had a dilated, non-collapsing IVC but had been volume-loaded as the LV was small and non-dilated. However, they did not respond to volume loading. (c) A4C view in a patient with cardiogenic shock. The LV is dilated, with regional wall thinning (basal septum, arrow) and apical thrombus (asterisk). Despite the dilated LV, the patient was profoundly hypovolaemic and responded well to volume resuscitation. (d) Short-axis view (TOE) of the LV in a patient resuscitated from cardiac arrest. The patient was hypovolaemic, but the LV remained small, as it was encased in tumour (T). IVC, inferior vena cava; LA, left atrium; LV, left ventricle; RA, right atrium; RV, right ventricle; T, tumour.

including PE, tamponade, or acute myocardial infarction. However, volume resuscitation may still be indicated. Where hypovolaemia is suspected, US can be used as an extension to clinical examination to search for potential causes, including examination of the thorax (haemothorax) and abdomen (aortic aneurysm/visceral injury). Figure 21.2 describes some of the potential pitfalls when assessing volaemic status with echo.

Cardiac tamponade

Cardiac tamponade arises from an increase in intrapericardial pressure, causing impaired chamber filling and/or emptying, thus negatively impacting cardiac function. As pressure (rather than volume) is important, development of tamponade relates to the rate of accumulation, rather than size of the collection per se. Although tamponade is a clinical diagnosis, the classical features of Beck's triad are rarely obvious during resuscitation. The use of echocardiography to demonstrate the presence of a pericardial collection and study its haemodynamic significance is well described in the cardiological literature. Features of tamponade include a swinging heart, right ventricular diastolic collapse, right atrial systolic collapse, pseudo-SAM, an enlarged and non-pulsatile IVC, and exaggerated respiratory variation of cardiac chamber size and transvalvular flows.

In non-arrested patients, abnormal flows correlate well with clinical features. However, these are affected by interventions, including positive pressure ventilation, and may not be present at all in certain circumstances such as post-cardiac surgery. Demonstration of a pericardial collection in a patient with cardiac arrest (unless it is very small and/or another cause for arrest is immediately apparent) should lead to consideration of immediate pericardiocentesis. Intravascular volume resuscitation should

be undertaken as a temporizing measure, even in the presence of a dilated and non-collapsing IVC.

Pericardiocentesis can be performed using echocardiographic guidance to determine the optimal approach, depth of the collection, and presence of the pericardiocentesis cannula in the pericardial space, confirmed with agitated saline (Figure 21.3). Finally, full aspiration of the collection can be monitored. Echocardiographic guidance is associated with fewer complications, although a major complication rate of 1.2% remains, including perforation of abdominal organs, coronary arteries, or cardiac chambers, pneumothorax, and death.

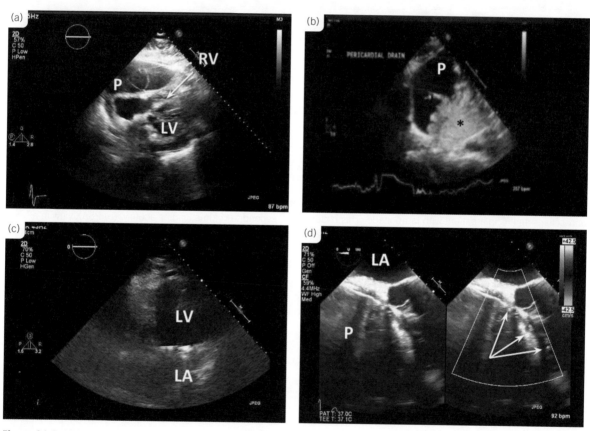

Figure 21.3 Echocardiography in tamponade. (a) Pericardial collection (P) compressing the whole heart, but in particular the RV which is slit-like. There are fibrinous strands seen within the collection, but when seen to this extent (minimal), they do not preclude attempted pericardiocentesis, in particular when associated with cardiac arrest. (b) Pericardiocentesis. A pericardial drain (arrowed) is seen in the pericardial collection (P), through which agitated saline has been injected (asterisk, *), confirming correct placement within the pericardial space. (c) TTE (A4C view) in a patient 12 hours post-mitral valve replacement. The mitral prosthesis is not clearly seen, and the right heart border is impossible to define. No echo features of tamponade were demonstrated using Doppler. TOE was performed to exclude a collection (see d). (d) TOE in the same patient as (c). A huge haematoma in the pericardial space (P) is seen compressing the right atrium and ventricle, so it becomes slit-like with functional tricuspid stenosis. Only a small amount of blood is seen passing into the right ventricle on colour Doppler (arrowed). LA, left atrium; LV, left ventricle; RV, right ventricle.

Myocardial infarction

Echocardiography is used in the diagnosis, monitoring, and risk stratification of coronary artery disease and its complications. With respect to cardiac arrest, certain situations warrant particular consideration. FoCUS may reveal RWMAs in the territory of one or more coronary arteries, suggesting new ischaemia (normal left ventricular wall thickness with hypokinesia, akinesia, or dyskinesia) or indicating prior myocardial infarction (left ventricular wall thinning, akinesia, or dyskinesia). Chest pain prior to arrest lasting >45 minutes with no RWMAs is unlikely to be of cardiac origin. By contrast, short episodes of ischaemia may not be associated with any RWMAs, and here echo cannot be used to exclude important coronary artery disease. Subtle RMWAs and advanced echo techniques (contrast/strain echo) are not the realm of FoCUS. However, obvious areas of non-functioning muscle within a suitable clinical context should raise the possibility of coronary artery thrombosis and consideration of urgent therapies such as PCI and avoidance of medications that increase cardiac oxygen demand. Important non-ischaemic conditions that may also be associated with RWMAs include dilated cardiomyopathy, pacing-induced dyskinesia, and Takotsubo cardiomyopathy.

Demonstration of a hyperdynamic LV in the context of a low output state raises the suspicion of a mechanical complication of acute myocardial infarction. Ventricular free wall rupture is a relatively rare complication, occurring in 0.2–2% of cases (Figure 21.4). However, it remains a catastrophic event, with a high mortality rate. Echo is the diagnostic tool of choice, but only a pericardial collection may be seen in up to 30%. Here careful scanning of the left ventricular free wall is indicated. Severe acute MR may result from acute myocardial infarction with PM rupture/dysfunction. The presence of a hyperdynamic LV in the context of cardiogenic shock and pulmonary oedema, together with a structurally abnormal MV (with the head of the PM visible prolapsing into the LA in systole), is diagnostic. Ventricular septal rupture may also complicate acute myocardial infarction. It is occasionally apparent using 2D echo, and colour Doppler is diagnostic. Isolated right ventricular infarction is uncommon, and features demonstrated using FoCUS are nonspecific. Findings of a dyskinetic/akinetic RV with/without dilatation suggest the diagnosis. However, more advanced echo techniques are needed, and differentiation from other causes of right ventricular dysfunction can be challenging.

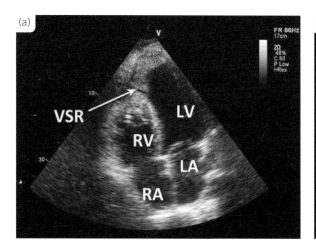 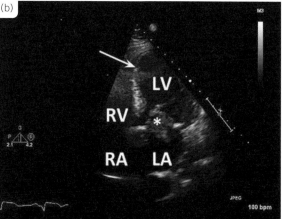

Figure 21.4 Cardiac rupture post-myocardial infarction. (a) Acute ventricular septal rupture (arrowed) in a patient post-cardiac arrest. (b) Ventricular free wall rupture in a patient post-acute myocardial infarction. The left ventricular wall (distal septum) is thinned and dyskinetic (arrowed). There is a small amount of fluid in the pericardial space. An incidental finding was a left atrial myxoma (asterisk) seen prolapsing across the mitral valve. LA, left atrium; LV, left ventricle; RA, right atrium; RV, right ventricle; VSR, ventricular septal rupture.

Pulmonary embolism

PE accounts for around 5% of cardiac arrests (13% of those from a non-cardiac cause). Diagnosis allows initiation of potentially lifesaving procedures but should only be utilized for the initial diagnosis where the patient is too unstable to transfer for CT. In the presence of severe haemodynamic compromise (including cardiac arrest), physicians may have to rely solely upon the findings of bedside echocardiography and proceed to thrombolytic treatment without further investigations. Signs indicating PE as a possible diagnosis include evidence of right ventricular strain (right ventricular dilatation/free wall hypokinesis) or pressure overload ('D-shaped' LV during systole with a dilated, non-collapsible IVC), in the absence of significant left-sided or pulmonary disease (Figure 21.5). Despite

clear limitations of FoCUS and echocardiography in the diagnosis of suspected acute PE in stable patients, PE leading to cardiac arrest is likely to be massive, resulting from occlusion of more than two-thirds of the pulmonary bed. Demonstration of a normal-sized and functioning RV in the context of cardiac arrest virtually excludes massive PE as the cause of arrest.

Pneumothorax

The sensitivity and specificity for LUS in the diagnosis/exclusion of pneumothorax exceeds that of plain chest radiography. Although if tension pneumothorax is suspected as a cause of cardiac arrest, this should be treated immediately by thoracocentesis; where the diagnosis is uncertain, then LUS can be

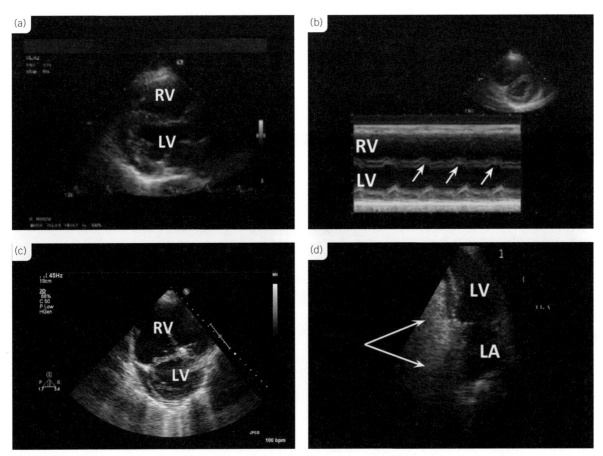

Figure 21.5 Right-sided pathology associated with cardiac arrest. (a) PLAX view demonstrating a dilated RV in acute PE. (b) M-mode showing a dilated RV and paradoxical septal motion (arrowed) in acute PE. (c) PSAX view demonstrating significant right ventricular dilatation, with a D-shaped septum. This patient had chronic right ventricular disease secondary to congenital heart disease. (d) A4C view immediately post-cardiac arrest showing opacification of the right heart due to massive air embolism (arrowed). LA, left atrium; LV, left ventricle; RA, right atrium; RV, right ventricle.

helpful. In addition, where central venous access has been obtained during cardiac arrest, LUS may be used to demonstrate/exclude the presence of an anterior pneumothorax after line insertion. Features that should be sought have been well described in published guidelines and are detailed in Chapter 15 and include demonstrating the presence/absence of pleural sliding, A-lines, B-lines, the lung pulse, and the lung point. As with any US, knowledge of the potential pitfalls is vital to avoid misinterpretation.

Echocardiography and lung ultrasound in post-resuscitation care

In addition to the use of echo and LUS to improve diagnostic accuracy in the ALS setting, these techniques can be used to guide therapy in the post-resuscitation setting. Here the techniques used will extend beyond those of FoCUS, to include the whole range of echocardiographic modalities. Echocardiography can be used to define not only the underlying cause of cardiac arrest (including myocardial ischaemia/infarction, underlying pre-excitation/predisposition to arrhythmia, and severe acute valvular, aortic, and/or pulmonary pathology) and guide catheter laboratory/operating theatre interventions, but also to determine the pathophysiological consequences of the primary pathology, as well as the post-cardiac arrest syndrome. This is characterized by a systemic inflammatory response, and the echo features that should be sought (in addition to the underlying cause) are outlined in Chapter 25. These include potential requirement/tolerance to volume loading, myocardial support (including requirement for inotropic agents/avoidance of beta agonists/heart rate optimization and/or extracorporeal support), as well as estimation of LAP, PAP, and pulmonary vascular resistance and demonstration of interstitial oedema and the response to any therapies/interventions. The applicability of these more advanced echocardiographic techniques to the hyper-acute setting is not well validated. Great care must be taken to interpret findings in the clinical and pharmacological context of the patient, while appreciating the limitations of the technique itself. Recommendations are therefore that all patients should undergo a comprehensive echocardiogram by an expert as soon as possible after successful resuscitation.

Conclusion

Echo performed during cardiac arrest will be focused and must not interfere with delivery of high-quality resuscitation. Novices can learn FoCUS with excellent correlation to that seen by experienced practitioners in the arrest scenario. Training involves attendance at an appropriate course, followed by mentored practice and maintenance of a logbook. Of note, even experienced sonographers/echocardiographers need training in ALS-compliant imaging, in order to minimize interruptions to chest compressions and optimize communication with the resuscitation team. Nonetheless, this adjunct to resuscitation provides all personnel with the ability to rapidly change the focus and management of the cardiac arrest scenario. When more time is available, comprehensive echocardiography should be performed to help clarify uncertainties and look more specifically at cardiac physiology, in particular in the post-arrest setting.

✅ Multiple choice questions

Interactive multiple choice questions to test your knowledge can be found in the Online appendix at www.oxfordmedicine.com/focusedicu. Please refer to your access card for further details.

Further reading

Breitkreutz R, Price S, Steiger HV, *et al*. Focused echocardiographic evaluation in life support and peri-resuscitation of emergency patients: a prospective trial. *Resuscitation* 2010;**81**:1527–33.

Lancellotti P, Price S, Edvardsen T, *et al*. The use of echocardiography in acute cardiovascular care: recommendations of the European Association of Cardiovascular Imaging and the Acute Cardiovascular Care Association. *European Heart Journal: Acute Cardiovascular Care* 2015;**4**:3–5.

Price S, Ilper H, Uddin S, *et al*. Peri-resuscitation echocardiography: training the novice practitioner. *Resuscitation* 2010;**81**:1534–9.

Soar J, Nolan JP, Böttiger BW, *et al*.; Adult advanced life support section Collaborators. European Resuscitation Council Guidelines for Resuscitation 2015: Section 3. Adult advanced life support. *Resuscitation* 2015;**95**:100–47.

Via G, Hussain A, Wells M, *et al*. International evidence-based recommendations for focused cardiac ultrasound. *Journal of the American Society of Echocardiography* 2014;**27**:683.e1–33.

22

Dyspnoea and hypoxaemia

Ashley Miller

Introduction

LUS can be used to diagnose most pathologies which cause respiratory failure. Pneumothorax, interstitial syndrome, and pleural effusion are all visible at the pleural line with US, while approximately 90% of alveolar consolidations extend to the pleura and will be detectable with US. This chapter will outline a systematic approach to assessing the patient presenting with acute respiratory failure. In addition, the role of US in assessing ventilated patients with established respiratory failure, monitoring fluid balance and pleural effusions, identifying ventilator-associated pneumonia (VAP), and monitoring lung recruitment will be reviewed.

Acute respiratory failure and the BLUE Protocol

A seminal study (Lichtenstein and Mezière, 2008) described how a protocolized LUS examination that took 5 minutes to perform was able to correctly identify the cause of acute respiratory failure in 90% of patients presenting with acute dyspnoea and hypoxaemia. This compared to a figure of around 75% with chest radiography and clinical examination. It was named the BLUE Protocol which stands for Bedside Lung Ultrasound in Emergency. This diagnostic accuracy was achieved solely using the blinded US findings, without taking into account any history, examination, blood results, or other imaging. This highlights the power of LUS as a bedside tool for assessing the patient presenting with acute respiratory failure. How this can be adapted for ventilated patients is described on

p. 194 and in Figure 22.1. Details of the technique of LUS, including where to place the probe, are described in Chapter 14.

Technique

A systematic approach to assessing the patient in acute respiratory failure is outlined in Table 22.1.

DVT scanning

If anterior scanning is normal (i.e. bilateral sliding and A-lines), then venous US should be performed to examine for a DVT. This is quick and simple to perform, using a modified 2-point compression test, which focuses on the areas of greatest probability for a thrombus and has a very high sensitivity and specificity for detecting a DVT (see Chapter 18 for further details). Briefly, the patient is positioned in a 30–40° reverse Trendelenburg position, with the hip externally rotated and flexed. Using a linear probe, the femoral vein is imaged 2 cm proximal to the junction of the saphenous and femoral veins. The examination should extend distally, encompassing the bifurcation of the saphenous and then deep femoral veins. All veins should be seen to compress with enough force to slightly compress the femoral artery. The second site, with the patient's knee flexed, is from the distal 2 cm of the popliteal vein to its trifurcation. Complete compression of the vein rules out a thrombus at the examination point, while incomplete compression rules one in. If a DVT is discovered, then the combination of acute respiratory failure and a normal anterior LUS makes a PE highly likely. Absence of a DVT means that the US examination of the lungs should continue to step

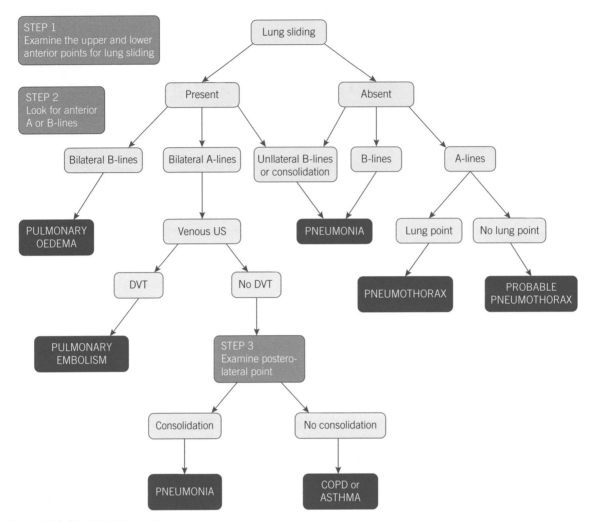

Figure 22.1 The BLUE Protocol.

3. It is worth noting that in Lichtenstein's study, while 20 out of 21 patients with a PE had a normal anterior LUS, half of them had postero-lateral consolidation (coexisting infection was common). This demonstrates the importance of the DVT examination.

Assessment of the ventilated patient

The BLUE Protocol was designed and validated for patients presenting acutely with respiratory failure. Most of the patients were spontaneously breathing; only a few (35 out of 260) had been intubated before the US exam took place. What does this mean for patients in critical care who are intubated and ventilated, perhaps for some time? The diagnostic accuracy of the BLUE Protocol will clearly be altered in these patients. The post-laparotomy patient with atelectasis would be identified as having pneumonia by the BLUE Protocol. In fact, it is unusual to perform an LUS on a ventilated patient and not find at least small amounts of pleural fluid and basal atelectasis. Also inflammation acute lung injury and fluid overload are common in ventilated patients. These will generate B-lines on US that are not the result of CPO. However, the BLUE Protocol, without necessarily drawing the same conclusions from its findings, can be extremely useful for assessing ventilated patients. LUS has been shown to have a higher diagnostic accuracy than chest radiography for interstitial syndrome, effusions, and consolidation and approaches the accuracy of the gold standard

Table 22.1 Examination of the upper and lower anterior points

Step 1	Look for lung sliding	Present: pneumothorax can be ruled out
		Absent: consider pneumothorax, ARDS, pneumonia, one-lung intubation, pneumonectomy
Step 2	Look for anterior A-lines or B-lines or consolidation	Bilateral A-lines with sliding: normal. Proceed to leg vein US to look for thrombus
		Bilateral B-lines: cardiogenic pulmonary oedema
		Unilateral B-lines: pneumonia
		A-lines without sliding: possible pneumothorax. Look for lung point to confirm pneumothorax. If absent, probable pneumothorax. Consider CT scan to confirm
A diagnosis may well have been reached by this point. Pulmonary oedema and pneumothorax are ruled in or out with anterior scanning, and pneumonia can be ruled in (but not out).		
Step 3	Examine postero-lateral points	Consolidation: pneumonia
		Normal: asthma or chronic obstructive pulmonary disease likely diagnosis (equivalent to a normal chest X-ray)

CT scanning. Most published assessments of LUS in ventilated patients have used six examination points on each hemi-thorax, but interestingly, region analysis confirmed that the diagnostic accuracy would have been just as good if only the three points from the BLUE Protocol had been used.

Perhaps the main difference between scanning acutely presenting patients and ventilated ones on ICU is the interpretation of the interstitial syndrome (the sign of which is B-lines).

Interstitial syndrome in ventilated patients

In the acutely presenting patient, interstitial syndrome will nearly always be due to CPO, whereas in the ventilated patient, it is a very common finding where it can be due to left ventricular failure, fluid overload, ARDS, or a combination of these. Lung fibrosis will also demonstrate B-lines. Advanced knowledge of LUS helps to distinguish between cardiogenic and non-cardiogenic pulmonary oedema (Table 22.2), but even without these, the identification of B-lines is very useful as it suggests that limiting fluid administration and establishing a diuresis may be beneficial to respiratory function, whatever the cause. Table 22.2 summarizes the US features which may be used to differentiate cardiogenic from other causes of pulmonary oedema.

Assessment of fluid balance

Simply put, A-lines mean the lungs are dry, while B-lines mean the lungs are wet (the exception to this is lung fibrosis). An important point to remember about B-lines is that they appear with interstitial oedema before alveolar oedema has occurred—the interlobular septa become engorged with fluid before the alveoli flood. This means interstitial oedema can be identified before the patient develops severe respiratory failure by the presence of a few discrete B-lines in the anterior chest. The absence of anterior B-lines has been shown to have a positive predictive value of 97% for a pulmonary artery occlusion pressure (PAOP) of <18 mmHg. If the B-lines are cardiogenic in origin (high PAOP), the presence of interstitial oedema on US suggests that the patient is on the flat portion of their Starling curve. They therefore provide a warning that respiratory failure will ensue if fluid resuscitation is administered. As alveoli start to flood, the LUS picture progresses to a white lung pattern where the B-lines become more numerous and confluent. This is a sign that the patient's condition will improve by using treatment to reduce lung water (diuresis, renal filtration, or PPV). Similarly, if the patient has B-lines from non-CPO, this is likely to get worse with fluid administration, regardless of the PAOP. The management here would be identical—avoidance of further IV resuscitation fluid, fluid removal, and PPV.

Table 22.2 Ultrasound features of cardiogenic and non-cardiogenic pulmonary oedema

Interstitial syndrome		
Ultrasound features	**Cardiogenic**	**ARDS/fibrosis**
Lung sliding	Normal	Reduced or absent
Pleural line	Normal	Irregular, thickened, coarse
		Often multiple small anterior subpleural consolidations
Distribution	Homogenous	Spared areas (normal pleura, no B-lines)
	Spread from postero-lateral to anterior, with increasing severity. No spared areas	More severe in dependent areas
Consolidation	No consolidation	Dependent consolidation
Lung pulse	Absent	Present in areas of reduced sliding
Pleural effusion	Common	Less common

Pleural effusions

More detailed information on the assessment of pleural effusions with LUS can be found in Chapter 15. US appearance can help discriminate between transudates and exudates, allows volume estimation, reveals any septations (Figure 22.2), and allows guided thoracocentesis for diagnosis or drainage.

Ventilator-associated pneumonia

LUS can help guide both the diagnosis and treatment of VAP. When there is deterioration in respiratory function in a ventilated patient, the differential diagnosis is broad. Other investigations are useful, but not very specific. Raised inflammatory markers, shadowing on a chest radiograph, and pyrexia, while suggestive, all have other causes. LUS will clearly demonstrate any new consolidation (Figure 22.3), as well as rule other causes in or out. Because basal consolidation and atelectasis are common in ventilated patients, it is important to regularly assess with LUS, so it is known whether a finding is new. A recent study compared various US features to assess their performance in detecting VAP and showed it to be superior to the Clinical Pulmonary Infection Score (CPIS). Lobar and semi-lobar consolidations were poor predictors (presumably because these were pre-existing atelectasis,

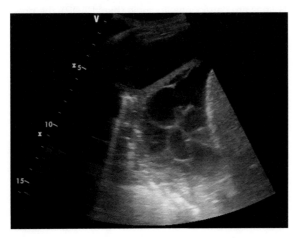

Figure 22.2 A septated parapneumonic effusion.

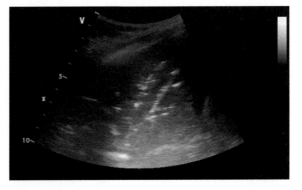

Figure 22.3 Linear air bronchograms in a consolidated lung base in a patient with VAP.

rather than consolidation or infiltrates from another cause). The two features most suggestive were dynamic air bronchograms and small subpleural consolidations, with dynamic air bronchograms performing the best. Demonstrating the presence of any associated effusion will allow a guided diagnostic tap to assess the nature of the effusion and provide a sample for microbiology.

Assessing response to treatment

Just as LUS has a high diagnostic accuracy, it can also be used for assessing response to treatment. B-lines in CPO will be seen to resolve quickly to therapy, whether that is preload reduction (venodilatation or positive airway pressure) or fluid removal (diuresis or filtration). ARDS will also be seen to resolve by the reduction in B-lines (albeit more slowly than with CPO). Aeration will be seen to increase, and consolidation decrease, with resolution of pneumonia. Parapneumonic effusions may be seen to resolve or become increasingly complicated, necessitating video-assisted thoracoscopic surgery (VATS). Lung can be seen to re-expand after pleural drainage. The size of pneumothoraces can be monitored by the location of the lung point, either in patients with chest drains or in those with pneumothoraces too small to drain.

Lung recruitment

Lung recruitment is straightforward to assess with LUS. Chapter 16 describes how consolidation and collapse have different features, depending on the proportion of air and fluid in the lung (fully consolidated and hepatized or the 'shred sign'). If alveoli are recruitable, then the US appearances will change to those of more aerated lung with increasing PEEP. Similarly, as pneumonia resolves, the lung will be seen to reaerate. A scoring system for assessing recruitment has been described by ascribing each area of the lung examined into one of four patterns of aeration: normal appearance, moderate loss of aeration (frequent B-lines), severe loss of aeration (confluent B-lines), and lung consolidation (see Chapter 23, table 23.1). The US score correlated well with lung recruitment induced by PEEP and quantified by changes to the pressure–volume curve and increases in PaO_2. An US scoring system has also been used to assess lung reaeration in VAP treated with antibiotics over 7 days. Highly significant correlation was found between US- and CT-assessed reaeration. It is very important to remember that hyperinflation cannot be assessed with LUS, which is a significant limitation. Aerated lung looks the same, whatever its volume. The principles of lung-protective ventilation strategies should still be employed.

When significant pleural effusions are present, it can be unclear whether the underlying lung is consolidated or collapsed (atelectatic). While there are some distinguishing features, it is only by draining the effusion that the underlying condition of the lung is revealed. A lung base that reaerates was simply squashed, while one that remains hepatized is consolidated.

Conclusion

LUS is a powerful tool in the diagnosis of respiratory failure. In acute presentations, the use of the BLUE protocol will rapidly and accurately yield the diagnosis. In ventilated patients, LUS can be used for diagnosis, to assess response to treatment and guide interventions. Any worsening of respiratory function in a ventilated patient should prompt an LUS, and progress should be reassessed. LUS is therefore a key tool in the emergency department, acute medical unit, and critical care.

✅ Multiple choice questions

Interactive multiple choice questions to test your knowledge can be found in the Online appendix at www.oxfordmedicine.com/focusedicu. Please refer to your access card for further details.

Further reading

Bouhemad B, Brisson H, Le-Guen M, Arbelot C, Lu Q, Rouby J-J. Bedside ultrasound assessment of PEEP induced lung recruitment. *American Journal of Respiratory and Critical Care Medicine* 2011;**183**:341–7.

Lichtenstein DA, Mezière GA. Relevance of lung ultrasound in the diagnosis of acute respiratory failure: the BLUE protocol. *Chest* 2008;**134**:117–25.

23

Failure to wean from mechanical ventilation

Andrew Walden

Introduction

Failure to wean from mechanical ventilation is a common problem in intensive care and represents a significant burden in terms of prolonged ICU stay with associated morbidity and mortality. US examination can aid the systematic assessment of the underlying pathophysiology that is often complex and multifactorial. This chapter reviews the role of US in assessing the contribution of inadequate lung aeration, pleural effusion, and diaphragmatic and cardiac function to weaning failure.

Clinical relevance

Weaning from mechanical to spontaneous ventilation is perhaps the most important first goal on recovery from critical illness. Failure to wean is defined as an inability to pass a spontaneous breathing trial (SBT) (either via a T-piece or by using a minimal setting of pressure support) or the need for re-intubation within 48 hours following extubation. This is known to occur in 20–30% of patients and represents a significant burden in terms of prolonged ICU stay with associated morbidity and mortality.

The pathophysiology of weaning failure is often complex and multifactorial—respiratory, cardiac, and neurological problems can all occur together, especially in patients who have had prolonged stays on intensive care. It is important therefore to take a structured approach, identifying each factor and addressing it in turn. US can greatly aid this approach. Identification of diaphragmatic weakness, unknown pleural collections or ongoing evidence of interstitial oedema, and impaired lung aeration are all identified with US, as are abnormalities of cardiac function.

Respiratory causes of failure to wean

Many factors relating to the lungs can lead to failed weaning, many of which are amenable to assessment with US. Neuromuscular weakness can be detected by dynamic US of diaphragmatic function. Impaired respiratory mechanics due to pleural collections are easily diagnosed with LUS, as is loss of lung aeration due to consolidation or interstitial oedema.

Ultrasound assessment of lung aeration

LUS can be used to assess changes in lung aeration during an SBT. Loss of lung aeration during a successful SBT has been shown to predict post-extubation respiratory distress. Loss of aeration represents the integrated effects of impaired cardiac, respiratory, and diaphragmatic function and reflects associated lung derecruitment and pulmonary oedema secondary to increased PAOP. Aeration is assessed by US with a semi-quantitative score that is determined by dividing each lung into six zones (Figure 23.1). The aeration of each zone is systematically assessed, and a score allocated of between 0 (normal aeration) to 3 (complete loss of aeration), which results in a maximum total US aeration score of 36 (Table 23.1).

A dynamic aeration score may be calculated from the change in aeration before and after start of SBT. A change in aeration by one category scores 1, by two categories scores 3, and by three categories scores 5.

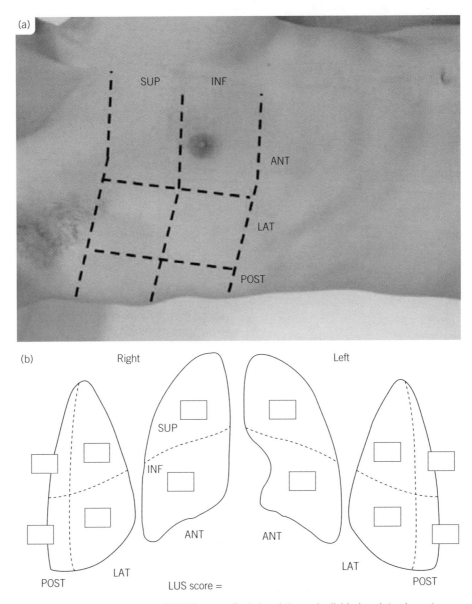

Figure 23.1 The regions of the lung ultrasound (LUS) score. Each hemi-thorax is divided up into six sectors, as shown.

Reproduced with permission from Bouhemad *et al.*, 'Ultrasound for "Lung Monitoring" of Ventilated Patients', *Anesthesiology*, **132**: 437–447. Copyright © 2015, Wolters Kluwer Health. http://anesthesiology.pubs.asahq.org/article.aspx?articleid=2091559

For instance, a change from normal to moderate, a score of 1 is added; for a change from normal to severe, a score of 3 is added; for a change of normal to total loss, a score of 5 is added. These scores are then subtracted from the total aeration score and added where there is improvement. During an SBT, a score of <13 predicts a very low chance of post-extubation failure, whereas a score of >17 identifies an 85% chance of post-extubation failure.

Aside from its utility in predicting post-extubation distress following an SBT, LUS may also identify other issues which may be addressed prior to weaning from mechanical ventilation, including pulmonary oedema and atelectasis, which may be associated with pleural effusion or mucus plugging. Interventions, including inducing diuresis, pleural drainage, and physiotherapy, may help to improve lung function prior to an SBT or extubation.

Table 23.1 Lung aeration score (each of the 12 sectors is scored according to the ultrasound appearance, resulting in a maximum possible total score of 36)

Number of points	Aeration	Description	Appearance
0	Normal	A line pattern with a maximum of two B-lines per sector	
1	Moderate loss	Multiple B-lines regularly spaced or coalescent B-lines within a limited portion of the sector	
2	Severe loss	Coalescent B-lines throughout sector	
3	Total loss	Consolidated lung	

Reproduced with permission from Soummer A *et al*. Ultrasound assessment of lung aeration loss during a successful weaning trial predicts postextubation distress *Crit Care Med* 2012; **40**:2064–2072.

Ultrasound assessment of pleural effusions

Pleural effusions are common in mechanically ventilated patients, with some studies reporting an incidence of over 50% in patients ventilated for >48 hours when examined with US. The physiological effects are varied but include:

- An increased pleural pressure, which increases the distending pressure of the chest wall and reduces that of the lung. This results in uncoupling of the normal volume relationship between the lung and chest wall, with an increase in chest wall volume and a reduction in lung volume. A restrictive ventilatory defect is predicted with reduced vital capacity, functional residual capacity, and total lung capacity, although the loss of lung volume may not be as large as expected from the size of the effusion, as the lung may be largely floating on the effusion. Uncoupled lung recruits and derecruits during the respiratory cycle, which increases the risk of ventilator-induced lung injury. This effect can be mitigated by the application of PEEP.

- Impaired chest wall and diaphragmatic mechanics due to outward and downward pressure—this leads to the muscles operating on an adverse portion of their length/tension curve and probably leads to subjective feelings of dyspnoea.

- Altered ventilation–perfusion matching due to compression atelectasis of the underlying lung and the development of a shunt.

Given these adverse effects, it is reasonable to assume that thoracocentesis or pleural drainage may help to improve overall lung function and thus make weaning from mechanical ventilation more successful. There is some evidence to support this, although based on case series and surrogate outcome measures. A meta-analysis of studies showed a consistent improvement in oxygenation, and another study has demonstrated a correlation between improvements in oxygenation and volume of pleural effusion drained.

US easily identifies pleural effusion (Figure 23.2) and can be used for both qualitative and quantitative assessments of when to drain.

If there is evidence of septation or organization, then there is a compelling reason to perform a diagnostic tap. A pleural fluid pH of <7.2 or aspiration of pus are indications to drain the effusion to prevent ongoing infection or chronic scarring and lung trapping. The presence of flattening, or even inversion, of the hemidiaphragm implies it will be on an adverse portion of the length/tension curve, so inefficient and prone to cause subjective dyspnoea.

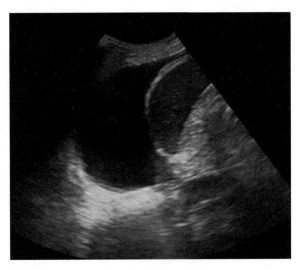

Figure 23.2 Large, free-flowing pleural effusion in a mechanically ventilated patient. The spleen and hemidiaphragm are clearly seen on the right-hand side of the image, with an extensive hypoechogenic area on the left-hand side of the image.

Quantitatively, it is possible to estimate the size of pleural effusions. The intra-pleural distance at the base of the lung (Figure 23.3) has been shown to correlate with volume of pleural fluid. In a supine patient, an intra-pleural distance at the base of the lung of 45 mm on the left or 50 mm on the right reliably predicts a pleural fluid volume of >800 mL. Similarly, with a patient supine with 15° elevation, the maximum

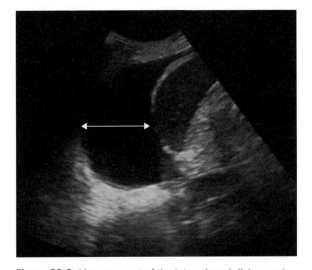

Figure 23.3 Measurement of the intra-pleural distance at the base of the lung.

intra-pleural distance when scanning in the posterior axillary line allows estimation of fluid volume. The volume approximates to the separation distance in millimetres multiplied by 20.

While there is no definitive volume identified at which to perform pleural drainage, the larger the effusion, the more likely there will be a benefit. There is no sense in draining small effusions, but where there is evidence of underlying lung collapse or a flattened hemidiaphragm associated with a moderate to large effusion, drainage is likely to improve respiratory mechanics, gas exchange, and subjective feelings of dyspnoea, which is likely to hasten weaning from mechanical ventilation. What is also clear is that pleural drainage using US in mechanically ventilated patients is a safe procedure with a low complication rate.

Diaphragmatic function

US visualization of the hemidiaphragm has been described in Chapter 16. There are two main ways of visualizing diaphragmatic function, either by examining the zone of apposition where the hemidiaphragm 'inserts' into the abdominal wall or by M-mode examination of the dome of the diaphragm over the liver and spleen in the mid-clavicular line. Dynamic visualization of the zone of apposition allows determination of the fractional thickening [(thickness at end-inspiration – thickness at end-expiration)/thickness at end-expiration]. Similarly, visualization of the dome of the hemidiaphragm allows an estimate of the total diaphragmatic excursion. Both these systems have been validated and perform well against correlates of diaphragmatic function, such as transdiaphragmatic pressure measurements, but notably this is in spontaneously breathing individuals. The application of PEEP increases lung volume and so affects the normal doming of the hemidiaphragm in expiration, thus limiting the utility of diaphragmatic excursion as a measure of function in mechanically ventilated patients. Fractional thickening probably remains a good measure of diaphragmatic efficiency, although at higher levels of PEEP and lung volume, it may become less useful.

Diaphragmatic US can be used to identify phrenic nerve injury, which may occur following cardiac surgery, by looking for asymmetric diaphragmatic dysfunction. During spontaneous breathing, the paralysed diaphragm will be noted to move cephalad during inspiration. If the function in the other hemidiaphragm is preserved, it appears that patients will still manage to wean successfully. A maximal diaphragmatic excursion of >25 mm in the non-affected diaphragm predicts a high likelihood of successful weaning, while if it is <25 mm, it suggests bilateral dysfunction and low likelihood of rapid weaning from mechanical ventilation.

In most other situations, diaphragmatic weakness is generalized due to systemic disorders. Critical illness polyneuromyopathy and specific neuromuscular disorders, such as Guillain–Barré syndrome, will lead to bilateral diaphragmatic weakness, meaning that unilateral assessment of function is adequate. Similarly, in conditions such as chronic obstructive pulmonary disease, high lung volumes due to gas trapping and increases in total thoracic capacity due to bullous disease can lead to impaired diaphragmatic function by placing the diaphragm on an adverse portion of the length/tension generation curve. In these situations, right-sided examination of the diaphragm can serve as an adequate proxy for whole diaphragmatic function.

Diaphragmatic excursion has been used in a general ICU population to predict successful weaning. In one study, a cut-off value of maximal excursion of 1.1 cm had a sensitivity of 84% and a specificity of 83% to predict re-intubation at 72 hours, and in another, a value of <10 mm for either hemidiaphragm defined dysfunction and was associated with a longer time to liberation from mechanical ventilation and re-intubation rates.

More recently, fractional thickening has been used as an effective tool to predict weaning failure. In patients with a fractional thickening of ≥30%, the positive predictive value for successful extubation was >90%, regardless of whether assessment was performed by SBT or on pressure support. Very similar results have been found using a cut-off value of 36% in patients with tracheostomy tubes in situ at being successfully weaned from respiratory support within 48 hours.

Cardiac failure—systolic and diastolic

A role for cardiac dysfunction in weaning failure is supported by evidence of a progressive reduction in mixed venous oxygen saturations, due to a fall in cardiac output, in patients who fail an SBT, compared to those who do not. The transition from PPV to spontaneous breathing is associated with a number of physiological effects that may predispose patients to a deterioration in cardiac function. The loss of positive intrathoracic pressure leads to an increase in venous return and ventricular preload, as well as effects on left ventricular wall stress that can lead to increases in afterload. This is often coupled with hypertension, as a patient's sedation is reduced or stopped, which, in turn, can lead to both systolic and diastolic dysfunction. It is difficult to be certain what role pure cardiac dysfunction has on weaning failure, as it is difficult to separate the effects on increased cardiac loading from the increases in respiratory loading, but it is certainly a factor in over 40% of cases.

TTE is useful in identifying both systolic and diastolic dysfunction, which can predict the likelihood of successful weaning or liberation from mechanical ventilation and may therefore indicate the need for diuretics, beta-blockers, or angiotensin-converting enzyme inhibitors to optimize cardiac function. Left ventricular systolic function has been discussed in Chapter 7 and is a skill that can be acquired relatively easily. Assessment of left ventricular diastolic function is an advanced echocardiographic skill, which involves spectral and tissue Doppler examination of MV inflow and annulus, respectively. PW Doppler of MV inflow in diastole provides information on the E wave during early diastole and the A wave due to atrial systole in late ventricular diastole. Tissue Doppler analysis of MV annulus allows determination of the e' wave of left ventricular relaxation. The E/e' ratio can then be calculated, which correlates with the left ventricular filling pressure (see Chapter 7 for more detailed explanation).

Several studies have examined the echocardiographic assessment of ventricular function prior to extubation and its relationship to failure of weaning.

The following are associated with a higher likelihood of failure of weaning:

- EF of <40%.
- E/A ratio of >2 in the presence of impaired left ventricular function.
- E/e' ratio of >12 in the presence of preserved left ventricular function.

Echocardiography undertaken during an SBT may demonstrate a cardiac cause for a failed trial of weaning that was not apparent when assessed while the patient was receiving ventilatory support due to the change in left ventricular loading conditions. Increases in E/A ratio and E/e' ratio correlate with measurement of increased PAOP, with a reasonable sensitivity and specificity, where the E/A ratio is >0.95 and the E/e' ratio >8.5.

✅ Multiple choice questions

Interactive multiple choice questions to test your knowledge can be found in the Online appendix at www.oxfordmedicine.com/focusedicu. Please refer to your access card for further details.

Further reading

Goligher E, Leis J, Fowler R, Pinto R, Adhikari N, Ferguson N. Utility and safety of draining pleural effusions in mechanically ventilated patients: a systematic review and meta-analysis. *Critical Care* 2011;**15**:R46.

Ho CY, Solomon SD. A clinician's guide to tissue Doppler imaging. *Circulation* 2006;113;**10**:e396–8.

Soummer A, Perbet S, Brisson H, *et al.* Ultrasound assessment of lung aeration loss during a successful weaning trial predicts postextubation distress. *Critical Care Medicine* 2012;**40**:2064–72.

Walden AP, Jones QC, Matsa R, Wise MP. Pleural effusions on the intensive care unit; hidden morbidity with therapeutic potential. *Respirology* 2013;**18**:246–54.

24

Trauma

Justin Kirk-Bayley and James Doyle

Introduction

US in trauma has become a mainstay of the management of the acute trauma patient over the last few decades, to the extent that it can almost be considered an extension of the physical examination performed in the primary survey. While practised for almost 40 years in continental Europe, it has taken a little longer for full integration in the UK and North America. While early CT scanning is a standard of care, focused US performed by trained operators remains an essential diagnostic tool because of its immediacy and low risk.

The FAST scan is very specifically a 'rule-in' scan. The detection of abnormal intra-abdominal free fluid is a supportive finding that may aid diagnostics. The absence of detection of fluid by the FAST scan does not mean that there is no fluid; it simply means that it has not been detected by the FAST scan. In this circumstance, clinical evaluation or alternative investigation modalities should be considered. This chapter describes how to undertake a FAST and an extended FAST scan, with examples of common pathology. The benefits, together with the limitations and pitfalls, are outlined.

Benefits of ultrasound

Patients who are victims of trauma have the potential to deteriorate rapidly. Any scanning modality used must provide useful information with a high degree of sensitivity and specificity and in a timely manner, without adding further risk to the patient. In this respect, focused US meets all these criteria. In the trauma patient who is hypotensive, is the recipient of abdominal trauma, or for whom an accurate history of the injury is unable to be provided by themselves or others, a FAST scan may be performed as an adjunct to the circulatory assessment. FAST scanning detects intra-abdominal free fluid, and in this context, the premise is that fluid is likely to represent haemorrhage and that, after injury, this fluid will collect with gravity into an area and volume that are adequate for detection. The quantity of fluid that can be seen relies on the speed of haemorrhage, the patient's position, and the operator's skill.

Clinical assessment alone has a poor sensitivity, as 20–43% of patients with significant abdominal injuries may have an initially normal physical examination.

By contrast, FAST has been demonstrated to have a sensitivity of 86–99% and a specificity of 90–99% for detecting haemoperitoneum.

FAST and CT scanning have largely replaced diagnostic peritoneal lavage (DPL) as the initial investigations of choice to detect intra-abdominal haemorrhage, although there remains a role for DPL in the unstable patient (Figure 24.1). The individual merits and drawbacks of the different investigations are outlined in Table 24.1.

Probe choice and settings

A low-frequency (2–5 MHz) curvilinear probe should be used. This gives the double benefit of a large, sector-shaped field of view and the ability to penetrate potentially to over 20 cm into the abdomen, depending on the habitus of the patient. While this probe has low temporal resolution when examining in the

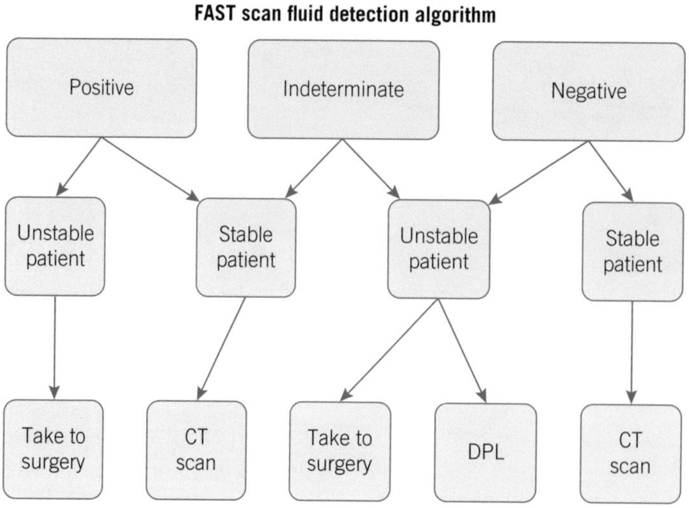

FAST scan fluid detection algorithm

Figure 24.1 Decision tree for the utility of FAST scanning in blunt abdominal trauma.

Adapted from Rozycki, Grace S. MD, FACS; Shackford, Steven R. MD, FACS, 'Ultrasound, What Every Trauma Surgeon Should Know', *Journal of Trauma and Acute Care Surgery*, Vol. **40**, Issue 1, pp. 1–4, © Williams & Wilkins 1996. All Rights Reserved.

Table 24.1 Advantages and disadvantages of investigations to detect intra-abdominal haemorrhage

Diagnostic peritoneal lavage	
Advantages	**Disadvantages**
• Can be performed at the bedside • Can be performed rapidly (10–15 minutes) • Very sensitive for identifying intra-peritoneal blood (approximately 20 mL with 100,000 red blood cells/mL)	• Invasive • Difficult in pregnancy or with many previous surgeries • Cannot be repeated • Overly sensitive and may result in an excessive laparotomy rate
CT scan	
Advantages	**Disadvantages**
• Good for hollow viscus and retroperitoneal injuries • Identifies specific injuries well • Both high sensitivity and specificity • Can detect free fluid ≥100 mL	• 30–60 minutes to complete a study • Requires a stable patient due to relative clinical isolation
FAST scan	
Advantages	**Disadvantages**
• Can be performed rapidly (<3 minutes) at the bedside • Non-invasive • Can be repeated (no ionizing radiation) • Sensitivity and specificity for free fluid similar to DPL and CT • Can detect free fluid ≥100–250 mL	• Operator-dependent • Poor detection for hollow viscus or retroperitoneal injuries • Obesity or subcutaneous air may hinder scanning • May not identify specific organ injuries as cause for haemorrhage

subcostal cardiac view, it is adequate for the detection of pericardial fluid.

Most US machines will likely default to an abdominal setting when this probe is selected, but if not, then this should be selected. The far gain or lower TGC sliders may need to be increased if there is significant adiposity causing US attenuation, in order to interrogate the intra-abdominal viscera.

Scanning technique

The FAST scan comprises four views, each of which seeks to detect the presence of abnormal, hypoechoic intra-abdominal free fluid, the presence of which may explain the trauma patient's clinical condition. The views may be undertaken in any order, but a complete scan must include an assessment in all four of them. Scanning convention is that the screen marker represents a right-sided or cephalad orientation, so the probe should be oriented thusly.

Additional views and assessments 'extend' the basic FAST assessment to become 'E-FAST'. These are essentially views of the lower thorax to look for signs that may indicate intrathoracic haemorrhage.

Right upper quadrant

Intra-abdominal fluid gathers between the liver and the right kidney, known as the hepatorenal angle or Morrison's pouch, and this is where this part of the examination is primarily focused (Figure 24.2a and b).

The US probe should be placed in the mid-axillary line at the level of the eleventh and twelfth ribs in a coronal plane; rotate the probe slightly to the plane of the kidney (the inferior pole of the kidney is slightly anterior), and then tilt the probe towards the retroperitoneum.

Once a view is obtained, the probe should be swept both perpendicular and parallel to the ribs to interrogate the whole of the hepatorenal space. If adequate views are really not available in this orientation, the probe may be moved anteromedially to a transabdominal orientation, with the US beam aimed laterally. It is often underappreciated just how posterior one needs to scan to adequately visualize the kidneys (a retroperitoneal organ).

Primary liver trauma may also be detected and lacerations seen with haematoma formation as abnormal hypoechoicities within the otherwise 'meaty' liver parenchyma. Haematomas may be seen to be confined by the liver capsule and contained, or extending into the peritoneal cavity.

Fluid in the dependent part of the pleural cavity may also be detected from this view and be seen as hypoechoic areas between the right lung and the liver (with the diaphragm above it). Where there is fluid present, an assessment of the diaphragm itself may be made (absent fluid, and hence fully aerated lung, precludes diaphragmatic visualization, except for lateral insertion). Detection of fluid here is sensitive, with detecting levels down to 20–50 mL in some studies, and its presence is supportive of a diagnosis of intrathoracic trauma with interpleural haemorrhage.

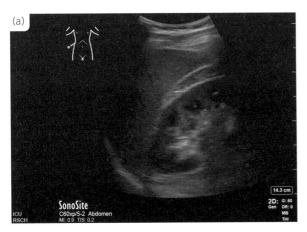
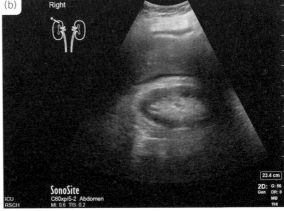

Figure 24.2 (a) Normal hepatorenal angle (Morrison's pouch). (b) Fluid in the hepatorenal angle (Morrison's pouch).

Left upper quadrant

Fluid may collect in the space between the spleen and the left kidney, the splenorenal angle, in a similar way to the right side, sitting between the two organs (Figure 24.3a and b). Scanning for it involves a similar process to that for the right, save that the left kidney sits more posteriorly and higher due to less displacement from the spleen, which may mean visualization is more hindered by the acoustic shadows cast by the ribs and require that the assessment be undertaken during inspiration by the patient, not forgetting again how posterior one must scan. Again a full examination will interrogate the whole of the space between the spleen and left kidney to look for fluid. In contradistinction to the right-sided examination, it is very common for fluid to sit between the spleen and the diaphragm, and this area must also be examined for a full assessment.

Injuries to the spleen may also be detected and have similar appearances to liver injuries.

Again fluid in the pleural cavity may be seen at the left lung base, and fluid, if present, will be seen as a hypoechoic area above the spleen and diaphragm.

Pelvic view

The transducer should be placed in a transverse orientation (marker to the right), just above the symphysis pubis. The beam should be angled down into the pelvis in order to demonstrate the bladder and rectum and the space between them, the rectovesical pouch (pouch of Douglas) (Figure 24.4). This is the lowest part of the pelvis in which free fluid will gather, having travelled down the paracolic gutters, and be seen as a hypoechoic area between the bladder and rectum on US.

The probe should be rotated into the sagittal plane, and the beam swept parasagittally to examine all these areas to look for free fluid. Views are best obtained when the bladder is full of urine, providing an acoustic window for the rest of the pelvis.

In male patients, fluid may also be found lateral to the prostate and superior to the seminal vesicles and bladder wall.

In female patients, fluid may also be found both superior and posterior to the uterus, as well as superior to the bladder. Note that the rectovesical pouch in the female extends deeper into the pelvis than in the male. Finally, one should also look at the uterus for the presence of a fetus.

Subxiphoid view

The probe is placed below the xiphoid process, with the probe held 'overhand', pointing almost parallel to the abdominal wall to insonate through the left lobe of the liver to the contents of the mediastinum. The probe may need to be angulated slightly towards the patient's left. In this view, fluid in the pericardial sac around the heart may be clearly seen as a

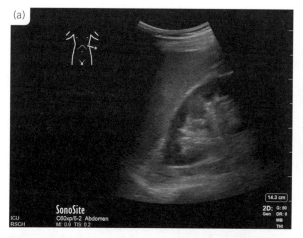
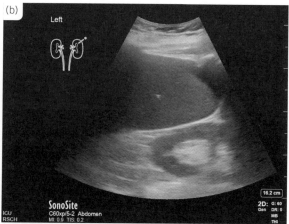

Figure 24.3 (a) Normal splenorenal angle. (b) Fluid around the spleen. A very thin rim of fluid in the splenorenal angle, with more obvious fluid between the spleen and diaphragm.

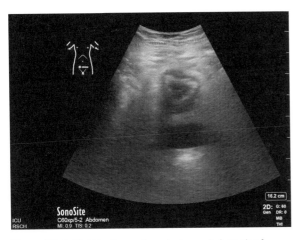

Figure 24.4 Fluid in the rectovesical pouch (pouch of Douglas). The bladder is empty due to catheterization.

hypoechoic rim (Figure 24.5). The fluid's effect on the (right) ventricle may be seen, although temporal resolution will be low, unless a formal echocardiography probe is used, and signs of ventricular compromise may confirm a clinical diagnosis of cardiac tamponade (Video 2.1.1 📷).

Anterior thorax

To complete the extended E-FAST scan, the anterior thorax is scanned bilaterally to exclude the presence of a pneumothorax. Depending on the body habitus of the patient, better resolution for assessment may be gained by switching to a high-frequency, high-resolution linear probe. Both lungs are assessed

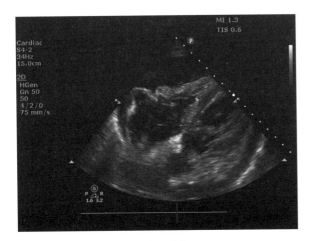

Figure 24.5 Fluid in the pericardial sac.

for the presence of lung sliding, which rules out a pneumothorax (Chapter 15). To confirm the diagnosis of pneumothorax, a lung point needs to be identified by moving the probe both inferiorly and laterally.

Pitfalls/limitations

Just as the absence of detectable free fluid does not indicate absence of haemorrhage, not all detected free fluid is haemorrhage. Intra-peritoneal fluid may also be a result of urine (bladder rupture), ascites (pre-existing comorbid disease), ruptured cyst fluid (e.g. of ovarian origin), bowel contents (from perforation or rupture), or amniotic fluid (in the pregnant trauma victim). It is normal for some menstruating women to have free fluid in the pelvis.

Interpleural fluid detected in an E-FAST scan may also represent the findings of pre-existing disease.

Any fluid detected must be considered in the clinical context.

In the right upper quadrant, the gall bladder, colonic hepatic flexure, IVC, and hepatic veins may be confused for fluid in the hands of an unskilled operator. On the left, a fluid-only-filled stomach may resemble free fluid, and in each case, care should be taken to describe the boundaries of the fluid. This is especially true with fluid around the diaphragm, the orientation of which must be discerned.

Obtaining subxiphoid views may be particularly challenging in the obese patient. A distended stomach, filled with air following overzealous bag–mask ventilation, can cause significant difficulty in this view, as will the presence of substantial intra-peritoneal air. Under these circumstances, recourse to formal echocardiography may have to be undertaken. Epicardial fat may sometimes be confused for pericardial fluid. It is not usually as echo-free as fluid and is generally seen anterior to the RV only.

Summary

FAST (and E-FAST) scanning is a valuable tool in the assessment of the trauma patient. It should be considered as an extension of physical examination, and when integrated with this, its immediacy and ability to detect the consequences of blunt and penetrating trauma have proven to reduce the time to commence surgery and improve survival.

✓ Multiple choice questions

Interactive multiple choice questions to test your knowledge can be found in the Online appendix at www.oxfordmedicine.com/focusedicu. Please refer to your access card for further details.

25

Advanced echocardiography: sepsis

Susanna Price and Guido Tavazzi

Introduction

Although superficially, some of the echocardiographic features of septic shock may resemble hypovolaemia, the pathophysiology is profoundly different. Echocardiography can be useful to evaluate the pathophysiological effects on the heart and circulation, as well as potentially demonstrate a cardiac source of sepsis, including infection related to intra-cardiac devices or endocarditis.

This chapter will introduce the key features to address in sepsis using echocardiography, including:

- Volaemic status: requirement for, and tolerance to, volume
- Alteration in myocardial function
- When sepsis is associated with ARDS, assessment of right heart function for potential extracorporeal support
- Differentiation of pulmonary oedema from ARDS
- Changes in PASP and/or pulmonary vascular resistance
- Exclusion/diagnosis of the underlying cause of sepsis, including endocarditis.

Hypovolaemia

A number of static and dynamic echocardiographic and US parameters may be used to suggest hypovolaemia and predict how the patient will respond to volume loading by increasing their cardiac output in response to a volume load. These include the static parameters of LVEDA (<5.5 cm²/m²) and IVC end-expiratory dimension of <1 cm in spontaneously breathing patients (or <1.5 cm with PPV). Dynamic echocardiographic parameters (Figure 25.1) include the respiratory variation in peak aortic velocities, the IVC distensibility index, and the SVC collapsibility

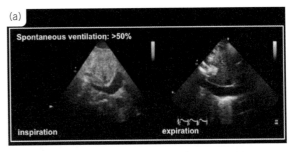

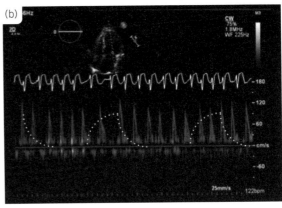

Figure 25.1 Echo parameters used to demonstrate potential responsiveness to volume loading in (a) spontaneous breathing and (b) positive pressure ventilation. (a) During inspiration, the IVC (subcostal view) collapses. Where this exceeds 50%, it may indicate that the patient will respond to volume loading by increasing cardiac output. (b) Trans-mitral PW Doppler (A4C view) in a patient with hypovolaemia. Note the increase in trans-mitral velocities shortly during inspiration (with a short delay for pulmonary transit time) shown in the green broken line. This is the opposite effect of that seen in spontaneous ventilation where left-sided Doppler velocities decrease with inspiration. For a colour version of this figure, please see colour plate section.

index. These have been mainly validated in the critical care patient population and are discussed further in Chapter 13. It is important, when using any such parameter, to consider the caveats/exclusions in their use, particularly in the presence of significant cardiac and/or respiratory disease, and also the mode of ventilation, in order to avoid misapplication and misinterpretation.

Tolerance to volume loading

Progressive volume resuscitation leads eventually to rising LAP (and pulmonary oedema), but with

no further increase in SV. A number of echocardiographic parameters have been used to substitute for LAP estimation, including the trans-mitral filling pattern: ratio of early/late diastolic flow (E/A), deceleration time of early diastolic flow (E deceleration time), ratio of peak early trans-mitral blood velocity/early systolic annular velocity (E/e'), pulmonary venous Doppler deceleration time, and M-mode colour Doppler propagation velocities (Figure 25.2). Although frequently used in the outpatient setting, they are not well validated in the critically ill where they are generally used in various combinations but still only provide

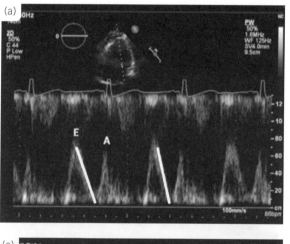

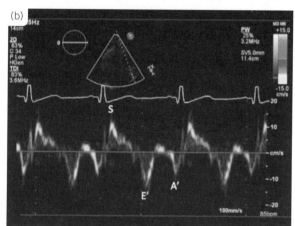

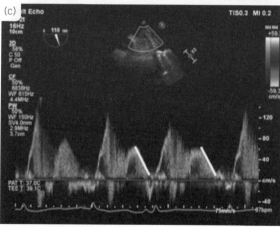

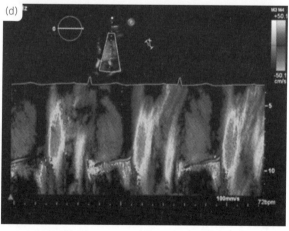

Figure 25.2 Echocardiographic modalities used for estimation of left atrial pressure in a patient with normal cardiac function. (a) Normal trans-mitral PW Doppler in a young patient, showing dominant early trans-mitral filling (E), compared with the peak late diastolic filling resulting from atrial contraction (A). The E deceleration time (red line) is normal (120–200 ms). (b) Tissue Doppler imaging of the lateral mitral annulus, showing the systolic velocity (S) and early (E') and late (A') annular diastolic velocities. The E'/A' is >1 and E/E' <8, consistent with non-elevated left atrial pressure. (c) Transoesophageal echo showing PW Doppler of the right upper pulmonary vein, with the deceleration slope of diastolic flow (solid white line) of >150 cm/s. (d) Trans-mitral M-mode colour velocity propagation time (transthoracic echo, A4C view), with the first aliasing velocity of >50 cm/s. These parameters are used in combination to support non-elevated versus elevated left atrial pressure estimation. For a colour version of this figure, please see colour plate section.

an estimate of a range of potential LAP measurements. In the presence of variable pulmonary inflammation, these parameters become even less helpful when trying to predict whether a patient may tolerate additional volume loading without developing pulmonary oedema, unless the LAP is clearly significantly elevated. Here, LUS may be used to detect the presence of interstitial oedema early, before radiographic changes and deterioration in oxygenation. It may also be used to help differentiate between pure CPO (homogenously distributed B-lines) and lung inflammation (inhomogenous presence of B-lines associated with subpleural and lobar consolidation). However, the two pathologies may coexist.

Ventricular function

Sepsis is frequently associated with a relatively high cardiac output and hyperkinetic biventricular systolic function. The LV is rarely dilated, except in the presence of underlying cardiac disease. Transient diffuse hypokinesia is occasionally observed, although the cardiac output usually remains elevated. If hyperdynamic biventricular function is not observed (i.e. measured ventricular function is 'normal'), this suggests relative myocardial functional impairment. Intrinsic depression of right ventricular function may be seen in up to 30% of patients, manifest by hypokinesia and associated with a variable degree of right ventricular dilatation. Where sepsis is associated with severe acute respiratory failure/ARDS, right ventricular function must be interpreted in the context of the current arterial blood gas analysis and increased intrathoracic pressure.

Emerging studies have suggested the potential use of speckle-tracking echocardiography (kinetic analysis of the myocardium's naturally occurring pattern) to detect ventricular dysfunction in septic shock when standard measures are normal, although this has been predominantly in the paediatric patient population. Here, abnormalities in circumferential and longitudinal strain, strain rate, rotational velocity, and radial displacement have been demonstrated, even in the presence of a normal EF. This remains a research tool at present, as its clinical application is unclear.

Systemic vascular resistance

A number of echocardiographic parameters have been proposed to estimate systemic vascular resistance in the outpatient population. However, there are no reliable and reproducible parameters applicable in the critically ill.

Pulmonary vascular resistance and pulmonary artery pressure

A degree of PHT (even if mild) and/or elevated pulmonary vascular resistance is common in sepsis, and when severe, these may result in acute right ventricular failure. This may occur in the context of normal PAPs, in particular where right ventricular failure is severe.

Estimation of pulmonary vascular resistance

Parameters used in critical care echocardiography have largely been extrapolated from the outpatient population (Figure 25.3). In patients with PHT, a pulmonary acceleration time (PAT) of <90 ms (normal 135 ms ± 25) is considered to be associated with elevated pulmonary vascular resistance. The presence of a mid-systolic notch on pulmonary artery Doppler, sampled using PW Doppler, is associated with severely raised PASP and pulmonary vascular resistance.

Estimation of pulmonary artery systolic pressure

The technique using echocardiographically derived TR velocities to estimate the PASP is widespread, whereby $PASP = 4(TR\ vel)^2 + RAP$, and is covered in Chapter 8. A number of caveats exist, including absence of TR, beam flow angulation, underestimation in the context of severe TR, and questionable accuracy in the context of arrhythmia. TR velocities must always be interpreted in terms of the right ventricular function and the estimated pulmonary vascular resistance, in particular, because they have only been validated in patients with normal right ventricular systolic function.

Sepsis and endocarditis

In addition to the cardiovascular effects of sepsis, echocardiography can be used to eliminate/diagnose

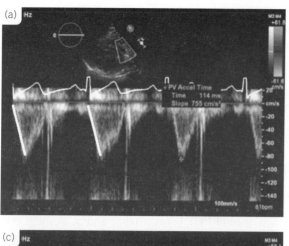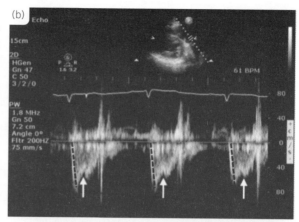
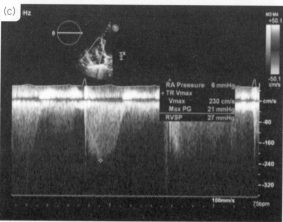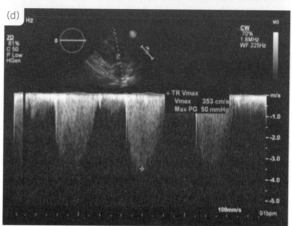

Figure 25.3 Doppler features of normal and elevated pulmonary vascular resistance and pulmonary hypertension. (a) PAT: the time from the onset of pulmonary flow to its peak is measured using PW Doppler (solid green line). An average of at least three beats (sinus rhythm) should be taken, with care not to overestimate the peak, in particular where the gain is too high. Here, the PAT is 114 ms, indicating normal pulmonary vascular resistance. (b) PAT in a patient with significantly elevated pulmonary vascular resistance. Note the very short PAT (<80 ms, broken green lines) and the mid-systolic notch (solid white arrow). (c) PASP estimated in a patient with normal pulmonary artery pressure undergoing positive pressure ventilation, measured by using CW Doppler across the tricuspid valve (A4C view). In the miniaturized 2D image, colour Doppler is used to align the CW Doppler to the regurgitant jet. Using the echo machine software, the peak velocity between the RV and RA is measured as 21 mmHg, and with an RAP of 6 mmHg, the PASP is estimated at 27 mmHg. (d) CW Doppler across the tricuspid valve of a patient with acute pulmonary hypertension. The pressure difference between the RV and RA is estimated at 50 mmHg, and with a measured RAP of 10 mmHg, the PASP is estimated at 60 mmHg. For a colour version of this figure, please see colour plate section.

intra-cardiac causes of sepsis, including endocarditis, and catheter-/device-related infection (Figure 25.4). The intensivist approaching any patient with sepsis should have a high index of suspicion of potential intra-cardiac infection, in particular in patients with valvular disease (including prosthetic valve replacement/implantation), those with intra-cardiac catheters/devices, and those with congenital heart disease. This is a highly specialized field, and echocardiography for confirmed or suspected endocarditis should be performed by an expert. However, there are certain important considerations regarding the interpretation of studies in this context:

- A negative TTE does not exclude endocarditis. Where suspected, but the TTE is non-diagnostic, expert TOE should be performed.

- There should be a low threshold for undertaking expert TOE, in particular in patients with catheter-related bloodstream *Staphylococcus aureus* infection, as it has a high propensity to cause endocarditis.

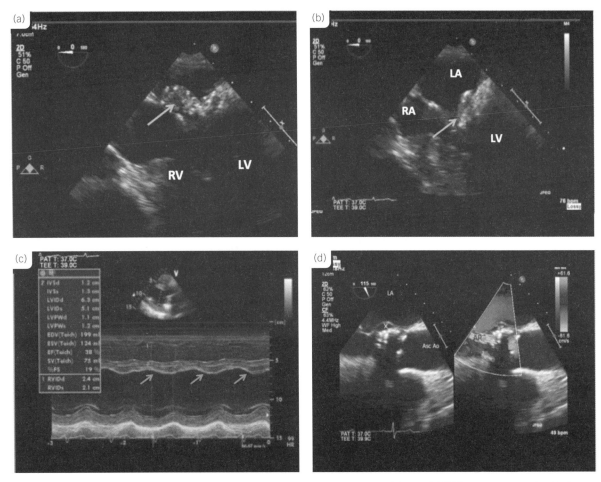

Figure 25.4 Some of the echocardiographic features of infective endocarditis. (a) and (b) TOE in a patient with mitral valve endocarditis, with a large vegetation (arrow) seen prolapsing into the LA during systole (a) and into the LV during diastole (b). (c) TTE parasternal long-axis view showing M-mode across the IVS and LV in a patient presenting with clinical features suggestive of pneumonia (bilateral pulmonary infiltrates on chest radiograph, hypoxia, elevated inflammatory markers). The patient had undergone mitral valve surgery 10 years previously. The septum shows normalization of movement (arrows), and in this clinical context, mitral valve dysfunction should be suspected and TOE performed to exclude endocarditis. (d) TOE (LVOT view, zoomed on the aortic valve) in a patient with aortic valve endocarditis and an associated root abscess (X). The valve is thickened and abnormal, and there is aortic regurgitation. Asc Ao, ascending aorta; LA, left atrium. For a colour version of this figure, please see colour plate section.

- Normalization of septal motion on TTE (parasternal long-axis M-mode) in a patient with previous AV and/or MV replacement should raise suspicion of valve malfunction. In the context of sepsis, paraprosthetic regurgitation due to endocarditis should be formally excluded, using expert TOE.

- In a patient with previous MV and/or AV replacement presenting with pneumonia and with a dynamic LV on TTE (with normalized septal motion), the diagnosis should be revised

to pulmonary oedema (infected) with valve malfunction, until proven otherwise. Expert TOE is indicated.

- Mobile masses are frequently seen with central cannulae and pacing systems. Their presence alone does not indicate line/system infection (echocardiography does not provide a histological or microbiological diagnosis), and expert consultation is warranted. In some patients where TOE is unhelpful, intra-cardiac echocardiography has been suggested.

• Non-valvular endocarditis is possible [aortic cannulation site, Eustachian valve, ventricular septal defect (VSD) patch]. For each, TOE to exclude/diagnose endocarditis/intra-cardiac infection and expert evaluation of the heart are indicated.

Approximately 0.8% of admissions to the general ICU are due to endocarditis, generally due to haemodynamic instability/heart failure related to sepsis and/or severe valvular pathology. Despite advances in treatment, mortality remains between 29% and 84% in critically ill patients. Guidelines exist for the investigation and management of patients with endocarditis (including suspected endocarditis). The diagnostic criteria for infective endocarditis in the ICU are identical to those in the non-ICU patient population. Echocardiography in this situation demands real expertise and should not be undertaken by a non-expert. Early discussion with the cardiology team, including review with high-quality imaging, is mandatory.

Conclusion

The potential applications for echocardiography in the evaluation of sepsis and septic shock are numerous. As with all echocardiography in the acute/critical context, it should be undertaken as an extension to clinical examination and always interpreted within the clinical context. There are, however, many potential pitfalls when applying standard echocardiography in this setting, and the user must be mindful of these when interpreting echo findings, in particular with respect to volaemic status and ventricular function. Finally,

evaluation of patients with valvular disease and sepsis is complex and demands an expert to perform and interpret, as endocarditis is a potentially lethal condition, which can be missed by the non-expert, with potentially lethal consequences to the patient.

✓ Multiple choice questions

Interactive multiple choice questions to test your knowledge can be found in the Online appendix at www.oxfordmedicine.com/focusedicu. Please refer to your access card for further details.

Further reading

Arkles JS, Opotowsky AR, Ojeda J, *et al*. Shape of the right ventricular Doppler envelope predicts hemodynamics and right heart function in pulmonary hypertension. *American Journal of Respiratory and Critical Care Medicine* 2011;**183**:268–76.

Charron C, Caille V, Jardin F, *et al*. Echocardiographic measurement of fluid responsiveness. *Current Opinion in Critical Care* 2006;**12**:249–54.

Habib G, Lancellotti P, Antunes MJ, *et al*. 2015 ESC Guidelines for the management of infective endocarditis: The Task Force for the Management of Infective Endocarditis of the European Society of Cardiology (ESC) Endorsed by: European Association for Cardio-Thoracic Surgery (EACTS), the European Association of Nuclear Medicine (EANM). *European Heart Journal* 2015;**36**:3075–128.

Oh JK, Park SJ, Nagueh SF. Established and novel clinical applications of diastolic function assessment by echocardiography. *Circulation: Cardiovascular Imaging* 2011;**4**:444–55.

Tossavainen E, Söderberg S, Grönlund C, *et al*. Pulmonary artery acceleration time in identifying pulmonary hypertension patients with raised pulmonary vascular resistance. *European Heart Journal: Cardiovascular Imaging* 2013;**14**:890–7.

26

Acute kidney injury

Alex Harrison

Introduction

US assessment of the urinary tract is frequently undertaken to identify post-renal or obstructive causes of renal failure. This chapter describes the normal renal sonoanatomy and the technique for scanning the renal tract, including the bladder. The sonographic features of the common pathology that may be identified are described, including the classification of hydronephrosis. The advanced section introduces the role of US in assessing renal perfusion.

Role of ultrasound

Acute kidney injury (AKI) is common in critical illness and is categorized by a change in serum creatinine levels or severity of oliguria (Table 26.1). The majority of AKI is due to 'pre-renal' factors such as sepsis, hypotension, and hypoperfusion. Therefore, in AKI, assessments of the patient's intravascular volume and cardiac output status are necessary (these are described in Chapter 13).

Up to 15% of AKI is 'post-renal' (i.e. due to obstruction to urinary flow and drainage). US is of critical use in the identification of this group of patients, as it can rapidly and effectively identify any distension of the renal tract, suggesting urinary obstruction. The main US signs of urinary obstruction are a distended bladder or hydronephrosis.

Basic sonoanatomy

The kidneys are retroperitoneal organs, sitting between T12 and L3. They are between 9 and 14 cm in

Table 26.1 Stages of acute kidney injury

Stage	Serum creatinine	Urine output
1	Rise of ≥26 μmol/L within 48 hours OR rise to ≥1.5–1.9 times baseline within 1 week	<0.5 mL/kg/hour For >6 consecutive hours
2	Rise to ≥2.0–2.9 times baseline	<0.5 mL/kg/hour For >12 hours
3	Rise to ≥3.0 times baseline OR rise to ≥354 μmol/L OR commenced on renal replacement therapy, irrespective of stage	<0.3 mL/kg/hour For >24 hours OR anuria for 12 hours

Reproduced from Springer *Nature: BMC, Critical Care*, **11**:R31, 'Acute Kidney Injury Network: report of an initiative to improve outcomes in acute kidney injury', Mehta *et al*. Copyright © 2007 Mehta *et al*.; licensee BioMed Central Ltd. Published under the terms of the creative Commons Attribution 2.0 Generic license (https://creativecommons.org/licenses/by/2.0/).

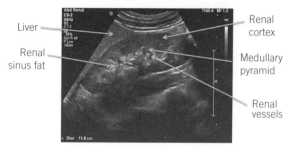

Figure 26.1 Ultrasound image showing a normal right kidney.

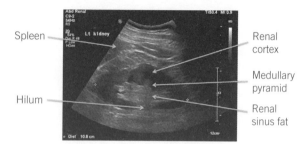

Figure 26.2 Ultrasound image showing a normal left kidney.

length. The left kidney is slightly bigger and is usually 1–2 cm higher than the right (the right being displaced downwards by the liver). A difference in >1.5 cm in length is significant.

The main vessels and ureter enter the kidney at the medial hilum.

On US, the kidney has a smooth outline and is surrounded by fat. Just under the capsule sits the renal cortex and medullary pyramids, with the highly echogenic renal sinus fat at the centre of the kidney (Figures 26.1 and 26.2). For reference, normal liver should be more echogenic than healthy renal cortex.

The renal pelvis is usually collapsed, and the ureter can be hard to identify on US.

Common anatomical variants

Renal cysts

Simple cysts are commonly seen on renal US. Simple cysts are associated with ageing and with CKD of any type.

They may vary in size and position, and their presence may confuse the inexperienced operator. Parapelvic cysts may mimic hydronephrosis.

Multiple cysts within enlarged kidneys are suggestive of polycystic kidney disease. There are associated liver cysts in up to 80% of cases.

Common congenital abnormalities

Duplex kidneys have two ureters and therefore often have two identifiable renal pelvices. There may be pathology affecting only one moiety.

In horseshoe kidney, there is midline fusion of the renal tissue. There may be other associated anatomical abnormalities, including duplex kidney.

Renal transplants

Renal transplants are usually grafted onto the external iliac vessels in the pelvis. There may be long-standing dilatation of the renal pelvis; find previous imaging for comparison.

Admission of a renal transplant recipient to a critical care environment should prompt a discussion with the local nephrology service.

Chronic kidney disease

Patients with CKD may have a normal renal US, although there may be increasing cortical echogenicity, loss of cortical thickness, and renal atrophy with advanced CKD. Small kidneys (<8 cm) are abnormal.

Imaging the kidneys

A formal US assessment of the kidneys would include imaging in a decubitus position, frequently with the ipsilateral arm over the head. This is often not possible in the critically ill patient; therefore, a technique appropriate for assessment of the supine patient is described.

Use a curved linear array probe with the highest frequency which achieves adequate views. In thin patients or children, a frequency of 7 MHz can be used, whereas 2–3 MHz may be required for larger patients. A phased array probe may be used if the acoustic window is very small.

Right kidney

Place the probe in an anterior subcostal position, and angle the transducer obliquely (posteromedially) to gain a longitudinal view of the kidney through the right

(a)

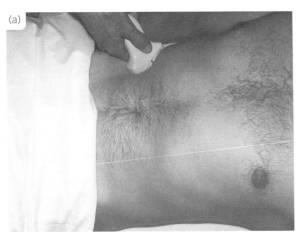

(b)

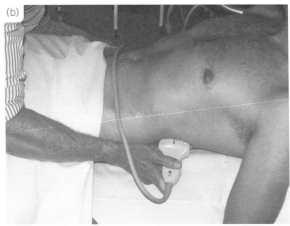

Figure 26.3 (a) Right anterior oblique probe position: provides a longitudinal image through the right lobe of the liver. (b) Left coronal probe position: recommended starting point to obtain a longitudinal image of the left kidney.

lobe of the liver (Figure 26.3a). The view may improve after inspiration, as the liver and kidney move down. The coronal view is gained by sliding the probe round laterally to between the iliac crest and costal margin. Scan the whole kidney from anterior to posterior.

From the position which gives the best longitudinal view, rotate the probe 90° to obtain views of the kidney in a transverse section, and scan the whole kidney from superior to inferior.

Left kidney

The left kidney can be harder to image with the patient supine. It is in a higher position, protected by the rib-cage, and there is a limited acoustic window afforded by the spleen.

Start with a coronal approach (as described in Right kidney, p. 221), and then scan between the ribs and through the spleen, varying the position until the kidney is visualized (Figure 26.3c). The view may be improved by a more posterior oblique approach (scan with the patient in right lateral tilt) or by extending the left arm above the head. Separate views of upper and lower poles may be needed. Scan the whole kidney from anterior to posterior.

Rotate the probe to gain transverse images, and scan the whole kidney from superior to inferior.

Renal length is determined by varying the view, so as to achieve the largest value, and is measured from capsule to capsule. Try not to accidentally foreshorten the kidney, as one pole may be easily obscured by bowel gas or overlying ribs.

Renal pathology in critical illness

The US images are normal in most cases of AKI. Increased cortical echogenicity is a non-specific sign which may be seen in AKI and CKD. Urinary obstruction is the most important renal diagnosis to make in the assessment of the anuric patient.

Hydronephrosis

Where there is obstruction to the flow of urine out of the kidneys, there is distension of the renal pelvis, termed hydronephrosis. The US appearance is an echo-free area in the centre of the kidney, surrounded by the echogenic renal sinus fat. Four grades of hydronephrosis are described (Table 26.2 and Figure 26.4).

Unilateral hydronephrosis should not cause anuria, unless the contralateral kidney is non-functioning. The absence of hydronephrosis and an empty bladder make obstruction unlikely.

Hydronephrosis may be absent where obstruction is of very recent onset or when there is associated oliguria from another cause (e.g. hypoperfusion). The relationship between severity of obstruction (and/or the degree of AKI) with the grade of hydronephrosis on US is not fixed, and any degree of hydronephrosis in this context should be taken seriously. Grade 4 hydronephrosis suggests long-standing obstruction, as there is evidence of cortical atrophy.

Percutaneous nephrostomy is facilitated by greater distension of the renal calyces.

Table 26.2 Progressive states of hydronephrosis

Grade	Ultrasonographic description
1	Mild dilatation of the renal pelvis; calyces remain normal
2	Mild dilatation of both pelvis and calyces; pelvicalyceal pattern is maintained
3	Moderate dilatation of both pelvis and calyces; blunting of the calyceal fornices and flattening of the papillae
4	Severe dilatation of both pelvis and calyces, with loss of borders between the pelvis and calyces; evidence of renal atrophy (cortical thinning)

© The Society of Fetal Urology.

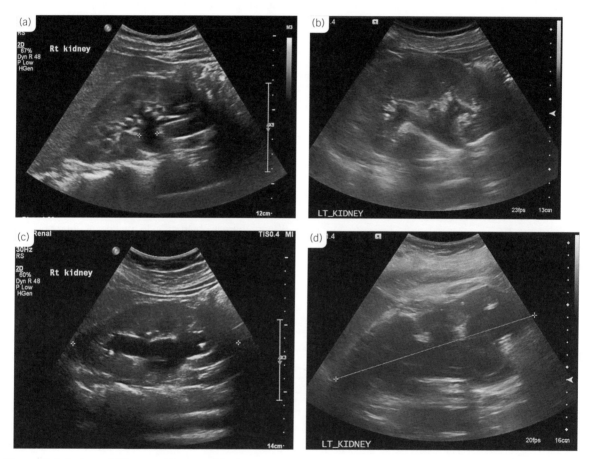

Figure 26.4 (a, b, c, d) Ultrasound images of the four stages of hydronephrosis.

If appearances of hydronephrosis are present and the bladder is empty, then the differential includes:

- Obstruction at the level of the ureter
- Recently relieved distal obstruction (e.g. by bladder catheterization)
- Extrarenal pelvis
- Parapelvic renal cyst
- Ureteric reflux
- Megaureter.

If hydronephrosis is identified, look for distension of the bladder and the presence of calculi in the kidney, ureter, or bladder.

Previous images are crucial for differentiating current anatomy from baseline. Prolonged obstruction leads to effacement of the calices and thinning of the renal cortex (Figure 26.4d). These kidneys may be of reduced function but could still be a cause for sepsis if there is associated pyonephrosis.

Pyonephrosis

The identification of low-level echoes in the distended renal pelvis of a septic patient, particularly with a tender kidney, suggests pyonephrosis. This should be urgently drained to provide source control and to prevent further renal parenchymal damage. Drainage can be achieved with either retrograde ureteric stenting or percutaneous nephrostomy.

Pyelonephritis

The US is often normal in ascending infection. Focal infection of renal tissue may lead to an area of decreased echogenicity with swelling and local tenderness. Renal abscesses are rarely echo-free. It may be impossible to distinguish an abscess with drainable pus from an area of inflammation.

Calculi

Calculi appear as echogenic foci with posterior acoustic shadowing, which is usually present once the stone is over 3–4 mm in width (Figure 26.5). It is easier to identify with a higher-frequency probe.

'Tumble artefact' or 'twinkle artefact', seen in approximately 80% of stones, is characteristic (a rapidly fluctuating mixture of colour Doppler signals occurring just behind a stone).

A staghorn calculus filling the renal pelvis is easily missed, as the echogenic stone is surrounded by similarly echogenic renal sinus tissue. The presence of deep acoustic shadowing should alert the operator to its presence.

Masses and tumours

Renal cell carcinoma is the most common malignancy of the kidney. These tumours are often found incidentally during imaging for another reason. The grey-scale appearances of renal cell carcinoma are similar to that of the renal cortex, and US is not the best modality for investigating renal masses. Therefore, clinical decisions should not be predicated on the nature of a renal mass identified by a non-expert.

Imaging the bladder and ureters

Ureters are hard to see with US, particularly in the supine patient.

The bladder is a muscular sac, with a wall that is usually 3 mm thick when the bladder is distended, but 5 mm or more when empty. The normal bladder capacity is 150–400 mL, and the bladder should empty almost completely. To image the bladder with US, it should be full.

Place a curved linear probe just above the symphysis pubis in the midline. Push firmly and angle

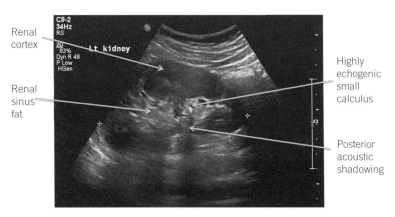

Figure 26.5 (a, b) Ultrasound image showing renal calculus with posterior acoustic shadowing.

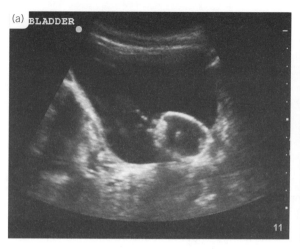 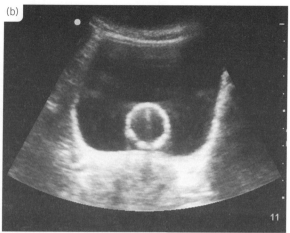

Figure 26.6 (a) Sagittal plane view of the bladder. (b) Transverse view of the bladder Urinary catheter balloon clearly visible.

down into the pelvis. Examine in both the transverse and sagittal planes (Figure 26.6a and b).

The bladder is roughly symmetrical and more or less square on transverse section and triangular on sagittal section. Bladder volume (cm³) may be estimated as (1/2 × width × depth × height) (each in centimetres).

A distended bladder suggests either neurogenic problems or obstruction of the urethra (e.g. by prostatic hypertrophy, blood clot, a blocked catheter, stone, or tumour). The balloon of a urinary catheter is easily identified (Figure 26.6 a and b).

The wall of the bladder should be smooth. On the posterior wall of the bladder, two small bumps may be identified on either side of the midline—these are the ureteric orifices.

Ureteric jets may be seen as the ureters empty urine (by peristalsis) into the bladder. These are symmetrical. They can be seen with power Doppler (a more sensitive type of colour Doppler) as small linear perturbations arising from the ureteric orifices in the otherwise echo-free space of the full bladder.

Advanced ultrasonography

Renal perfusion assessment

The majority of AKI is 'pre-renal' in nature. Biochemical markers and urine output measurements provide only limited information about kidney function, and particularly which treatment strategies are likely to result in resolution of AKI. US techniques that incorporate the Doppler principle may offer additional information with regard to renal perfusion. Currently, they remain largely research tools and are not recommended for routine use in the management of AKI in critically ill patients (Ichai *et al.*, 2016).

Arterial occlusion will lead to absent perfusion. Power Doppler gives the simplest images of absent renal perfusion. The most common cause for this is embolism, but it may also occur in prothrombotic states, in trauma, or as a consequence of arterial dissection.

Venous occlusion may cause reversal of arterial flow during diastole.

Any pathology within the kidney may affect blood flow through the kidney. Renal blood flow is measured using PW Doppler (the artery being identified with colour Doppler) and described as the resistive index (RI). RI is a measure of pulsatile blood flow that

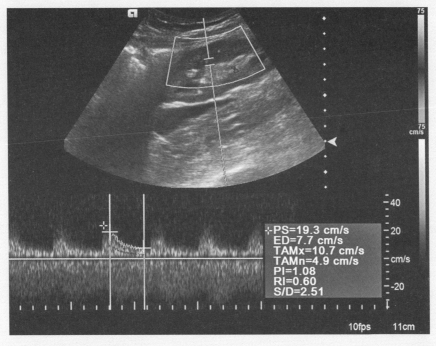

PS=19.3 cm/s
ED=7.7 cm/s
TAMx=10.7 cm/s
TAMn=4.9 cm/s
PI=1.08
RI=0.60
S/D=2.51

Figure 26.7 Renal RI measurement and the waveform produced. For a colour version of this figure, please see colour plate section.

reflects the downstream resistance to flow within the microcirculation (Figure 26.7).

Unfortunately, the movement of the kidney with respiration can make assessment of the waveform challenging, particularly in critically ill patients.

Resistive index
= (peak systolic velocity – end-diastolic velocity)
/peak systolic velocity

This should be calculated from assessment of interlobar arterial waveforms in the upper, middle, and lower poles of the kidney and averaged. A normal RI is 0.60, and most authorities would agree that values over 0.70 are abnormal.

Many conditions causing AKI can cause a rise in the RI. For example, in septic AKI, there is usually a reduction in peak systolic velocity, with an increase in diastolic velocity, resulting in an overall rise in RI (to perhaps 0.72–0.85). However, an increase in the interstitial pressure within the (encapsulated) kidney may lead to reduction in overall perfusion, particularly during diastole. This occurs commonly with intra-abdominal hypertension, fluid overload, and hydronephrosis, which have all been associated with an elevated RI.

Measured RI early on in critical illness has been shown to be associated with subsequent development of AKI, and additionally, some correlation has been demonstrated between a rise in RI and the need for renal replacement therapy and also the likelihood of quick recovery of AKI (Ninet *et al.*, 2015). Clinical and experimental studies have suggested that the correlation between RI and true vascular resistance or actual renal blood flow is weak. Most studies on RI are small, single-centre observational studies by enthusiasts. There is significant heterogeneity in their results and the cut-off values of RI used to differentiate patient groups.

Doppler studies of the kidney have several limitations. They are operator-dependent yet seem to have good inter-observer reliability between experts, but less so between inexperienced operators. In addition, there is significant potential for confounding here. The same numerical RI may be manifested by varying combinations of flow and resistance. Age and previous renal disease may affect vascular compliance, and RI is affected by interstitial renal pressure and intra-abdominal pressure. Hypoxia increases RI, and the relationship between RI and mean arterial pressure is variable. Furthermore, the arterial waveform may be affected by reduced left ventricular function leading to reduced peak systolic velocity, and in tachycardic states, the end-diastolic velocity is overestimated. Nonetheless, this is an area of potential future research.

An alternative technique to assess renal cortical perfusion makes use of contrast-enhanced US. This technique may be more accurate than Doppler-based tools but requires administration of microbubble US contrast agents and more advanced scanning software and hardware. However, the predictive value of these tools remain to be validated in clinical practice (Schnell and Darmon, 2015).

✅ Multiple choice questions

Interactive multiple choice questions to test your knowledge can be found in the Online appendix at www.oxfordmedicine.com/focusedicu. Please refer to your access card for further details.

Further reading

Ichai C, Vinsonneau C, Souweine B, *et al*. Acute kidney injury in the perioperative period and in intensive care units (excluding renal replacement therapies). *Annals of Intensive Care* 2016;**6**:48.

Ninet S, Schnell D, Dewitte A, Zeni F, Meziani F, Darmon M. Doppler-based renal resistive index for prediction of renal dysfunction reversibility: a systematic review and meta-analysis. *Journal of Critical Care* 2015;**30**:629–35.

Schnell D, Darmon M. Bedside Doppler ultrasound for the assessment of renal perfusion in the ICU: advantages and limitations of the available techniques. *Critical Ultrasound Journal* 2015;**7**:24.

27

Acute respiratory distress syndrome

Kelly Victor, Justin Kirk-Bayley, and Nicholas Ioannou

Introduction

ARDS is an acute, diffuse, inflammatory lung injury, characterized by bilateral pulmonary infiltrates, increased pulmonary vascular permeability, and reduced lung compliance, that is not fully explained by cardiac failure or fluid overload and results in significant hypoxaemia.

Both echocardiography and LUS can play a significant role in the assessment of ARDS, both in terms of diagnosis and its complications, and an integrative approach can be extremely useful.

This chapter will review the targets for US assessment, including biventricular function, extravascular water, and systemic volume assessment. Importantly, it will discuss how to differentiate CPO from non-CPO, how to recognize ACP, and when to look for a PFO. The advanced section will introduce Doppler-based methods to evaluate right ventricular systolic function and PASP, which can both become compromised in ARDS.

Echocardiography in ARDS

In critically ill patients with ARDS, echocardiography can be used to evaluate right ventricular and right atrial size and function, estimate PA pressures, assess volume status and fluid responsiveness, monitor left ventricular function, and adapt the mechanical ventilation strategy. Echocardiography also has an important role in assessing, establishing, and monitoring patients with severe ARDS on extracorporeal support.

In critically ill patients with ARDS, obtaining good acoustic windows using TTE is often considered to be technically challenging. This may be attributed to high

levels of PEEP, heavily consolidated lung, fluid overload, patient positioning (e.g. prone position), and patient immobility. However, in experienced hands, adequate images can be obtained, and most critically ill patients will, at the very least, have a good-quality subcostal window that allows for direct visualization of the atria, ventricles, valves, pericardium, and IVC, albeit with limited capacity to perform haemodynamic measurements. Compared to TTE, TOE (Chapter 6) may provide better image quality of some cardiac structures. However, this is a more invasive technique that requires a higher level of technical expertise.

Lung ultrasound in ARDS

LUS (Chapter 16) can be used to identify the presence of pulmonary interstitial syndrome, evaluate extravascular lung water, and assist in differentiating between CPO and non-CPO.

Pulmonary interstitial syndrome is not a diagnosis, but a term given to a group of ultrasonographic features

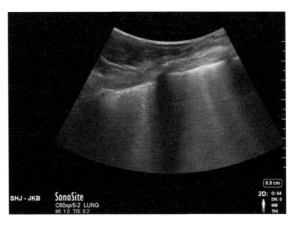

Figure 27.1 B-lines in ARDS.

> **Box 27.1** Defining features of B-lines
>
> - Hyperechoic (white) and clearly arise from the pleura
> - Narrow with clear definition
> - They spread out, without fading, as they descend down the screen
> - They obliterate 'A'-lines (pleural reverberation artefacts)
> - They move with the pleura, as it slides with respiration

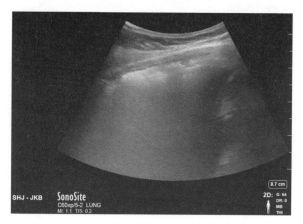

Figure 27.2 Subpleural consolidation in ARDS.

that indicate thickening of the interlobular septa, by increased extravascular lung water (from ARDS or CPO), inflammation, or fibrosis. The syndrome is characterized by the presence of multiple 'B-lines' on an US scan of the pleura (Figure 27.1 and Video 2.2.1 ⦿). These lines are entirely artefactual in origin and are of the 'comet tail' variety, but to be classified as B-lines, they must fulfil the strict criteria seen in Box 27.1.

The number of B-lines seen in one intercostal space may vary. While solitary B-lines may occur at normal lung bases, in interstitial syndrome, their number within each field and the number of intercostal spaces in which they are seen increase, such that they become almost confluent throughout the lungs, generating echogenic homogeneity throughout the lung field.

Diagnosing ARDS

While the diagnostic criteria of ARDS does not currently include US, the following LUS features are supportive in a patient with acute hypoxaemic respiratory failure:

1. B-lines. As alveolar permeability varies throughout the lung fields, so do the number and distribution of B-lines, equating to significant heterogeneity in the B-line pattern seen when scanning throughout the lung fields. There will be areas with none and adjacent intercostal spaces where many are seen (Figure 27.1).

2. Subpleural consolidation. Small areas of subpleural consolidation in the anterior of the lungs are frequently seen in ARDS. They too are

patchy and seen as hyperechoic, punctiform, or hepatized areas just below the pleural line (Figure 27.2 and Video 2.2.2 ⦿).

3. Pleural abnormalities. Pleural sliding is reduced in ARDS. This may be a feature of subpleural consolidation with locally restricted movement, but it may also relate to reduced lung compliance with generalized reduction in expansion seen at the pleural margin. In addition, the pleural line itself may be thickened, fragmented, and irregular (Figure 27.3 and Video 2.2.2 ⦿).

While posterior, dependent consolidation is often apparent in ARDS; its presence does not contribute to the diagnosis.

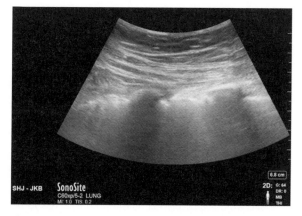

Figure 27.3 Pleural irregularity in ARDS.

Differentiating cardiogenic from non-cardiogenic pulmonary oedema

The diagnosis of ARDS relies on the exclusion of raised left ventricular filling pressure, which is usually associated with a dilated and poorly contractile LV. However, impaired left ventricular performance is also commonly seen in patients with ARDS. Therefore, left ventricular function should be assessed using echocardiography in all patients who develop severe respiratory failure.

Assessment of left ventricular contractility (Chapter 7) should include a visual estimate of EF (LVEF), using multiple echocardiographic windows. Left ventricular function can be graded as normal, hyperdynamic, or mildly, moderately, or severely impaired. In experienced hands, visual assessment can be made quickly and easily, and it correlates well with quantitative measurements.

Linear left ventricular dimensions, using 2D measurements taken in the PLAX view, can be used to calculate FS and LVEF. The modified Simpson's biplane method and 3D echocardiography both provide accurate and reproducible estimations of LVEF. However, these are rarely used in practice because they require good endocardial border delineation in the apical window, which often proves difficult in ARDS patients.

Left ventricular dysfunction may occur in ARDS patients as a result of severe hypoxaemia, pre-existing coronary disease, or underlying cardiomyopathy, secondary to right ventricular dysfunction due to ventricular interdependence, and as a consequence of metabolic acidaemia associated with severe organ failure. In such cases, LUS and the distribution and morphology of B-lines can help differentiate between CPO and ARDS.

The hydrostatic pressure transmitted from the left heart is uniform throughout the pulmonary venous system, save for the additional effects of gravity upon it. Consequently, cardiogenic oedema is homogenous and gravity-dependent. By contrast, pulmonary oedema seen in ARDS is heterogenous, as exhibited by patchy opacifications on chest X-ray and CT scans. B-line distribution reflects these differences.

The distance between individual B-lines at the pleural line also varies according to the pathology. B-lines separated by 7 mm (the distance equivalent to that of the superficial pleural projections of interlobular septa) correlate with the incidence of Kerley B-lines seen on chest X-ray and suggest CPO. B-lines separated by 3 mm correlate with ground-glass shadowing seen on CT and suggest ARDS.

Recognizing complications of ARDS

Acute cor pulmonale

ACP is defined as an acute increase in right ventricular afterload, characterized echocardiographically by right ventricular dilatation, impaired systolic function, and dyskinesia (paradoxical motion) of the IVS. ACP is common in patients with severe ARDS, with a historically reported incidence of 50–60%. However, the widespread use of lung-protective ventilation strategies appears to have reduced this incidence to approximately 20–30%. In patients with ARDS, ACP is independently associated with increased mortality, and if not reversed, ACP will cause progressive left ventricular failure, resulting in reduced cardiac output, systemic hypotension, and ultimately circulatory failure.

Echocardiographic assessment and diagnosis of ACP (Chapter 8) in patients with ARDS should include assessment of right atrial and right ventricular size, assessment of right ventricular systolic function, and estimation of PASP.

Right atrial dilatation

Under normal circumstances, the LA should be larger than the RA. The presence of a dilated RA with an IAS that bulges towards the LA is a useful indicator of right heart overload. This can be assessed using 2D echocardiography in A4C and subcostal views (Chapter 9).

Right ventricular dilatation

The RV is a thin-walled structure, and this reflects its relationship to the pulmonary circulation, which has low resistance and high capacitance. Small changes in pressure within the pulmonary circulation can have significant effects on the right heart; thus, both pulmonary disease and positive pressure mechanical ventilation may have adverse effects on the RV.

ARDS causes acute pressure overload of the RV, resulting in ACP (massive PE also causes this picture). Rapid and early right ventricular dilatation is associated with flattening of the IVS during early diastole, and a characteristic D-shaped appearance of the LV is seen on echocardiography. In the acute setting, the RV does not have time to hypertrophy, and acute pressure overload is indistinguishable echocardiographically from volume overload (as seen in tricuspid or pulmonary regurgitation or ASDs/VSDs). By contrast, chronic pressure overload (as seen in chronic respiratory disease) results in flattening of the IVS throughout diastole and systole; the RV becomes thickened and is able to generate much higher systolic pressures. A PSAX view at the level of the PMs should be obtained to fully assess IVS flattening and timing during the cardiac cycle (Figure 27.4 and Video 2.2.3 ■).

The RV has a complex crescent shape, with distinct structural and functional parts, requiring multiple acoustic windows and imaging planes to assess it comprehensively.

When assessing the RV, both its absolute and comparative size with the LV should be considered. An RV that appears the same size or larger than the LV is indicative of right ventricular dilatation. Furthermore, the position of the right ventricular apex can be used as an indicator of right ventricular enlargement. In a normal heart, the LV forms the cardiac apex. However,

in severe right ventricular enlargement, the RV may become the apex-forming ventricle. With this change in geometry, there may be a concomitant loss in the characteristic triangular shape of the RV in A4C (Figure 27.5, and Videos 2.2.4 and 2.2.5 ■).

Right ventricular systolic dysfunction

In critically ill patients, right ventricular systolic dysfunction most commonly occurs as a consequence of acute or chronic pulmonary disease, mechanical ventilation, and/or left ventricular dysfunction.

An initial estimate of right ventricular systolic function should be made visually, using multiple acoustic windows to assess longitudinal and radial contractility, in addition to both global and regional function.

In contrast to the LV, longitudinal contractility contributes to right ventricular emptying to a significantly greater extent than radial contractility. TAPSE is a useful and easy-to-obtain quantitative marker of right ventricular systolic function, performed in the A4C view. However, it should always be used in conjunction with other 2D signs such as FAC and septal motion.

Systemic hypovolaemia

Inadequate fluid resuscitation early in critical illness can be detrimental due to tissue hypoperfusion and organ dysfunction.

In the absence of hypertrophy, a small, vigorously contracting ('hyperdynamic') LV usually indicates low left ventricular preload (Chapter 13). In this setting, both LVEDA and LVESA (assessed in PLAX or PSAX view at PM level) are reduced, and when hypovolaemia is severe, 'kissing' PMs (or even complete obliteration of the left ventricular cavity) may also be seen at end-systole. Coexisting echocardiographic signs of low right ventricular preload will help to identify hypovolaemia and differentiate this from ACP.

The IVC can provide information regarding right ventricular preload in critically ill patients. This can be assessed using 2D imaging or M-mode (Figure 27.6 and Video 2.2.6 ■); if the latter is used, it is important to ensure that the changes in IVC diameter are genuinely indicative of respiratory variation, rather than movement artefact of the M-mode cursor away from the true midline axis of the IVC.

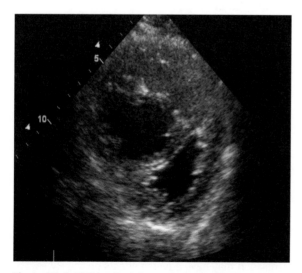

Figure 27.4 PLAX at the left ventricular papillary muscle level, demonstrating a dilated right ventricle and flattening of the interventricular septum.

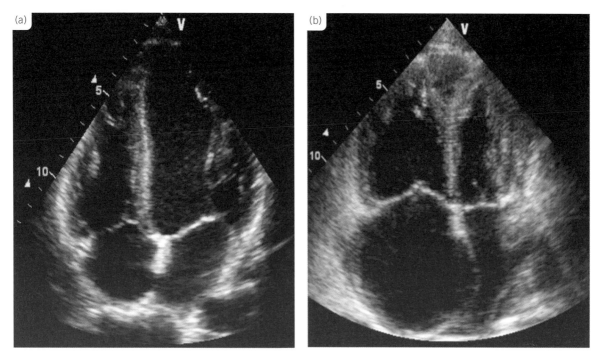

Figure 27.5 A4C images demonstrating: (a) normal-sized ventricles with normal systolic function; (b) a dilated right ventricle with low left ventricular preload.

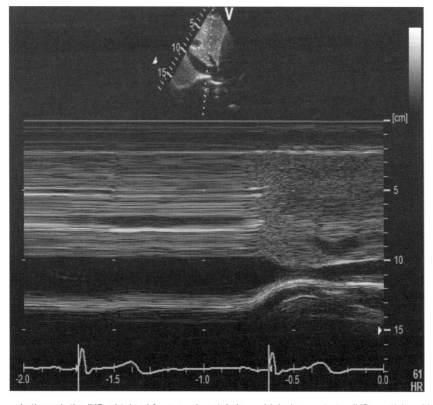

Figure 27.6 M-mode through the IVC, obtained from a subcostal view, which demonstrates IVC reactivity with respiration.

In patients mechanically ventilated with positive pressure, the IVC increases in diameter during inspiration and decreases in diameter during expiration; this is in contrast to spontaneously breathing patients when the opposite is true. Importantly, in mechanically ventilated patients, measurement of IVC diameter does not accurately reflect RAP, and respiratory reactivity of the IVC is often only seen in the context of a low or normal RAP.

An IVC distensibility index has been suggested to predict fluid responsiveness in mechanically ventilated patients. However, as a general rule, a small, collapsed IVC that increases in diameter during inspiration is likely to indicate fluid responsiveness and a large, dilated IVC (>2 cm) with no respiratory variability is likely to indicate a lack of fluid responsiveness.

Excessive fluid therapy

Excessive fluid administration can result in increased extravascular lung water and impaired right ventricular performance. In patients with ARDS, this is associated with increased morbidity, prolonged length of intensive care stay, and increased duration of mechanical ventilation; thus, a conservative approach to fluid therapy is recommended in the management of ARDS.

Though limited work is published specifically on ARDS, emerging evidence shows that B-line quantification and qualitative analysis correlate with extravascular lung water in a number of models and that there may be a linear relationship with the PaO_2/FiO_2 ratio. US can also demonstrate the response to fluid removal in ARDS by diminution in the numbers of B-lines and the areas containing them. These are all areas of current research, and LUS may go on to form part of critical care fluid de-resuscitation.

Assessing response to interventions

PEEP setting in lung-protective ventilation

Utilizing low-tidal volume ventilation (4–6 mL/kg ideal body weight) with a plateau pressure of <30 cmH$_2$O and a high PEEP to keep the lung 'open' is associated with improved survival in patients with ARDS.

However, although beneficial for lung recruitment, this strategy may have a detrimental effect on the pulmonary circulation, RV, and haemodynamics, which is reflected in the fact that the incidence of ACP remains high.

Using echocardiography to evaluate and monitor the RV may allow titration of mechanical ventilatory support, in order to find the optimal balance between beneficial recruitment of the lungs and overdistension, with its adverse effects on the heart and vasculature.

LUS may demonstrate areas of recruitment in response to titrated PEEP changes by demonstrating resolution of signs compatible with high extravascular lung water and resolution of areas showing atelectasis. However, as yet, it cannot be used to assess accurately for areas of hyperinflation.

Prone positioning

This has been shown to have a significant mortality benefit in critically ill patients with severe ARDS. In addition to improving lung recruitment, oxygenation, and carbon dioxide clearance, the prone position has also been shown to have beneficial effects on the pulmonary circulation and the RV.

Pulmonary vasoconstriction is decreased, thus reducing right ventricular afterload and improving right ventricular function. By identifying and evaluating right ventricular dysfunction echocardiographically in patients with ARDS, the use of the prone position may be considered earlier and provide beneficial effects for both the lungs and the RV.

Inhaled nitric oxide

Inhaled nitric oxide (iNO) causes preferential pulmonary vasodilatation and reduced pulmonary vascular resistance. Although iNO has been shown to improve oxygenation in patients with ARDS, it does not provide a mortality benefit and may cause harm. Its use should be limited to the management of PHT; serial echocardiography can be used to monitor the right ventricular response to treatment in this setting.

Advanced echocardiography

Right ventricular systolic function

Right ventricular TDI can provide information relating to systolic function in the longitudinal plane. An A4C view should be acquired, with the cursor aligned parallel to the right ventricular free wall, and the peak systolic integral of the tricuspid lateral annular plane should be obtained and measured using TDI (RV TDI S') (Figure 27.7). An RV TDI S' of <10 cm/s is considered abnormal.

Estimating pulmonary arterial pressure

The pressure gradient between the RA and the RV can be estimated by measuring the peak TR velocity using CW Doppler (Figure 27.8; also Chapter 8). If present, TR can be detected in multiple acoustic windows (RVI, PSAX at AV level, A4C, and subcostal views) using colour flow Doppler imaging. Adding RAP to the

calculated peak pressure gradient allows estimation of the right ventricular systolic pressure (RVSP) that, in the absence of RVOT obstruction or pulmonary valve stenosis, provides an estimate of PASP.

Using the presence of TR to estimate RVSP is useful in critically ill patients with ARDS; it is a marker of disease severity, and serial echocardiography may provide valuable information regarding the effects of interventions (PEEP setting and prone positioning) on the pulmonary circulation and the RV as clinical improvement is often associated with a decreasing PASP.

Doppler assessment of intravascular volume status

A small, hypovolaemic left ventricular cavity may result in high-velocity, turbulent flow in the LVOT, causing a

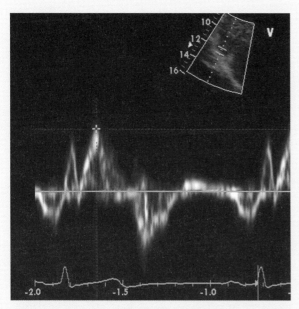

Figure 27.7 Tissue Doppler imaging of the right ventricle from an A4C view, with measurement of the peak systolic wave (RV TDI S'). For a colour version of this figure, please see colour plate section.

Reproduced from Victor K, Harden F, Mengersen K, Howard J, Chambers J. B., 'Echocardiographic measures of pulmonary hypertension and the prediction of end-points in sickle cell disease.', *Sonography*, Vol. **3**, Issue 1, © 2016 Australasian Sonographers Association, published by John Wiley and Sons.

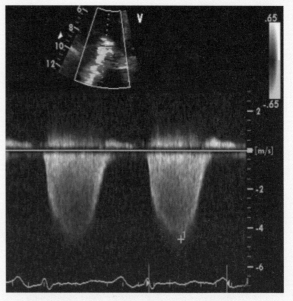

Figure 27.8 Continuous wave Doppler of tricuspid regurgitation from an A4C view, with measurement of the peak velocity. For a colour version of this figure, please see colour plate section.

Reproduced from Victor K, Harden F, Mengersen K, Howard J, Chambers J. B., 'Echocardiographic measures of pulmonary hypertension and the prediction of end-points in sickle cell disease.', *Sonography*, Vol. **3**, Issue 1, © 2016 Australasian Sonographers Association, published by John Wiley and Sons.

disorganized and mosaic-like appearance when colour flow Doppler imaging is applied.

SVV with both respiration and PLR has been evaluated echocardiographically as a means to assess fluid responsiveness. SV is calculated following measurement of the LVOT diameter and the left ventricular VTI (A5C or A3C view), using PW Doppler.

Furthermore, in mechanically ventilated patients with a pulse pressure variation of >12% (i.e. patients predicted to be responsive to fluid), a tricuspid annular systolic velocity (RV TDI S') of <15 cm/s, determined by TDI, has been shown to identify patients who are unlikely to respond to a fluid challenge.

Diagnosing a patent foramen ovale

ACP may lead to the opening of a PFO due to raised RAP, resulting in a right-to-left shunt and worsening hypoxaemia. Colour flow Doppler imaging of the IAS may reveal the presence of a PFO with a right-to-left shunt (Chapter 9). This is best visualized in the subcostal view, using colour flow Doppler imaging with a reduced scale. A PFO is present in up to 25% of the general population as a normal variant; therefore, a contrast bubble study using agitated saline should only be performed to confirm the presence of a PFO if it is suspected based on clinical findings and the diagnosis is likely to change the patient's medical management (Figure 27.9).

Extracorporeal membrane oxygenation

Veno-venous extracorporeal membrane oxygenation (ECMO) is an advanced form of organ support indicated in selected cases of ARDS refractory to conventional management.

Echocardiography can be used to facilitate decision-making regarding the appropriateness of ECMO, to guide ECMO cannula insertion and confirm the position, to identify potential complications of ECMO, and finally to assess clinical progress and suitability for weaning (Figure 27.10).

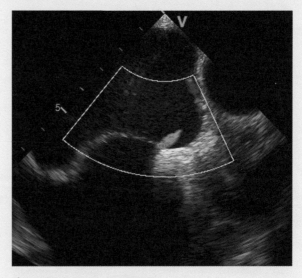

Figure 27.9 Mid-oesophageal-level TOE image focusing on the IAS. The image demonstrates right-to-left shunting across a PFO and an IAS that bows to the left, consistent with raised right atrial pressures. For a colour version of this figure, please see colour plate section.

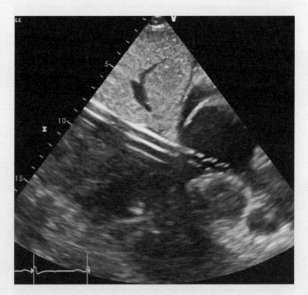

Figure 27.10 Subcostal view focusing on the IVC. ECMO cannulae can be visualized in the IVC and right atrium.

✓ Multiple choice questions

Interactive multiple choice questions to test your knowledge can be found in the Online appendix at www.oxfordmedicine.com/focusedicu. Please refer to your access card for further details.

Further reading

Corradi F, Brusasco C, Pelosi P. Chest ultrasound in acute respiratory distress syndrome. *Current Opinion in Critical Care* 2014;**20**:98–103.

Lazzeri C, Cianchi G, Bonizzoli M, Batacchi S, Peris A, Gensini GF. The potential role and limitations of echocardiography in acute respiratory distress syndrome. *Therapeutic Advances in Respiratory Disease* 2016;**10**:136–48.

Mandeville JC, Colebourn CL. Can transthoracic echocardiography be used to predict fluid responsiveness in the critically ill patient? A systematic review. *Critical Care Research and Practice* 2012;**2012**:513480.

Repessé X, Charron C, Vieillard-Baron A. Acute cor pulmonale in ARDS: rationale for protecting the right ventricle. *Chest* 2015;**147**:259–65.

Shyamsundar M, Attwood B, Keating L, Walden AP. Clinical review: the role of ultrasound in estimating extra-vascular lung water. *Critical Care* 2013;**17**:237.

28

Vascular access

Ahmed Labib and Andrew R Bodenham

Introduction

Hospitalized patients, and particularly critically ill patients, usually require vascular access in the form of peripheral venous, short-term (non-tunnelled), and/or long-term (tunnelled) access to central veins and arterial cannulation.

Vascular access is a fundamental clinical skill and is undertaken by multiple medical disciplines in a variety of clinical environments. Annually, over 5 million CVCs are inserted in the United States, with complications observed in up to 15% of the procedures.

US guidance has become a standard of care when undertaking vascular access for central venous cannulation and is increasingly used for peripheral procedures in challenging patients (obesity, coagulopathy, blocked veins, and repeated cannulation). This chapter describes how to use US to guide central venous, peripheral venous, and arterial cannulation, using both in-plane and out-of-plane techniques. The sonoanatomy of the common areas for vascular access are described and any pitfalls highlighted.

Advantages of ultrasound-guided vascular access

Real-time US-guided vascular access (USGVA) offers several advantages over both traditional landmark technique and static pre-procedural vascular scanning. Clear benefits of US include higher success and faster access at first attempt, fewer mechanical and infectious complications, and reduced cost.

Extensive medical literature favours the use of US in vascular access, in particular for the IJV. Although less well documented, US is likely to be equally beneficial at other CVC access sites.

Central venous cannulation can cause significant and potentially life-threatening mechanical complications, including pneumothorax, haemothorax, cardiac tamponade, and carotid cannulation. Furthermore, inadvertent venous or arterial puncture can cause a haematoma or an arteriovenous fistula and increase the risk of infection and thrombosis. Collateral damage, such as injury to nerves, can be minimized or avoided by use of US.

Critically ill patients with coagulopathy and patients requiring repeated vascular access are particularly likely to benefit from USGVA. ICU patients can be difficult to reposition or have limited access site(s) because of previous catheters, drains, or trauma; USGVA can help direct the practitioner to alternative and more appropriate access site(s).

US facilitates novel access sites for the central venous circulation. Axillary vein cannulation, rather than the SCV, supraclavicular subclavian venous access, and external jugular and innominate vein catheterization are possible with the help of US. Upper arm veins are extensively used for PICCs.

Prior to creating a sterile field, a pre-procedural scan of the area of interest and other potential vascular access sites is recommended but should not replace real-time guidance. A pre-procedural scan will help the operator decide on the most appropriate patent vessel to cannulate and minimize delays, risks, and patient discomfort. Unanticipated thrombus, narrowing, or blockage may be evident.

US assessment can depict the size, depth, and patency of the target vessel and the presence of thrombus, and inform the choice of catheter size. To reduce the risk of venous thrombosis, the CVC outer diameter should ideally not exceed one-third of the vessel diameter.

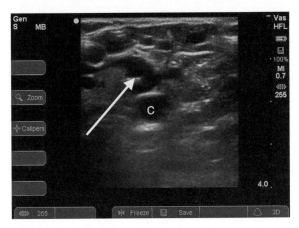

Figure 28.1 Transverse mid-neck view of the left carotid (C), with abnormal configuration of veins anterior to the artery. These represent multiple collaterals after prolonged catheterization at this site. One of the veins (arrow) anterior to the carotid probably is a scarred remnant of the original jugular vein.

Confirming the presence of the target vessel is crucial because absence of the target vein and venous anomalies can be found in a significant number of patients.

US demonstration of a filling defect suggestive of thrombosis, reverse venous flow on Doppler examination, narrowing or atheroma, or engorged superficial collaterals alerts the practitioner of difficult or impossible cannulation (Figure 28.1).

Practical approach and general recommendations for USGVA

Choice of ultrasound probe

A high-resolution 5–15 MHz linear array probe is typically used. This allows depiction of superficial and small structures, e.g. arteries and nerves, and offers adequate tissue penetration. Small footprint or hockey stick-style transducers are suitable for confined areas and children. A microconvex probe provides adequate imaging of the supraclavicular region. Full asepsis should be maintained throughout the procedure with the use of a sterile sheath and sterile US gel.

Scanning technique

The spatial relationship between the transducer and the target blood vessel determines the obtained image. Accordingly, a transverse, oblique, or longitudinal vascular view is displayed. The transverse (short-axis)

view is easier to learn and ensures visualization of surrounding at-risk structures, as well as the posterior vessel wall. However, posterior wall perforation remains a risk with all approaches.

The orientation of the needle axis in relation to the plane of the US beam defines needle visualization. Either a part of the, or the entire, needle trajectory can be visualized, giving rise to out-of-plane and in-plane needle images, respectively.

The main disadvantage of the out-of-plane approach (transverse view) is poor confirmation of needle tip position. A less experienced operator may misinterpret the needle shaft for the tip, with subsequent unnecessary needle advancement and potential collateral damage. The depth of the vein can be measured in the transverse view at the outset, in order to avoid undue needle advancement.

Despite limitations, a transverse view with an out-of-plane approach is commonly used. A longitudinal scan and an in-plane orientation provide more precise needle control and venous puncture but are more difficult to learn. Hybrid approaches with the vein in cross-section and an in-plane needle are useful.

When inserting catheters with the Seldinger technique, a scan should be undertaken to confirm that the guidewire is in the target vein and following the correct path before proceeding to vessel dilatation.

Specific access sites

Internal jugular vein

The IJV is usually the first choice in acute situations. Compared to femoral veins, IJV catheterization is associated with less thrombosis and fewer mechanical and infectious complications. The right IJV traverses a straight course. A left IJV catheter crosses two corners and can be more difficult to site in a good central position.

Out-of-plane-approach

A transverse out-of-plane approach is commonly used (Figure 28.2a, b, and c). The operator should be aware of the possibility of posterior wall perforation and potential damage to vital structures, e.g. a posterior-lying carotid artery, subclavian artery, and its branches

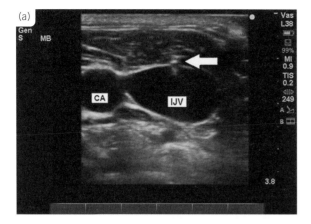

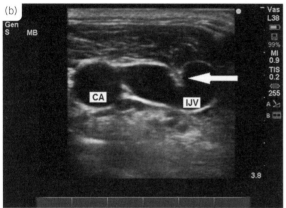

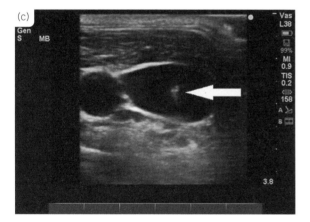

Figure 28.2 (a–c) Short-axis view out-of-plane needle puncture of the right IJV. The white arrow represents the tip of the cannulation needle. Note venous wall indentation and collapse followed by expansion. CA, carotid artery; IJV, internal jugular vein.

(vertebral and thyrocervical trunk). A steeper approach than the classical landmark technique will ensure that the needle tip is close to the US plane, while the operator should scan along the length of the needle to visualize the tip as it is advanced into the vein.

In-plane approach

To obtain a longitudinal image of the IJV, the transducer is first positioned in a transverse orientation on the patient's neck, 1–2 cm above the clavicle, to capture the vein in transverse view. While ensuring that the vein is in the centre of the US field, the probe is rotated through 90° to lie parallel to the course of the vein. If the vein image is lost, the operator should return to the transverse view for confirmation before proceeding further. Use the non-dominant hand to maintain the probe in a longitudinal orientation over the patient neck, with the caudal end of the probe adjacent to the clavicle.

To access the vein, insert the needle in-plane in the middle of the cephalic end of the probe at a shallower angle, typically at 45° to the skin. Needle insertion causes distortion of adjacent tissues; further advancement of the needle within the US beam allows visualization of the entire needle (Figure 28.3a). Anterior vascular wall indentation is observed (Figure 28.3b), due to pressure from the needle tip. Penetration of the wall is associated with a 'give', followed by re-expansion of the vein. Failure to aspirate blood may be caused by apposition of the venous walls; careful withdrawal of the needle allows entry into the vein and free flow aspiration. Visualization of the intraluminal tip position should be ascertained before insertion of the guidewire (Figure 28.3c).

The in-plane approach allows visualization of the tip and shaft and offers better control of the tip and venous puncture, provided that both the needle and vein are kept in view at all times. A major limitation of this approach is a lack of visualization of adjacent structures such as the carotid artery and the thyroid gland. Another practical difficulty may arise in patients with a short neck, due to limited space for probe position, when a smaller footprint linear array transducer may be useful. Because the probe is positioned perpendicular to the direction of blood flow, it may be difficult to capture colour or spectral waveform Doppler analysis—another limitation of this technique.

Lateral transverse in-plane approach

The IJV can be accessed via the lateral wall, using a lateral transverse in-plane approach. Combining a transverse view of the IJV and real-time in-plane visualization of the entire needle trajectory has several

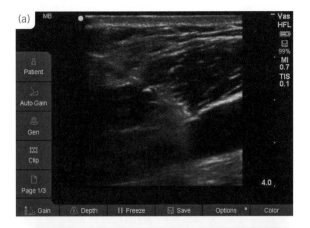

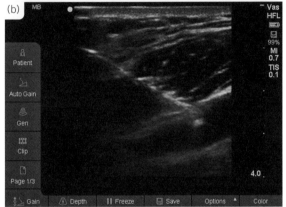

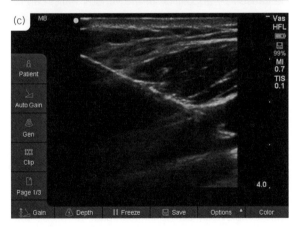

Figure 28.3 Long-axis view in-plane sequence of a left IJV puncture. (a) The entire needle is visualized. (b) Puncture of the anterior wall and intraluminal tip confirmation. (c) Guidewire visualized inside the vessel, with acoustic shadow caused by the wire.

advantages. For example, display of surrounding structures, visualization of the entire needle, and control of needle tip position suggest this approach may further improve safety and accuracy.

Patients with carotid artery disease, atheroma, or graft may be at particular risk from inadvertent carotid puncture. In case of inadvertent carotid artery cannulation, the operator should leave the catheter in place and seek urgent advice from interventional radiology and vascular surgery.

> **Pitfall**
>
> Inadvertent carotid perforation or cannulation can cause significant bleeding or thrombosis (resulting in ischaemic stroke). Removal of large-bore arterial catheters requires careful consideration.

Subclavian vein

Lower infection rates, greater patient comfort, better cosmetic site, and easier dressing and securement are the main advantages of SCV access, which makes it an attractive site for both short- and long-term (tunnelled) catheters, e.g. Hickman lines and implanted ports.

Serious mechanical complications, including haemo- and/or pneumothorax, are potential risks. Due to close approximation of the SCV and the clavicle, the SCV is not easily imaged for USGVA and novel approaches have been developed.

Infraclavicular axillary venous cannulation is an appealing alternative. US scanning of the lateral chest wall at the delto-pectoral groove allows visualization of the axillary vessels, cephalic vein, brachial plexus, adjacent chest wall, and underlying pleura. A more lateral approach is potentially safer, as the target vein and pleura become more separated and effective pressure and surgical access are possible, if required. Arterial branches from the thoraco-acromial trunk cross the vein and should be identified and avoided. Similarly, the brachial plexus can be identified and injury avoided. This approach is an advanced skill and requires additional training and practice. The patient is placed in a neutral supine position, with 15° Trendelenburg tilt, with the arms by the side. A high-frequency linear array probe is placed inferior to the mid-clavicular point in a longitudinal orientation, with the probe marker pointing cephalad (Figure 28.4a). The axillary vessels are identified as two hypoechoic structures, with the artery typically sited cephalad to the vein. Other important structures to identify are branches of the axillary artery, the first and second ribs, and the pleura (Figure 28.4b).

The probe is then rotated through 90° to obtain a long-axis view of the axillary vessels. This enables visualization of branches of the axillary artery, which may cross in front of the axillary vein. The probe is then returned to the short-axis view, and an optimum puncture site chosen. The operator adjusts the image (depth, gain, and width), so that the vein is seen at the centre of the screen. The needle is advanced out-of-plane at a steep angle towards the vein, avoiding the pleura and surrounding structures. Vascular wall indentation precedes venous puncture. Gentle probe manipulation may be needed to enable visualization of the intraluminal tip position, which is then confirmed by free aspiration of venous blood. A guidewire is passed through the needle, and cannulation is performed in a standard fashion (Figure 28.4c).

Infraclavicular axillary cannulation of the SCV is a safe alternative to the traditional approach. In case of inadvertent arterial puncture and uncontrolled bleeding, both vascular compression and surgical access are much easier, compared to the subclavian artery. However, this approach is challenging in the muscular and morbidly obese, due to deep location of the axillary veins.

The supraclavicular view avoids the acoustic shadow of the clavicle and allows for in-plane needle visualization and imaging of the distal part of the SCV and brachio-cephalic vein. This approach is popular in paediatric practice, as the vein is larger than the jugular.

Femoral vessels

The femoral vessels, along with other sites, may have variable anatomy. Variants include an anteriorly lying long saphenous vein (LSV), a posterior common femoral artery (CFA), and an aberrant superficial femoral artery (SFA). US allows the operator to access the common femoral vein close to the inguinal ligament, while avoiding a higher puncture with the risk of abdominal injury (Figure 28.5a and b).

Vascular mechanical complications, including arteriovenous fistula and pseudo-aneurysm, are more prevalent at the femoral site. US enables visualization of the target vessel, choice of optimal puncture site, and avoidance of inadvertent arterial injury. Real-time US is valuable, particularly in obesity, coagulopathy, and extensive tissue oedema. Femoral access is increasingly used for veno-venous and/or veno-arterial ECMO where US is used to ascertain vessel patency, measure the vessel diameter, inform cannula size

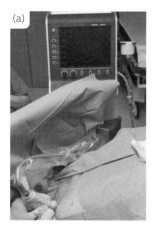 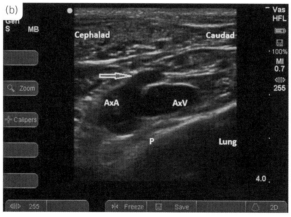 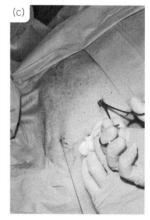

Figure 28.4 (a) Right axillary vein puncture with vessels in transverse view, with short-axis out-of-plane view of the needle. The operator needs good 3D orientation to adjust for the angle of the probe and maintain good needle visualization at all times. The ultrasound machine is directly opposite the operator to allow easy vision. (b) The right infraclavicular axillary vein (AxV) is seen to the right, while the axillary artery (AxA) is seen to the left. A major arterial branch—the thoraco-acromial trunk (arrow)—is seen anterior to the vein; this should be looked for and avoided. The pleura (P) and lung are seen inferiorly. (c) Note the relatively lateral position of the skin puncture site where the guidewire passes through the skin into the vein. This patient is having a tunnelled Hickman-type device inserted, hence the second lower puncture on the chest wall.

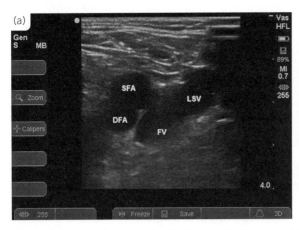 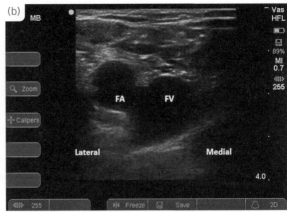

Figure 28.5 Femoral vessels visualized caudal to the inguinal ligament. (a) Superficial (SFA) and deep (DFA) femoral arteries. Note the long saphenous vein (LSV) as it joins the femoral vein (FV). (b) Sliding the probe cephalad allows identification of the common femoral vein (FV), avoiding cannulation of the LSV.

selection, and for real-time guidance. USGVA of the femoral vein is usually undertaken with a transverse out-of-plane technique, in a similar manner to accessing the jugular vein.

Femoral vein access is associated with more thrombosis and mechanical and infectious complications than other CVC sites. Repeated unsuccessful attempts increase the frequency of complications and should be avoided.

Peripherally inserted central catheters

The use of US guidance has resulted in PICCs being a practical alternative route of vascular access in ICU for total parenteral nutrition (TPN) and for patients requiring ongoing central access. Advantages of PICCs include an appropriate route for long-term vascular access, a lower infection rate, and fewer and less serious immediate and delayed complications. US guidance enables PICC insertion via the upper arm cephalic, basilic, or brachial vein, away from the elbow flexure.

Using USGVA, operators can identify and visualize patent veins, measure the vein diameter, and choose an appropriate catheter size and the most appropriate puncture site away from the elbow crease. The brachial artery, median, and ulnar nerves can be identified and injury avoided (Figure 28.6). US allows cannulation in the mid-upper arm, which avoids the risk of catheter damage from elbow flexion, provides optimal securement and device fixation, and is more comfortable for the patient.

The basilic vein has the least tortuous route to the central veins and is the favoured site for PICC placement due to the ease of catheter advancement. Transverse in-plane or longitudinal out-of-plane US techniques are both used, depending on the operator's experience, although the latter will reduce the risk of needle passage through the posterior vessel wall. US is used to guide placement of a micro-Seldinger peel-away introducer cannula, through which the PICC line (cut to an appropriate length for the site of

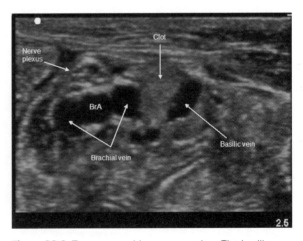

Figure 28.6 Transverse mid-upper arm view. The basilic vein is partially occluded by a clot. Move to another site, and consider the need for anticoagulation, depending on the extent of the clot and the status of the arm. Note the nerve plexus anterior to the brachial artery (BrA). Note two brachial veins (white arrows) on each side of the BrA.

cannulation and patient size) is advanced. Scanning of the ipsilateral IJV by an assistant can demonstrate inadvertent catheter misplacement, allowing further attempts to advance the catheter while maintaining asepsis. Rapid injection of 10 mL of agitated saline as a bubble contrast through the line will increase sensitivity for identifying a misplaced catheter tip in the jugular vein.

A midline catheter is inserted in an identical way to a PICC but is shorter (20–25 cm) and is an alternative method of access for up to 4 weeks for the administration of non-irritant drugs such as antibiotics. Double- and triple-lumen PICC lines are now available and are used increasingly for longer-term access in the ICU, in order to reduce the risk of infectious complications.

Peripheral venous access

Challenging adult and paediatric patients are likely to benefit from USGVA. Upper arm cephalic, basilic, or brachial veins can be used in the short term in the difficult-to-cannulate patient. A short-axis view and an out-of-plane needle approach is typically used for this procedure.

Long-term ICU patients often need repeated cannulation. Multiple blind attempts at arterial and venous cannulation is distressing to patients, relatives, and care providers and should be discouraged where trained personnel and appropriate equipment are available.

USGVA increases patient comfort, reduces failure rate and cost, and enables faster access. Recent literature suggests an increased success rate and a reduced need for CVC insertions in the emergency department.

Arterial cannulation

Arterial catheterization can be challenging in patients with shock, trauma, significant arrhythmia, vascular disease, coagulopathy, and obesity. For advanced cardiovascular monitoring, larger arterial catheters may be inserted in the femoral, brachial, or axillary artery, often in unstable patients. Repeated blind attempts relying on palpation or external landmarks should be minimized and avoided.

Advantages of US in arterial cannulation include verification of the presence of a healthy patent artery and absence of clots, atheroma, or anatomical anomalies. US facilitates access to less commonly used arteries, e.g. mid forearm radial and ulnar, axillary, and posterior tibial arteries. Real-time US arterial cannulation is recommended as the standard technique for shocked patients A small, high-frequency transducer and an out-of-plane short-axis view are typically employed for arterial cannulation.

Adjuncts to USGVA

Echogenic needle tips enhance visualization and more accurate needle tip localization. This technology may benefit the novice. In expert hands, its superiority over standard needles is questionable.

Less experienced operators may struggle with eye–hand coordination. Maintaining the US probe in a steady position with the non-dominant hand may be difficult for beginners. A hands-free probe holder is available and may help overcome these issues. A needle guide can be used to secure the needle trajectory towards the target vein. There is not enough evidence to support routine application of these devices. Self-aspirating bulbs (e.g. Raulerson-type) can be used to free up the hand and allow the needle to be held directly.

Doppler US provides diagnostics to flow and direction but requires additional experience and is not associated with improved procedure outcome. 3D technology is not supported in current guidelines.

Post-procedure ultrasound

US confirmation of intraluminal placement of a CVC, together with free aspiration of low-pressure venous blood, permits immediate use of the CVC. Following the procedure, the operator should rule out pulmonary complications and ascertain the CVC tip position. Ideally, the catheter tip should be positioned in low SVC or at the cavo-atrial junction.

A post-insertion chest X-ray is routinely requested to rule out CVC malposition and an immediate pneumothorax. Disadvantages of a chest X-ray include: patient and staff exposure to radiation, a need for patient repositioning, staff and resource cost, plus limited information on the catheter (only confirms central passage and lack of kinking).

Post-placement US examination of the pleura can reliably exclude a pneumothorax and is more sensitive than a standard chest X-ray. US lung examination is simple, easy to learn, and repeatable and attaches no added cost. The same probe used for catheterization is utilized to demonstrate pleural sliding (Chapter 15).

In addition, studies are reported imaging the CVC position within the right side of the heart, to rule out CVC malposition or contralateral cannulation. TTE with a microconvex probe in the subcostal area is performed to visualize right heart cavities, the vena cava, and the CVC. A longitudinal view of the SVC is obtained via a suprasternal scan.

TTE assessment with microbubbles and/or contrast enhancement can reliably confirm the CVC tip position within the RA. This requires advanced training and contrast injection and is less precise if the tip lies in the SVC. TOE is more accurate in delineating the CVC tip position. However, TOE is invasive and requires specific equipment and expertise.

Pitfalls of USGVA

- Operator dependency. More experienced operators obtain better images and safer needle placement.

- May give a false sense of reassurance. Further checks of venous placement and the central tip are required. US only helps with the initial steps of vascular access.

- Does not entirely prevent inadvertent arterial puncture or cannulation.

- Does not entirely prevent posterior vein wall perforation or collateral damage.

- Does not allow easy central tip visualization to avoid CVC malposition.

- Cannot substitute thorough anatomical knowledge and sound clinical judgement.

- Some approaches require additional training and are more difficult skills to acquire.

✓ Multiple choice questions

Interactive multiple choice questions to test your knowledge can be found in the Online appendix at www.oxfordmedicine.com/focusedicu. Please refer to your access card for further details.

Further reading

American Society of Anesthesiologists Task Force on Central Venous Access, Rupp SM, Apfelbaum JL, Blitt C, *et al.* Practice guidelines for central venous access: a report by the American Society of Anesthesiologists Task Force on Central Venous Access. *Anesthesiology* 2012;**116**:539–73.

Bedel J, Vallée F, Mari A, *et al.* Guidewire localization by transthoracic echocardiography during central venous catheter insertion: a peri- procedural method to evaluate catheter placement. *Intensive Care Medicine* 2013;**39**:1932–7.

Chapman GA, Johnson D, Bodenham AR. Visualisation of needle position using ultrasonography. *Anaesthesia* 2006;**61**:148–58.

Fragou M, Gravvanis A, Dimitriou V, *et al.* Real-time ultrasound-guided subclavian vein cannulation versus the landmark method in critical care patients: a prospective randomized study. *Critical Care Medicine* 2011;**39**:1607–12.

Lamperti M, Bodenham AR, Pittiruti M, *et al.* International evidence-based recommendations on ultrasound-guided vascular access. *Intensive Care Medicine* 2012;**38**: 1105–17.

O'Leary R, Ahmed SM, McLure H, *et al.* Ultrasound-guided infraclavicular axillary vein cannulation: a useful alternative to the internal jugular vein. *Br J Anaesthesia* 2012;**109**:762–8.

29

Percutaneous tracheostomy

Ahmed Labib and Andrew R Bodenham

Introduction

Percutaneous dilatational tracheostomy (PDT) is a common procedure in the ICU. The UK 2014 National Confidential Enquiry into Patient Outcome and Death (NCEPOD) report estimated that up to 15,000 tracheostomy procedures are undertaken annually, with over two-thirds performed percutaneously in ICU.

Recent advances in technology and equipment design, coupled with increasing experience and structured training, have contributed to improved safety and success of PDT. This chapter outlines the use of point-of-care US in PDT in order to improve the safety and success of the procedure. This chapter reviews the role of a pre-procedural US examination and describes the technique and the normal sonoanatomy. The use of US to guide tracheal cannulation during percutaneous tracheostomy and cricothyrotomy is also described.

Role of ultrasound

Historically, access to the trachea was performed in the operating theatre via open surgical approaches. In the 1985, Ciaglia introduced elective PDT as a safe alternative to surgical tracheostomy. Increasing medical literature supports the safety, outcome, and cost-effectiveness of PDT.

PDT is usually performed under endoscopic guidance via an orotracheal tube, and the stoma site is chosen after palpation of external anatomical landmarks (thyroid and cricoid cartilage, tracheal rings, and suprasternal notch). This approach has several limitations, including a lack of identification of aberrant blood vessels and suboptimal puncture site, particularly when there are inadequate surface landmarks such as in obesity and burns.

Pre-procedural US examination of the anterior neck is easy to learn and perform and offers several advantages, including (Figures 29.1, 29.2, and 29.3):

- Confirmation of the position and direction of the trachea. This is useful in obesity, limited neck extension, goitre, local surgery or radiotherapy, burns, and previous tracheostomy.

- Measurement of the depth of the trachea to choose an appropriate-length tracheostomy tube (TT). A thick pre-tracheal fat pad, local swelling or oedema, or a deep-sited stoma necessitates the use of an extended-length or adjustable-flange TT. Inadequate TT length increases the

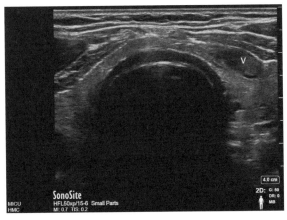

Figure 29.1 A relatively superficial trachea, a normal isthmus, and a prominent vein (v). Typically, the trachea is <2 cm deep to the skin surface.

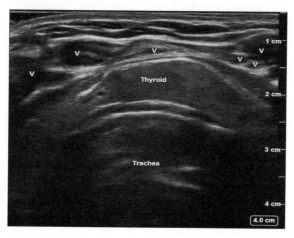

Figure 29.2 Multiple superficial veins (v) overlying the thyroid isthmus and the trachea. Careful US examination and appropriate puncture site selection may avoid peri-procedural bleeding.

risk of tube dislodgement and misplacement, especially in the morbidly obese patient, which can cause significant morbidity and mortality. Assessment of trachea depth is performed, with the neck in a neutral position, at the optimal puncture site.

• Evaluation of the transverse tracheal diameter. The outer diameter of the TT should not exceed three-quarters of the internal tracheal diameter. This facilitates airflow on cuff deflation and minimizes insertion trauma.

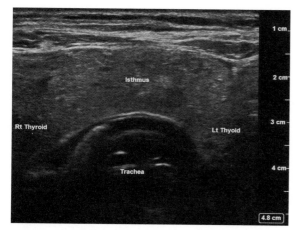

Figure 29.3 A thick thyroid isthmus measuring approximately 2 cm without major vessels visible on ultrasound is noted. This patient was referred for a surgical tracheostomy. Note the trachea >3.5 cm deep to the skin.

• Visualization of prominent and aberrant blood vessels, including the anterior jugular veins and inferior thyroid and thyroid ima arteries.

• Assessment of thyroid gland size and vascularity.

• Identification of abnormal anatomy.

> **Pitfall**
>
> US reveals aberrant and at-risk blood vessels. Excessive skin compression should be avoided to ensure they are identified.

The UK Intensive Care Society (ICS) guidelines allude to the benefits of US in PDT; however, a lack of randomized controlled trials and robust evidence does not permit a strong recommendation. Some European guidelines suggest routine US for PDT and cite evidence of higher quality, compared to the evidence supporting the routine use of endoscopy.

Ultrasound technique

A high-frequency 5–15 MHz vascular-style linear array probe is typically used for US assessment of the neck. A 38-mm transducer allows visualization of a wider area of the neck, with adequate penetration which is ideal for pre-procedural evaluation. However, it is not suitable for real-time intra-procedural guidance because it will occupy a small operating field, and a smaller 25-mm transducer may be more convenient.

The operator should set the US display screen at a suitable height on the opposite side of the patient. Having confirmed the correct image orientation and appropriate gain, adjust the depth, so that the trachea is seen central at the bottom of the screen on the transverse/axial view.

Sonoanatomy of the anterior neck

Transverse view

The thyroid cartilage (TC) is identified as an inverted, 'V'-shaped, hypoechoic structure, anterior to the air shadow (Figure 29.4). Immediately caudal to the TC lies the cricothyroid membrane (CTM), followed by the arch-shaped cricoid cartilage (CC) (Figure 29.5). The CC is thicker, more superficial, and bigger than the tracheal rings.

Scanning towards the suprasternal notch allows visualization of individual tracheal rings. Typically,

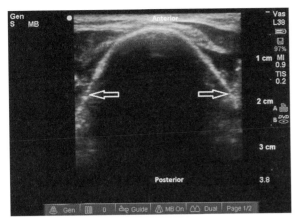

Figure 29.4 A midline cross-sectional view with a high-frequency linear transducer. The thyroid cartilage is a superficial inverted, U-shaped structure (white arrows) overlying the air-filled upper airway. Calcification of the thyroid cartilage is common in the elderly.

tracheal rings are superficial, round, and hypoechoic. The thyroid isthmus and at-risk midline blood vessels can be visualized (Figures 29.1, 29.2, and 29.3). Moving the probe laterally enables visualization of thyroid lobes and major vessels.

Longitudinal sagittal/parasagittal view

This view delineates the cartilaginous structure of the larynx and trachea. The air–mucosa interface is depicted as a hyperechoic line immediately posterior to the hypoechoic cartilaginous framework. The resulting

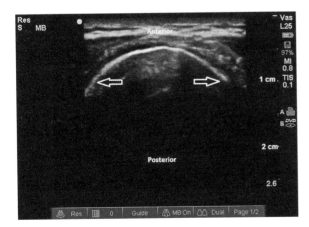

Figure 29.5 By sliding the probe caudally, the cricoid cartilage is visualized. The cricoid cartilage is typically <1 cm deep to the body surface, hypoechoic, and arch-like. The image displays a hyperechoic calcified cricoid (white arrows).

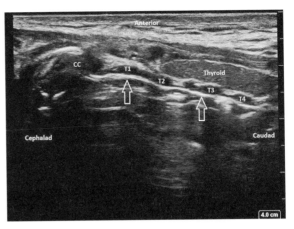

Figure 29.6 A longitudinal parasagittal view of the neck with the same probe depicting the cricoid cartilage (CC). Three tracheal rings (T1, 2, 3) are visualized as dark, hypoechoic structures. The white arrows point to the hyperechoic line that defines the air–mucosa interface. This image is typically referred to as 'pearls on a string'. Note the thyroid gland overlying the tracheal rings and the relatively superficial trachea. The posterior tracheal wall cannot be visualized.

image is referred to as 'pearls on a string' (Figure 29.6). Air artefacts and an endotracheal tube (ETT) can be visualized. This view allows identification and counting of individual tracheal rings. A skin mark is drawn, overlying the most appropriate puncture site.

Ultrasound-guided PDT

Real-time intra-procedural US guidance can be performed, with full asepsis, to visualize tracheal cannulation in real time. A pre-procedural scan is performed, and the operator identifies a satisfactory stoma site.

Patient preparation, positioning, monitoring, sedation, and local anaesthesia are as per standard practice. The ETT is withdrawn under direct laryngoscopy, so the cuff lies immediately above the vocal cords. Alternatively, the ETT is replaced with a supraglottic airway device.

The operator places the US transducer in a sterile probe sheath and, holding the transducer with the non-dominant hand, localizes the inter-cartilaginous space of interest. The introducer needle attached to a saline-filled syringe is then advanced in the midline, perpendicular to the skin, and observed on the US monitor.

In the transverse view, indentation of the anterior tracheal wall is observed, followed occasionally by tracheal collapse and finally expansion after correct

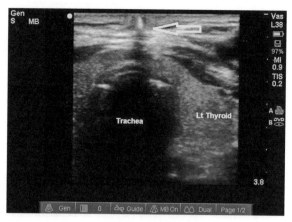

Figure 29.7 A cross-sectional midline display with a high-frequency linear transducer of real-time ultrasound-guided percutaneous tracheostomy. The puncture needle is visualized as a hyperechoic structure (arrow), with tissue artefacts ahead of the advancing needle.

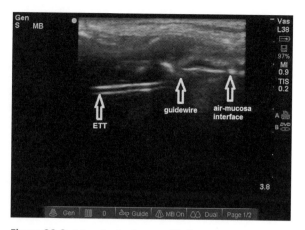

Figure 29.9 A longitudinal scan with the same probe. Note the double hyperechoic lines of the ETT on the left side of the screen. The guidewire is seen in the middle of the screen below the hyperechoic air–mucosa interface.

needle placement. The hyperechoic needle tip is then visualized within the trachea. Jiggling the needle sometimes helps to appreciate the needle tip position. Aspiration of air confirms correct intraluminal position (Figures 29.7 and 29.8).

US does not allow visualization of the posterior wall of an air-filled trachea. Pre-procedural measurement of the tracheal depth should alert operators of excessive needle advancement.

The operator advances the guidewire and confirms the intraluminal position in both transverse and longitudinal views (Figure 29.9). Following confirmation of correct placement of the guidewire, the operator

follows standard practice to complete the procedure. Immediately after the procedure, the same transducer used for US guidance can be used to rule out a pneumothorax. US images may be stored and/or printed out and filed in the patient's notes for procedural documentation. Although studies have been published showing that tracheostomy can be performed safely under US guidance alone, it is recommended that endoscopy is undertaken in addition, in order to confirm an anterior midline puncture without posterior wall injury or tracheal ring damage.

> **Pitfall**
>
> The posterior tracheal wall cannot be visualized with US. The risk of posterior wall perforation is minimized by measurement of the tracheal depth.

Ultrasound-guided cricothyrotomy

A large UK audit of major airway complications reported that failure of rescue airway techniques and serious complications were observed more frequently in critical care and morbid obesity. US-assisted airway management allows identification of the CTM in the challenging patient with difficult anatomy or morbid obesity and may be included in the failed intubation plan for undertaking emergency cricothyroidotomy.

When a difficult airway is anticipated, the clinician can utilize US to localize the CTM before induction

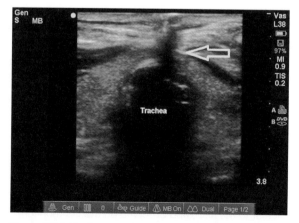

Figure 29.8 Further needle advancement into the trachea with wider acoustic shadow (arrow) and indentation of the tracheal wall. This was confirmed with free air aspiration.

of anaesthesia, to ensure preparation for a failed intubation.

On the sagittal/parasagittal view, the CTM is visualized as a hypoechoic structure spanning between the thyroid and cricoid cartilage. The location of the CTM is then marked on the skin (Figure 29.6).

A 'can't intubate, can't ventilate' (CICV) scenario is a very stressful situation, and timely intervention is paramount to avoiding a catastrophic outcome. To make the most of real-time US-guided cricothyrotomy, adequate preparation is fundamental. Prior to induction of anaesthesia, the clinician has to ensure US is readily available and switched on and with the appropriate settings for the patient. A cricothyrotomy kit should be immediately available.

Pitfalls

- The posterior tracheal wall cannot be visualized with US, which does not eliminate the risk of posterior wall perforation or tracheal ring damage.

- Limited evidence comparing US versus endoscopy guidance does not support a US-only approach. They should be seen as complementary methods, with US readily identifying the site and depth of cannulation, while endoscopy confirms intraluminal placement and prevents posterior wall perforation.

- A small operating field hinders the use of a standard probe for real-time guidance.

- Superficial venous vessels may not be visualized due to excess compression.

- Operator experience and familiarity with airway sonoanatomy are essential.

✔ Multiple choice questions

Interactive multiple choice questions to test your knowledge can be found in the Online appendix at www.oxfordmedicine.com/focusedicu. Please refer to your access card for further details.

30

Pleural drainage

Jennie Stephens

Introduction

US guidance is recommended by the British Thoracic Society (BTS) when undertaking any procedure on a pleural effusion in order to reduce complications. This chapter outlines the indications for draining a pleural effusion and describes the technique for using US to identify a safe site for drainage. A detailed description of how to undertake an US-guided pleural aspiration, thoracocentesis, and insertion of chest drain follows.

Role of ultrasound

Pleural effusions are frequent in the critical care setting, and pleural US is the ideal bedside imaging modality for the assessment and drainage of pleural effusions. In addition, real-time imaging of the hemidiaphragm provides information about any restriction of movement secondary to the effusion. The depth of the effusion at the most postero-lateral point allows estimation of the effusion volume (Figure 30.1), and the US characteristics of the effusion can indicate the type of fluid (transudate, exudate, empyema). Of most significance, the use of real-time US guidance to drain effusions significantly reduces the complication and failure rates of the procedure. Complications of pleural drainage include pneumothorax, procedure failure, pain, haemorrhage, and visceral injury.

The BTS guidelines recommend that all drainage procedures for pleural fluid are undertaken using US guidance. An 'X marks the spot' technique that is undertaken remote in time and place from the drainage procedure carries the same complication rate as performing blind drainage and should not be undertaken.

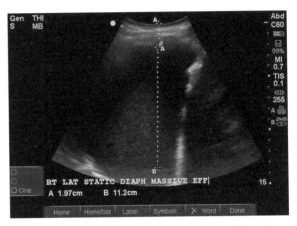

Figure 30.1 Massive pleural effusion. Note the flattened appearance of the hemidiaphragm in this image. Despite spontaneous respiration, diaphragmatic movement was significantly limited by the effusion.

Indications for drainage

It is rare to find a patient on the critical care unit without a small pleural effusion. The decision about whether to drain or sample the pleural fluid is patient-specific and not always dependent on the effusion size. Pleural aspiration and insertion of intercostal drains are invasive procedures with associated risks; neither should be undertaken without careful clinical consideration. Common indications for drainage are discussed in the following sections.

Respiratory compromise

Bedside observations, arterial blood gas results, and clinical examination indicate whether a patient is compromised by a pleural effusion. Direct observation of the movement of the hemidiaphragm on the affected side will also aid this decision (Video 3.1.1 📹). Although a larger-volume effusion is more likely to compromise an individual, a pleural effusion should not be drained because of size alone. Smaller effusions (e.g. <400 mL) are unlikely to have a significant effect on respiratory function.

Suspicion of empyema

An empyema should always be drained to dryness, using an adequately sized intercostal chest drain. US assessment can aid in the differentiation between purulent fluid and a simple transudate. A diagnostic tap under US guidance can provide the definitive answer. The pH of non-purulent fluid should be measured, with a value of <7.2 indicating an empyema and the need for tube drainage of a parapneumonic effusion.

Diagnostic uncertainty

Pleural drainage can help diagnostically. Pleural fluid can be sent for microbiology, biochemistry, and cytology, all of which can provide vital diagnostic information. Light's criteria from the results of lactate dehydrogenase (LDH) and total protein measurements in pleural fluid and serum are used to differentiate a transudate from an exudate (Box 30.1).

With atelectatic lung surrounded by effusion, drainage of the fluid will reveal if the lung is solely compressed by the surrounding fluid or if there is a proximal bronchial obstruction causing lobar collapse.

Ultrasound assessment

US assessment of the pleural effusion can contribute to the decision to drain. Use US to answer the following questions:

- How large is the effusion, and is it compromising diaphragmatic movement (Figure 30.1 and Video 3.1.1 📹)? Comparison of both sides will highlight the effect of a unilateral effusion.
- What type of fluid makes up the effusion (purulent, exudate, transudate)?
- Is there a suitable and safe site to drain the fluid (Box 30.2)?

Assessment of site for drainage

It is recommended that the minimal fluid depth for safe drainage is at least 10 mm. A puncture site should be chosen which is not impinged by the underlying lung during inspiration. Identify any structures which may be in proximity such as the liver, spleen, or LV and it's associated vasculature (Figure 30.2 and Videos 3.1.2 and 3.1.3 📹). If loculations are present, identify the largest locule for symptomatic drainage or diagnostic sampling (Figure 30.3). Referral for video-assisted thoracoscopy may be necessary for breaking up the locules and a safer and more effective method of drainage.

The ideal site for insertion without US guidance is within the 'safe triangle', defined by the lateral border of the pectoralis major, the anterior border of the latissimus dorsi, and the fifth intercostal space. US imaging may identify a safe and appropriate place to access a pleural effusion which is outside the 'safe triangle'. However, the neurovascular bundle may not lie under the inferior border of the

---

Box 30.1 Light's criteria: pleural fluid is an exudate if one or more of the criteria are met

- Pleural fluid protein divided by serum protein is >0.5
- Pleural fluid LDH divided by serum LDH is >0.6
- Pleural fluid LDH >2/3 the upper limits of laboratory normal value for serum LDH

Box 30.2 Safe site for pleural drainage

- Fluid depth >10 mm
- No lung incursion during inspiration
- Adequate clearance from adjacent structures (diaphragm, liver, spleen, ventricle)

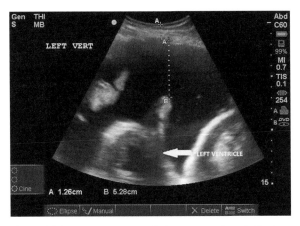

Figure 30.2 Left ventricle visible beneath a pleural effusion. It is important to identify visceral structures that may be in close proximity to the puncture site.

rib posteriorly, but in the middle of the intercostal space, such that very posterior sites of drainage should be avoided.

Although US is very sensitive at identifying loculated effusions, if there is any uncertainty regarding the nature of a pleural effusion, CT imaging should be undertaken prior to any intervention. Differentiating a complex loculated effusion from consolidated lung can be very difficult, and the CT scan remains the gold standard imaging modality for the lung.

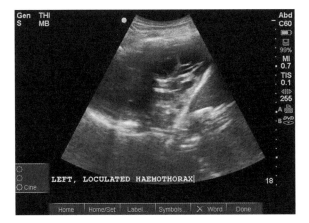

Figure 30.3 Loculated posterior effusion. There are multiple superficial locules within this effusion; it would be difficult to drain the effusion completely, but it might be possible to access some of the larger locules for a diagnostic tap.

Technique

Choice of procedure and size of drain

This will depend on the nature and estimated volume of the pleural collection. If drainage over a number of days is required, a large-gauge surgical drain is inserted for a haemothorax, while a small-gauge Seldinger drain is used to drain transudates. Traditionally, larger-gauge drains are inserted to manage an empyema, although BTS guidance recommends insertion of an image-guided small-gauge Seldinger drain in the first instance. The Seldinger technique is not recommended for large drains (24 French gauge and above) when a surgical blunt dissection method is most appropriate. Treatment of smaller effusions and diagnostic sampling are undertaken by aspiration, using a small-gauge needle or cannula without placement of a drain.

Preparation and consent

Documented consent should be obtained prior to all pleural procedures, which should encompass the indications for the procedure and all common or serious possible complications. All equipment should be collected and prepared in advance. Pleural drainage is an invasive procedure and should follow locally developed standards to ensure safe practice that are based on national safety standards. A peri-procedural checklist, equivalent to the World Health Organization surgical safety checklist that is now a standard of care for all surgical procedures, can ensure compliance with local standards and improve safety.

Clotting disorders and anticoagulation

Any non-urgent pleural procedures should wait until the patient's international normalized ratio (INR) is below 1.5 and the platelet count is above 50. For patients on direct-acting oral anticoagulants, ensure an appropriate delay since the last dose. Advice should be sought about the best way to correct any coagulation abnormalities, if they exist, prior to attempting pleural aspiration or chest drain insertion.

'X marks the spot' ultrasound technique

Carefully position the patient in the position you will be performing the diagnostic tap. Using US, identify the safest and most appropriate areas to puncture and drain, identifying the characteristics previously described. Using a curvilinear probe, obtain a still image in the longitudinal plane at the proposed puncture site, and measure the depth of the skin and the depth of the effusion. Now obtain a transverse still at the proposed puncture site by rotating the probe 90 degrees, and measure the depth of the skin and the depth of the effusion. Carefully note any significant changes in measurements, and also look for solid structures within the pleural fluid that were not visible in the alternative plane. Mark the site using an indelible pen or by applying pressure with a narrow, blunt object.

Ensure the patient remains in the same position.

Direct real-time ultrasound technique

For loculated or small effusions, it is recommended that aspiration is performed under direct US guidance, visualizing the needle as it is advanced into the pleural space. Use a sterile probe cover and sterile US gel. An 'in-plane' approach, using a high-frequency linear array probe, is recommended for most patients.

Equipment

Diagnostic aspiration and therapeutic drainage are undertaken as an aseptic technique, using sterile gloves, a sterile dressing pack, cleaning solution (chlorhexidine in alcohol), and an appropriate range of syringes and an aspiration kit, if planned. Insertion of a chest drain is undertaken with full aseptic barrier precautions (surgical gown, hat, face mask, sterile gloves), using a proprietary Seldinger chest drain insertion kit or with surgical blunt dissection.

Procedure

1. Diagnostic aspiration

Ensuring that the patient is in the same position as when the US was performed and using an aseptic technique, a 20-mL syringe with a 21G needle attached is passed through the skin at the marked site. Once the skin is punctured, advance the needle, keeping the syringe under negative pressure. On puncturing the pleura, there will be a rush of fluid. Do not advance the needle any further. Obtain an adequate sample for diagnostic purposes (20–50 mL).

Apply a sterile dressing to the puncture site.

2. Therapeutic aspiration (thoracocentesis)

The aspiration kit should be put together before scanning the patient, in order to minimize the time between US and puncture. US scan is undertaken as described previously, and ensure that the patient's position remains unchanged.

Infiltrate local anaesthetic down to the pleura (pleural puncture is painful) until pleural fluid is aspirated. Using a 5- or 10-mL syringe attached to the intravenous cannula, puncture the skin at the marked and anaesthetized site. Advance the cannula, keeping the syringe under negative pressure. On puncturing the pleura, there will be a rush of fluid. Advance the cannula over the needle into the pleural space. Remove the needle and attach the three-way tap. Using the 50-mL syringe, withdraw pleural fluid and flush it away through the free port of the three-way tap attached to intravenous infusion giving-set tubing. Ensure that a sample is taken for analysis. Once an adequate amount of fluid has been drained, remove the cannula from the pleural space and apply a sterile dressing.

Therapeutic aspiration can also be performed by inserting a small-gauge chest drain that is removed immediately after the effusion has been drained. The puncture site is larger than with using a cannula, thereby increasing the risk of pneumothorax. It will need closing with a suture. Following completion of therapeutic aspiration, repeat the US examination and store an image to allow comparison with pre-procedure images (Figure 30.4).

3. Chest drain insertion

The technique of US-guided Seldinger drain insertion is similar to that described previously for therapeutic aspiration. Once the pleural space is entered, a guidewire is passed through the cannulating needle. Direct real-time US may be used to allow confirmation of the correct guidewire position within the pleural space before proceeding to dilatation and chest drain insertion. The dilator should be inserted with caution to ensure that it just enters the pleural space when a distinct 'give' will be felt. Inserting an excessive length of dilator may damage the underlying lung. Following dilatation, the chest drain with a stiffening insert is passed over the guidewire. The distal end of the guidewire must be visible at all times to prevent inadvertent loss into the

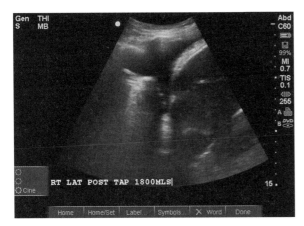

RT LAT POST TAP 1800MLS

Figure 30.4 Appearance of Figure 30.1 following therapeutic aspiration. Note the significant reduction in the depth of the pleural effusion following the therapeutic tap. Although there is still a small effusion present, the diaphragm is now convincingly convex.

thoracic cavity. Once the drain is inserted to an appropriate length, the guidewire and stiffening insert are withdrawn together. The drain should then be attached to an appropriate drainage system, including an underwater seal. The volume of fluid drained should be monitored and drainage temporarily stopped if >1500 mL is drained or the patient develops chest pain or cough. A detailed explanation of the insertion technique for both types of chest drain can be found within the BTS pleural procedures and thoracic US pleural disease guideline 2010. Insertion of chest drains should only be performed by staff who have been trained and assessed as competent in the procedure.

Pitfalls

Pleural drainage using US guidance has been shown to be considerably safer than using a blind technique. The benefit of US in these circumstances is determined by the ability of the observer to accurately interpret the US images obtained in order to correctly identify the presence of pleural fluid.

Potential pitfalls in US interpretation include:

- Differentiating pleural effusion from pleural thickening
- Differentiating complicated pleural effusions from consolidated lung
- Mistaking ascitic for pleural fluid.

The size of an effusion may be overestimated if the plane of the US scan is not perpendicular to the chest wall, but angled posteriorly to cut through a dependent posterior collection. Always obtain views in two planes (longitudinal and transverse) when assessing the size of an effusion.

Once the US has identified the appropriate site for drainage, ensure that the patient's position is not changed before completing the drainage procedure. Fluid will move under the effect of gravity, and changes in posture can have a marked effect on the depth and position of an effusion.

When undertaking chest drain insertion for a pleural effusion, it is essential that pleural fluid is aspirated during the infiltration with the local anaesthetic agent as a confirmatory step prior to proceeding. If no pleural fluid is obtained, stop and re-evaluate.

✓ Multiple choice questions

Interactive multiple choice questions to test your knowledge can be found in the Online appendix at www.oxfordmedicine.com/focusedicu. Please refer to your access card for further details.

Further reading

Havelock T, Teoh R, Laws D, Gleeson F; BTS Pleural Guideline Group. Pleural procedures and thoracic ultrasound: British Thoracic Society Pleural Disease Guideline 2010. *Thorax* 2010;**65**(Suppl 2):ii61–76.

Hooper C, Lee YCG, Maskell N; BTS Pleural Guideline Group. Investigation of a unilateral pleural effusion in adults: British Thoracic Society Pleural Disease Guideline 2010. *Thorax* 2010;**65**(Suppl 2):ii4–17.

31

Pericardial drainage

Shirjel Alam and Michael Gillies

Introduction

Percutaneous drainage may be indicated in 'medical' causes of tamponade or emergency situations. Surgical drainage is preferable in post-operative or traumatic causes, as well as regional collections not amenable to a percutaneous approach.

Where time permits, expert help should be sought from either a cardiologist or a cardiac surgeon before performing this procedure. However, there may be occasions when urgent drainage by an intensivist is required (i.e. cardiac arrest in a patient with a significant pericardial collection). This chapter will explain how it can be done using echocardiographic guidance and will discuss indications, contraindications, monitoring and equipment, positioning and approach, technical aspects of the procedure using US, and post-procedure care.

Indications

Percutaneous pericardiocentesis is indicated in patients with cardiac tamponade (Chapter 10) and may be lifesaving, so all its contraindications are relative.

Some causes of tamponade (e.g. post-operative haemopericardium, aortic dissections, and myocardial rupture) are best treated with immediate surgery, which should not be delayed. Percutaneous pericardiocentesis may be indicated as a temporizing measure in traumatic tamponade, but emergency thoracotomy is usually indicated, particularly in cardiac arrest.

Emergency pericardiocentesis is not indicated in a haemodynamically stable patient with a pericardial

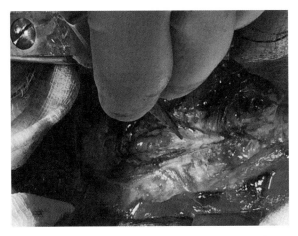

Figure 31.1 Thickened pericardium being opened during pericardectomy.

effusion but no signs of tamponade. Instead, expert guidance on clinical management should be sought. Coagulopathy should be corrected whenever time permits. Blood, pus, and effusions following recent surgery or trauma are better treated with open drainage in the operating theatre (Figure 31.1).

Monitoring and equipment

Full monitoring is advisable, ECG and invasive blood pressure in particular, and resuscitation equipment should be immediately available. Echocardiography increases the chances of successful and uncomplicated drainage. Where possible, full aseptic precautions should be taken, including a sterile cover for the echo probe. A Seldinger pericardiocentesis kit is ideal. However, in emergency situations, other needles of suitable gauge and length may be used, along with a three-way tap and a syringe.

Positioning and approach

Several approaches for percutaneous pericardiocentesis have been described. Ideally, the patient should be positioned at approximately 45°, to strike a good balance between optimum echo windows and needle approach. The subcostal approach is often technically easier, but it risks trauma to the liver and diaphragm. An apical approach avoids this but risks laceration of the left anterior descending artery at the apex, or iatrogenic pneumothorax. Ultimately, the decision depends on the location and depth of the effusion.

Echocardiographic measurements

The following useful echocardiographic measurements should be made (Figure 31.2):

1. The distance from skin to effusion—this is the length a needle must be inserted before fluid is aspirated

2. The distance from pericardium to apex (for apical approach) or RV (for subcostal approach)—this is the length the needle can be inserted after first aspiration of fluid before the myocardium is reached

3. The distance from skin to apex of RV—this is the total length the needle can be inserted before the myocardium is reached.

These measurements are useful to guide the procedure and help to prevent accidental damage to adjacent structures (e.g. perforation of the myocardium).

Percutaneous drainage of a pericardial collection

If possible, a Seldinger (needle-over-wire) drainage kit and real-time echocardiographic guidance should be used. With a sterile sheath over the US probe, a needle is inserted into the pericardial cavity under direct imaging, and a guidewire passed. Imaging is used to ensure that the guidewire is correctly placed (i.e. not in the pleural space or ventricle) before the drain is inserted (Figure 31.3).

It may not always be possible to advance the needle constantly within the echo plane, in which case imaging can only advise direction and depth of needle advancement. In such cases, correct placement of the needle or pericardial drain can be confirmed with agitated saline (1 mL air and 9 mL saline), which is injected directly into the pericardial cavity and visualized with echo (Figure 31.4). If there is concern about placement prior to dilatation of a tract, the aspiration needle can be used to inject agitated saline.

Aspiration of pericardial fluid or blood (using a syringe) should continue via the needle or drain until no more can be withdrawn. After drainage of the effusion, echocardiography should be repeated. The location and depth of any residual fluid should be identified and measured; subsequent echocardiography can then monitor for re-accumulation.

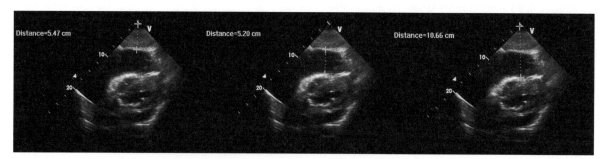

Figure 31.2 A subcostal view demonstrating depth of probe to effusion (left), depth from pericardium to myocardium (middle), and total distance from probe to myocardium (right).

(a)

(b)

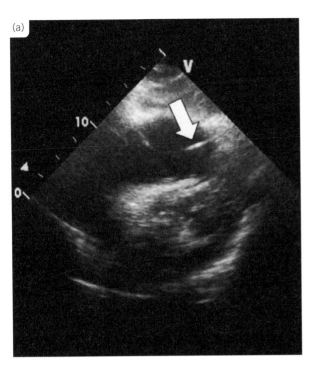

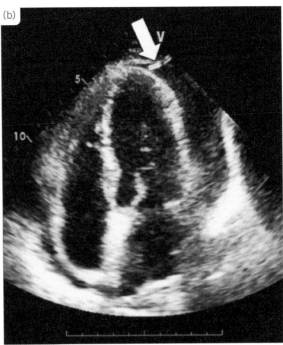

Figure 31.3 A guidewire (arrowed) in the pericardial cavity, inserted via the apical approach. (a) Subcostal view. (b) Apical view.

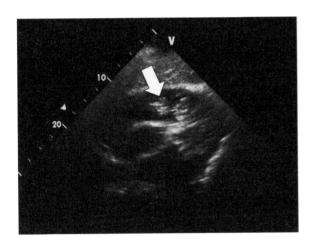

Figure 31.4 Correct placement of a pericardial drain, confirmed by injection of agitated saline.

Post-procedure care

Resuscitation must continue until the patient is haemodynamically stable. Continuous drainage of blood should raise the suspicion of right or left ventricular perforation and necessitate emergency cardiothoracic assessment. Fluid should be sent for biochemical, microbiological, and cytological examination. Depending on the clinical scenario, urgent Gram stain, mycobacterial or fungal culture, or viral polymerase chain reaction (PCR) may be appropriate. Following the procedure, chest X-ray should be performed to exclude pneumothorax. Monitoring of blood pressure, ECG, and oxygen saturations should continue. The catheter is usually left in situ on continuous drainage overnight or until the clinical team is satisfied that there is no re-accumulation of fluid (echocardiography is performed prior to confirm this); it can then be removed.

✅ Multiple choice questions

Interactive multiple choice questions to test your knowledge can be found in the Online appendix at www.oxfordmedicine.com/focusedicu. Please refer to your access card for further details.

Further reading

Fitch MT, Nick BA, Pariyadath M, McGinnis HD, Manthey DE. Emergency pericardiocentesis. *New England Journal of Medicine* 2012;**366**:e17.

Honda S, Asaumi Y, Yamane T, *et al*. Trends in the clinical and pathological characteristics of cardiac rupture in patients with acute myocardial infarction over 35 years. *Journal of the American Heart Association* 2014;**3**:e000984.

Huang YK, Lu MS, Liu KS, *et al*. Traumatic pericardial effusion: impact of diagnostic and surgical approaches. *Resuscitation* 2010;**81**:1682–6.

Kuvin JT, Harati NA, Pandian NG, *et al*. Postoperative cardiac tamponade in the modern surgical era. *Annals of Thoracic Surgery* 2002;**74**:1148–53.

Price S, Prout J, Jaggar SI, *et al*. 'Tamponade' following cardiac surgery: terminology and echocardiography may both mislead. *European Journal of Cardio-Thoracic Surgery* 2004;**26**:1156–60.

32

Paracentesis

David Ashton-Cleary

Introduction

US readily identifies ascites and is used to improve the safety and success of performing therapeutic and diagnostic paracentesis, when compared to a technique based on clinical signs. This chapter outlines the indications, preparation, and technique for undertaking US-guided paracentesis.

Indications for procedure and the role of ultrasound

Accumulated intra-abdominal fluid may represent a variety of underlying disease processes (Table 32.1) and result in a significant spectrum of symptoms, ranging from an asymptomatic state to an abdominal compartment syndrome. Sampling this fluid for diagnostic purposes or draining for therapeutic relief is a common procedure (Table 32.2). Traditionally, this has relied on landmark approaches, but US guidance can improve success and reduce complications.

The ability to safely aspirate fluid for either diagnostic or therapeutic paracentesis depends on being able to locate and access the deepest collection of fluid. Knowledge of the extraperitoneal anatomy traditionally suggests a point within either lower quadrants or just caudad to the umbilicus as safely offering the best access to a likely sump of fluid, while avoiding the inferior epigastric vessels in particular (Figure 32.1).

Table 32.1 Causes of ascites

Cause	Proportion of ascites admissions (%)
Cirrhosis	62
Malignancy	13
Non-alcoholic cirrhosis	5
Malignancy with cirrhosis	5
Others—cardiac failure, tuberculosis, pancreatitis	15

Data from Khan J, Pikkarainen P, Karvonen A-L, Makela T, Peraaho M, Pehkonen E, Collin P. Ascites: Aetiology, mortality and the prevalence of spontaneous, bacterial peritonitis. *Scand J Gastroenterol* 2009;**44**(8):970–4.

Table 32.2 Indications and contraindications for paracentesis

Indications	Contraindications
Diagnosis of new-onset ascites	Disseminated intravascular coagulopathy (A)
Exclude spontaneous bacterial peritonitis in pre-existing ascites	Cellulitis/local infection at puncture site (A)
Relieve discomfort or respiratory compromise in tense ascites	Bowel obstruction (R)
	Organomegaly (R)
	Pregnancy (R)

A = absolute; R = relative for contraindications.

Data from Nazeer SR, Dewbre H, Miller AH. Ultrasound-assisted paracentesis performed by emergency physicians vs the traditional technique: a prospective, randomized study. *Am J Emerg Med.* 2005;**23**(3):363–7.

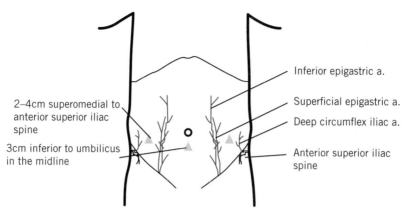

Figure 32.1 Vascular anatomy of the anterior abdominal wall and traditional landmark puncture sites.

Clinical signs frequently misdiagnose the presence of ascites. In one study of 100 patients undergoing paracentesis in the emergency department, US-guided drainage was successful in 95% with confirmed ascites, compared to 61% in the landmark group. US identified that 25% did not have ascites despite this being clinically suspected.

The most commonly reported complications following paracentesis include haematoma, seroma, and infection. More serious complications, such as bowel perforation and haemoperitoneum, are rare (<1:1000 procedures). US guidance has been associated with reduced complications and hospitalization costs, compared to landmark-based procedures. In addition, there are case report data for fatal outcomes from inferior epigastric artery laceration in landmark procedures. The anatomical landmark for these vessels is the lateral edge of the rectus muscle, but this procedure is rarely performed on those with clear muscular definition. The blood vessels can be easily visualized, and therefore potentially avoided, under US guidance.

Patient selection

Contraindications to paracentesis are summarized in Table 32.2. Although many patients will have a baseline coagulopathy, bleeding complications are rare (<1 in 1000 procedures). In the majority of patients, prophylactic fresh frozen plasma is not indicated, although most clinicians would administer platelets to patients with severe thrombocytopenia (e.g. platelet

count <40x109/L). Severe coagulopathy, as occurs in disseminated intravascular coagulopathy, is considered an absolute contraindication to the procedure.

Consideration should also be given to relative contraindications. The bladder should be empty, and in patients with bowel obstruction, a nasogastric tube passed to decompress the stomach. Those with organomegaly and pregnant patients are at an increased risk of solid organ injury.

Preparation

The patient should be positioned supine, with a 15° head-up tilt, to pool fluid within the lower abdomen. Ultrasonography should then be performed with an abdominal curvilinear probe in the lower quadrants to confirm the presence of fluid. The fluid will appear as an anechoic region below the abdominal wall structures (Figure 32.2). A safe point for drainage should be identified with an appropriate depth of fluid (ideally at least 2–3 cm), no vessels under the proposed needle pathway, and no bowel between the peritoneal wall and fluid. Bowel tends to float and move around in ascites and can be close to the abdominal wall (Video 3.2.1 ▢). If scanning reveals insufficient fluid or the possibility of an alternative diagnosis, abandon the procedure and seek specialist opinion, as required.

Paracentesis should be undertaken using a full aseptic technique, including skin preparation and sterile gown, gloves, mask, and drapes. Sterile draping of the US probe should be completed if

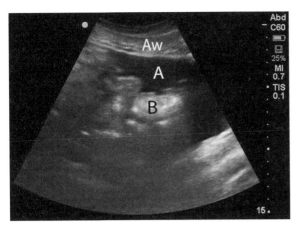

Figure 32.2 Typical appearance of ascites. A, ascites; Aw, abdominal wall; B, bowel.

real-time US guidance is planned Equipment requirements will be dictated by the procedure. A diagnostic tap requires a 20-mL syringe, a suitable needle (a 38-mm, 19G needle will permit aspiration of viscid ascites, while minimizing the size of an inadvertent bowel or vascular puncture), and an array of specimen tubes (see Post-procedure care, p. 266). For therapeutic drainage, a suitable drainage kit will be required, with a means by which to collect large volumes; either evacuated bottles or a drainage bag. Although various kits exist, a Seldinger technique is increasingly used due to its inherent safety, compared to catheter-over-needle techniques such as the pigtail catheter. A Veress needle-based approach is another suitable alternative, as this avoids the presence of a sharp point within the abdomen once the peritoneum has been punctured. The choice will depend on operator familiarity and local availability and practice.

For drainage of >5 L or in those with pre-existing renal impairment, consideration should be given to human albumin solution replacement. Transfusion of 100 mL of 20% albumin per 2.5 L reduces the incidence of post-procedural cardiovascular decompensation, re-accumulation of ascites, and development of type 2 hepatorenal syndrome.

The procedure

In the conscious patient, a wheal of local anaesthetic solution should be raised in the skin with a 25G needle before anaesthetizing the proposed tract of the puncture. A further 5–10 mL of lidocaine can be instilled within the peritoneum once breached, as this can alleviate discomfort further.

Due to the mobility of bowel within ascites (Video 3.2.1), a blind approach using US to mark a point for subsequent insertion is not generally recommended. In-plane continual visualization of the needle using US throughout insertion is the technique of choice (Video 3.2.2). Either a curvilinear or linear array probe may be used.

Two techniques for paracentesis which minimize post-procedural fluid leak and consequent infection risk are described (Figure 32.3). The anterior abdominal wall can be punctured tangentially or the Z-tract approach can be used. Both aim to ensure that the skin and peritoneal punctures are not directly adjacent. In the Z-tract approach, the skin is held under tension and the needle inserted perpendicularly. When the needle or drainage tube are finally removed, the skin returns to its resting position, and so the puncture sites are offset from one another. For the US-guided technique, a Z-tract will require an assistant to apply skin tension, as the operator has both hands occupied with the US probe and the needle; this is therefore generally impractical. In addition, the perpendicular trajectory makes in-plane visualization impossible, and this is one of the key advantages offered by real-time ultrasonography for this procedure. In-plane visualization necessitates a tangential trajectory, and so this technique, rather than an attempt at Z-tract, should be utilized. In addition, a tangential approach affords additional safety from bowel injury, particularly for more shallow collections or where bowel distension ablates a deep sump of fluid (Video 3.2.2). The needle trajectory relative to the bowel surface is nearing parallel, rather than in the perpendicular entry seen in a Z-tract, which may be associated with a greater risk of bowel injury.

Once the peritoneum is breached and ascitic fluid successfully aspirated, a diagnostic procedure is completed simply by removing 20 mL of fluid for analysis and applying a small dressing to the skin puncture site. For a therapeutic procedure, the drain should be inserted and secured, according to the manufacturer's instructions. Evacuated bottles or conventional drainage bags can be used to collect the fluid.

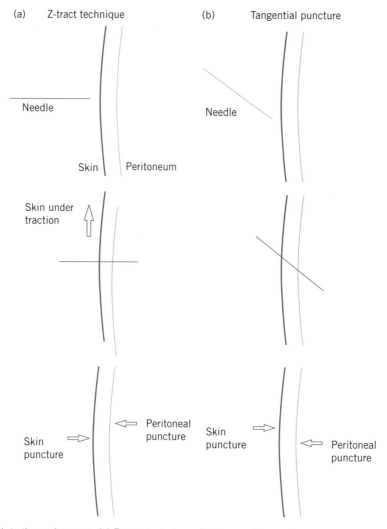

Figure 32.3 Approach to the peritoneum. (a) Z-tract technique. (b) Tangential puncture.

Post-procedure care

Once the procedure is complete and the patient made comfortable, attention should turn to analysis of the fluid. Tests should include a minimum of culture, cell count, and protein/albumin assay (with a corresponding serum albumin sample). Other tests can be requested on the basis of clinical suspicion (Table 32.3). Arguably of most value is the serum-ascites albumin gradient (SAAG), which is determined by subtracting the ascitic value from concurrent serum value. The differential diagnosis when the gradient is <1.1 g/dL is relatively broad and includes nephrotic syndrome, pancreatitis, carcinomatosis, and tuberculosis. However, for a gradient greater than or equal to 1.1 g/dL, the diagnostic accuracy for portal hypertension as the cause is 97%.

Once drained to the desired effect (usually to dryness), drains should be removed promptly to minimize the risk of infection. Usually this is within 6 hours; however, small studies have demonstrated no infective complications with large-volume drainage over 72 hours.

Pitfalls

- Bleeding due to inadvertent damage to inferior epigastric vessels

- Mistaking bladder or cystic masses (e.g. ovarian cyst) for ascites

- Bowel perforation due to insertion of the needle too close to bowel.

Table 32.3 Analysis of ascitic fluid

Possible diagnosis	Test	Result	Comment
Portal hypertension	SAAG	>1.1 g/dL	For example, cirrhosis, portal thrombosis, cardiac failure, alcoholic hepatitis
Spontaneous bacterial peritonitis	Glucose	>2.8 mmol/L	
	LDH	Within normal lab range	
	Total protein	<1 g/dL	
	Cell count/differential	>250 polymorphonuclear white cells per mm^3	And no potential cause of secondary peritonitis
Perforated viscus	Alkaline phosphatase	>240 IU/L	
	Carcinoembryonic antigen	>5 ng/mL	
	Glucose	<2.8 mmol/L	
	LDH	Above normal lab range upper limit	
	Total protein	>1 g/dL	
	Amylase	>2000 IU/L	May also suggest pancreatitis
Carcinomatosis	Fluid smear		Usually from breast, colon, pancreas, or gastric primaries

Data from: Thomsen TW, Shaffer RW, White B, Setnik GS. Paracentesis. *N Engl J Med* 2006;**355**(19):e21; and Runyon BA. Management of adult patients with ascites due to cirrhosis. *Hepatology* 2004;**39**(3):841–56.

✓ Multiple choice questions

Interactive multiple choice questions to test your knowledge can be found in the Online appendix at www.oxfordmedicine.com/focusedicu. Please refer to your access card for further details.

Further reading

Cervini P, Hesley GK, Thompson RL, Sampathkumar P, Knudsen JM. Incidence of infectious complications after an ultrasound-guided intervention. *American Journal of Roentgenology* 2010;**195**:846–50.

Francesco Salerno F, Guevara M, Bernardi M, *et al.* Refractory ascites: pathogenesis, definition and therapy of a severe complication in patients with cirrhosis. *Liver International* 2010;**30**:937–47.

Khan J, Pikkarainen P, Karvonen A-L, *et al.* Ascites: aetiology, mortality and the prevalence of spontaneous, bacterial peritonitis. *Scandinavian Journal of Gastroenterology* 2009;**44**:970–4.

Nazeer SR, Dewbre H, Miller AH. Ultrasound-assisted paracentesis performed by emergency physicians vs the traditional technique: a prospective, randomized study. *American Journal of Emergency Medicine* 2005;**23**:363–7.

Patel PA, Ernst FR, Gunnarsson CL. Evaluation of hospital complications and costs associated with using ultrasound guidance during abdominal paracentesis procedures. *Journal of Medical Economics* 2012;**15**:1–7.

Runyon BA. Management of adult patients with ascites due to cirrhosis. *Hepatology* 2004;**39**:841–56.

Sekiguchi H, Suzuki J, Daniels CE. Making paracentesis safer a proposal for the use of bedside abdominal and vascular ultrasonography to prevent a fatal complication. *Chest* 2013;**143**:1136–9.

Skovgaard Wiese S, Christian Mortensen C, Bendtsen F. Few complications after paracentesis in patients with cirrhosis and refractory ascites. *Danish Medical Bulletin* 2011;**58**:A4212.

Thomsen TW, Shaffer RW, White B, Setnik GS. Paracentesis. *New England Journal of Medicine* 2006;**355**:e21.

Van Thiel DH, Moore CM, Garcia M, George M, Nadir A. Continuous peritoneal drainage of large-volume ascites. *Digestive Diseases and Sciences* 2011;**56**:2723–7.

33

Lumbar puncture

Paul Margetts

Introduction

Undertaking lumbar puncture (LP) in the ICU patient can be technically challenging due to patient positioning and body habitus. US guidance can improve the success rate and is relatively easy to learn. This chapter describes the normal sonoanatomy of the lumbar spine and how to use US to guide LP.

Benefits of ultrasound

LP is usually performed by a landmark technique, but in the critically ill, this can be considerably more challenging than in the general hospital population. Patients are frequently sedated and ventilated, which, combined with the need to measure cerebrospinal fluid (CSF) opening pressure, mandates performing LP in the lateral position. Prior to the procedure, the patient needs to be positioned on the edge of the bed, with his or her knees drawn up to the chest, in order to maximally open up the lumbar interspinous spaces. This represents a minor manual handling challenge in the sedated and ventilated patient, and optimal positioning is often not satisfactorily achieved. In addition, the increasing prevalence of obesity in the general population can make palpation of the bony landmarks for LP unreliable and occasionally even impossible. Often simply establishing the anatomical midline can be a challenge. In this context, US assistance can be invaluable, saving time, minimizing unsuccessful attempts at blind needling, and improving the success rate and safety of the procedure. US-guided LP is a relatively easy procedure to perform and learn.

Probe choice

In the lumbar region, the subarachnoid space is generally located at a depth of between 4 and 8 cm from the surface of the skin, though it can be deeper in obese individuals. For this reason, lumbar spinal US is best performed with a curvilinear transducer with a frequency range of between 3 and 8 MHz. Higher-frequency linear array probes may improve resolution in thin patients or children, but landmark techniques are generally less of a challenge in these groups, except in the presence of spinal disease such as severe osteoarthritis or previous trauma.

Sonoanatomy

Several US views of the lumbar spine have been described, but all are essentially variations of the following approach. The US survey should begin with a paramedian sagittal view, to establish the correct lumbar interspace for puncture, before rotating the probe to a transverse view and identifying the anatomical midline and the depth from the skin to the ligamentum flavum.

Paramedian sagittal oblique view

With the patient in the left lateral position, the probe is orientated in a longitudinal plane, with the direction marker pointed towards the patient's head. Place the probe on the patient's lumbar region, 2–3 cm from the estimated midline, with the beam direction angled in towards it. Adjust the degree of angulation and distance from the midline until the sawtooth pattern of the underlying laminae is visualized (Figure 33.1). Between, and deep to, the laminae will be visible the

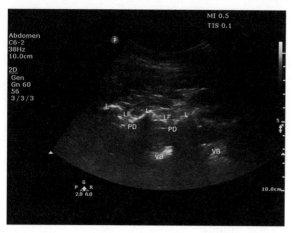

Figure 33.1 Paramedian sagittal oblique view of lumbar vertebrae. L, laminae; LF, ligamentum flavum; PD, posterior dura; VB, vertebral body.

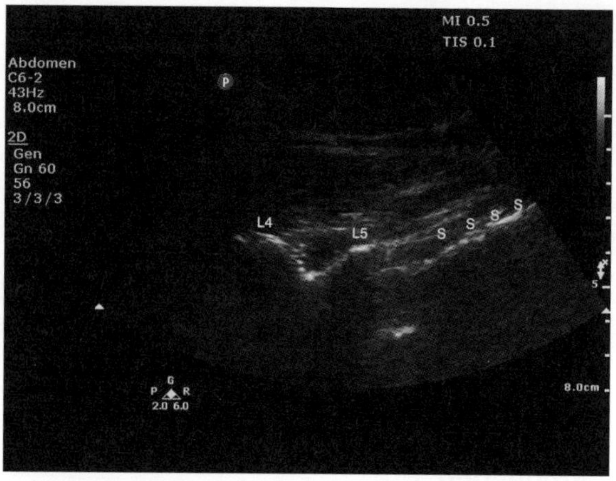

Figure 33.2 Paramedian sagittal oblique view of lumbo-sacral junction. L4 lamina; L5 lamina; S, sacrum.

ligamentum flavum and the posterior dura, separated by the narrow, hypoechoic epidural space.

Having identified the laminae, slide the probe caudally to find the sacrum. This will appear as a continuous, hyperechoic line, caudal to the interrupted pattern of the laminae (Figure 33.2). Once the sacrum is located, slide the probe cranially again, counting the vertebral levels until the L3/4 interspace is identified.

Transverse view

At the level of the L3/4 interspace, rotate the probe through 90° to obtain a transverse view (Figures 33.3 and 33.4). The probe will usually need to be angulated slightly cranially to align with the downward sloping spinous processes. Superficially, the interspinous ligament will appear as a bright, hyperechoic line, with the ligamentum flavum and posterior dura visible below. Unlike in the parasagittal view, where the ligamentum flavum and posterior dura are often identifiable as separate structures, in the transverse view, these generally appear as a single complex, marking the posterior border of the hypoechoic intrathecal space. If the probe slides cranially or caudally off the vertebral interspace, the interspinous ligament will be replaced with the more echogenic spinous process, obscuring all deeper structures with its dense acoustic shadow.

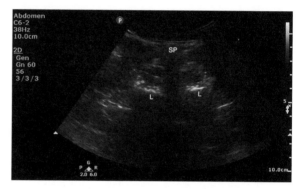

Figure 33.3 Transverse view of the fourth lumbar spinous process. L, lamina; SP, spinous process.

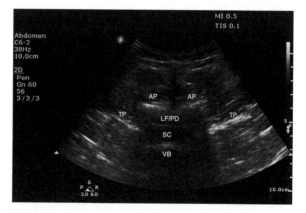

Figure 33.4 Transverse view of lumbar 3/4 interspace. AP, articular process; LF/PD, ligamentum flavum/posterior dura; SC, spinal canal; TP, transverse process; VB, vertebral body.

Techniques

US-assisted LP is most often performed with a pre-procedural scan method. The target L3/4 interspace, and point of needle entry, is marked prior to performing the LP 'blind'. This technique is well suited to the critical care setting, as the common problem of patients altering position between scan and LP is generally eliminated by sedation. Real-time US guidance of LP is also possible, but it is a difficult procedure and offers few advantages over the pre-procedural scan method in the sedated patient.

Pre-procedural scan technique

The pre-procedural scan should be performed immediately prior to the LP to ensure the patient's position does not change. Ideally the same operator should perform both the US scan and the procedure, as the subtleties of probe angulation for optimally visualizing the interspace is a useful guide for subsequently directing the spinal needle. Establish the indications and absence of contraindications for LP, and then position the patient in the left lateral position, flexing the lumbar spine as much as possible. Start scanning in the paramedian sagittal oblique view, and identify the sacrum and L5/S1 interspace. Then move the probe cephalad, marking the interspace levels with a surgical skin marker until the L2/3 interspace is identified.

Rotate the probe to the transverse view and position it, so the L3/4 interspace is in the centre of the probe. Mark this midline on the skin, and repeat at a level above and below the target. Returning to the L3/4 interspace, identify the ligamentum flavum/dura complex and measure its depth below the skin with the US machine's calipers. This is a useful guide to how far to insert the spinal needle, although the actual depth of insertion required will usually be slightly less due to compression of subcutaneous tissues.

Real-time technique

This is an advanced technique as it requires visualizing, with a curvilinear probe, a thin needle inserted at a steep angle. This can be very challenging, even for those with extensive previous experience of US-guided procedures. Various methods have been described, mostly variations on the paramedian approach to the

intrathecal space and utilizing both in-plane and out-of-plane needle visualization. No convincing evidence yet exists to recommend one method over another, but the following is perhaps the most logical and easiest to learn.

Having established the indications and lack of contraindications for LP, position the patient in the left lateral position, with the lumbar spine maximally flexed. Full aseptic precautions should be taken, with the US probe covered in a sterile sheath. Disinfect and drape the patient's lower back, and perform an initial longitudinal paramedian scan, as per the pre-procedural method, to establish the correct level for LP.

Once the L3/4 level has been identified, position the probe in the paramedian sagittal plane, visualizing the laminae above and below the intervertebral space. From this point, try to maintain the caudal aspect of the probe fixed over the L4 lamina, and by rotating the probe around this point, move the cranial aspect of the probe towards the midline until the spinous process of the L3 vertebra comes into view. Between these points, the hypoechoic line of the ligamentum flavum/dura complex may be visible but is usually hard to identify (Figure 33.5). The spinal needle is then directed in-plane, with the US beam into the interlaminar space. It is often difficult to maintain good needle visualization at the steep angle required, and the tip may disappear into the acoustic shadow of the L3 spinous process before penetrating the ligamentum flavum, usually felt by a palpable give or click as the needle is advanced.

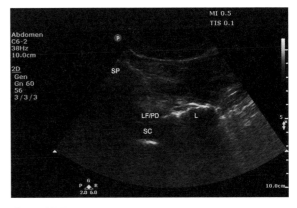

Figure 33.5 Rotated paramedian oblique view for real-time in-plane ultrasound-guided technique. L, lamina; LF/PD, ligamentum flavum/posterior dura; SC, spinal canal; SP, spinous process.

Pitfalls and pearls

As the intrathecal effects of US gel are unknown, it is important that none contaminates the needle during LP. All gel must be thoroughly removed from the site of skin puncture prior to needle entry. If performing real-time US guidance, sterile saline may be used as a safe alternative acoustic coupling agent.

It can be hard to prevent skin markings made during pre-procedural scanning from being erased when removing the US gel and disinfecting the back prior to LP. Reinforcing the markings between these stages may help, as can gently indenting the patient's skin at the point of intended needle insertion with a blunt circular object such as the hub of a drawing-up needle or the tip of a non-luer lock syringe.

If performing the real-time US technique, a larger 22G spinal needle may be more easily visualized than the commonly used 25G and does not need a separate introducer needle.

✔ Multiple choice questions

Interactive multiple choice questions to test your knowledge can be found in the Online appendix at www.oxfordmedicine.com/focusedicu. Please refer to your access card for further details.

SECTION 5

Governance-based

34

Governance in point-of-care ultrasound

Peter Macnaughton and Marcus Peck

Introduction

Technological advances have resulted in a proliferation of relatively cheap, portable, easy-to-use, and high-quality US machines. This has resulted in the rapid uptake of this modality by healthcare professionals who have incorporated it into their clinical practice but were not traditionally trained in imaging. While there are undoubted benefits of point-of-care US (POCUS), numerous authorities have raised concerns about its potential for patient harm, as performance and interpretation of US are user-dependent and require significant training and experience. Use of US by clinicians who have not had adequate training and experience potentially exposes patients to the risk of incorrect diagnosis and inappropriate management.

The safe use of POCUS, including focused echocardiography, is not limited to ensuring that practitioners have undertaken appropriate training. Each ICU using US needs to establish a quality assurance programme to ensure that equipment is fit for purpose and well maintained, studies are appropriately reported and documented, and there is continuing audit of practice, a process for peer review, and continuing professional development of all practitioners.

It is recommended that each ICU has a clinical lead for POCUS, with responsibility for training and quality assurance.

Training

Correct use of US is dependent on the skills of the operator, which only come with adequate training.

There is widespread consensus that focused ultrasound should be a core skill for all intensive care clinicians, although it has not, to date, been included in national training programmes. A number of organizations have published recommendations for POCUS training programmes, with largely similar outlines (Box 34.1). The UK Intensive Care Society has established training recommendations and accreditation pathways for focused echocardiography [known as Focused Intensive Care Echo (FICE)] and POCUS [known as Core Ultrasound in Intensive Care (CUSIC)], which includes vascular access, lung, and abdominal imaging.

Theoretical training should include the basic physics and principles of US, how to obtain images, normal sonoanatomy, relevant pathology, and initial hands-on supervised practice using normal models; for focused echocardiography, this is typically around 10 hours in duration.

Directly supervised practice should continue until the trainee has demonstrated competence in obtaining and saving satisfactory images. Then follows mentored practice, when the trainee may undertake examinations without direct supervision but saves their

---

Box 34.1 Structural outline of an ultrasound training programme

- Theoretical training
- Supervised practice
- Mentored practice, with generation of logbook
- Confirmation of satisfactory experience in logbook
- Summative assessment of competence

---

images for later review by their training supervisor. Details of each examination, and the trainee's interpretation, are recorded in their logbook. Their findings must be reviewed and verified by their mentor, before being recorded in the patient's clinical record and used to influence clinical care.

In order to gain experience and competence, the trainee needs to undertake an appropriate number of investigations with a representative range of pathology. It is important that the logbook of examinations should be those undertaken on critically ill patients, and not stable outpatients or normal subjects.

Once trainees have demonstrated a satisfactory number of examinations with an appropriate range of pathology, as assessed by their supervisor, a summative competency assessment should take place before sign-off and completion of training (Box 34.2).

There is a lack of consensus on the number of examinations that need to be completed during training to gain competence. It is clear that this will vary between trainees and the modalities being assessed. There are transferrable skills between different areas of US practice, which may influence the number of examinations that need to be completed. Overall, emphasis should be on demonstrating competence, rather than achieving absolute numbers, although supervisors must be satisfied that the trainee has gained appropriate experience in the range of pathology that is likely to be encountered. Table 34.1 summarizes the typical number of examinations that will need to be

Table 34.1 Typical number of examinations required for training

Ultrasound modality	Suggested logbook numbers
Focused echo	50
Lung ultrasound	30
Basic abdominal	25
Vascular access	10

completed in each area in order to gain competence and experience.

Revalidation

The pathway for re-accreditation is not always as clear as accreditation, but revalidation is increasingly important in modern healthcare. Demonstrating ongoing involvement with POCUS by collecting a logbook of clinical practice and attendance at relevant local and national meetings should become part of each practitioner's portfolio.

Required case numbers for POCUS re-accreditation have not been suggested as yet. The British Society of Echocardiography expects a minimum of 100 cases per year for critical care echo re-accreditation; however, this is advanced-level practice. Locally, the POCUS clinical lead may become an increasingly important link in the revalidation process.

Distinction between POCUS and diagnostic ultrasound

POCUS and comprehensive US are fundamentally different. POCUS only assesses the presence or absence of a limited number of specific US findings, while comprehensive US is a comprehensive, systematic examination of anatomy and function (Box 34.3).

POCUS does not replace a comprehensive examination. Other healthcare professionals, as well as patients and their families, need to be made aware of the distinction between POCUS and a comprehensive examination, as misinterpretation of this may prevent

---

Box 34.2 Definition of competence in POCUS

- Demonstrates a patient-centred approach
- Uses the ultrasound machine safely
- Uses appropriate functions of the machine correctly, including image optimization
- Reproducibly obtains good-quality and correctly orientated images
- Labels, records, and stores images correctly
- Identifies normal and abnormal scans
- Interprets findings correctly, in keeping with the clinical situation
- Demonstrates good infection control practice
- Understands the limitations of focused ultrasound, and their scope of practice

> **Box 34.3** Features of a POCUS examination
>
> - Undertaken by the primary care provider
> - Used as an adjunct to clinical examination
> - Identifies the presence or absence of a limited number of ultrasound findings
> - Does not replace comprehensive diagnostic ultrasound
> - Used to clarify clinical findings and identify important (often life-threatening) conditions in acute care
> - Used to guide invasive procedures to improve patient safety

further appropriate investigation. A 'negative' POCUS examination is not the same as a normal comprehensive diagnostic examination, as it does not exclude all pathology in the area examined.

Reporting, documentation, and image storage

When scans are verified and used to change clinical management, it is essential that representative images are stored and an appropriate report is documented in the patient's medical record. This should ensure proper communication with other healthcare professionals and enable quality assessment at a later date. The report should be limited to the specific US findings assessed and not be over-interpreted, and any limitations of the examination should be highlighted. A standardized reporting format is encouraged (Figures 34.1 and 34.2).

> **Pitfall**
>
> Negative findings should not be reported as a normal scan.

Whenever a POCUS examination is undertaken, the practitioner should start by ensuring that the patient details are entered (e.g. name, date of birth, and identifying number), together with details of the examiner, in order that images can be saved and retrieved for peer review and medico-legal purposes. Representative images should be recorded throughout the examination. As US is a dynamic modality, it is recommended that short video clips are stored and combined with still images when any measurements are undertaken. Images should be stored in a format that is permanent. Ideally, this should be undertaken by uploading to the existing hospital digital storage system, usually managed by either cardiology or radiology. If this is not possible, there should be a process for confidential, secure, and permanent storage. North American practice requires that US images that lead to a change in clinical practice are stored for at least 7 years. Use of the storage within an US machine is not adequate alone, as it is not permanent, secure, or backed up. Machine hard drive memory is of limited size, and when this is reached, data can be irretrievably lost. Whenever images are copied for the purposes of teaching or training logbooks, they must be anonymized to maintain confidentiality. Some US machines offer an option for downloading images without patient details, and this should be selected whenever possible.

Quality assurance

A robust quality assurance programme is essential to ensure delivery of a safe and high-quality POCUS service.

Equipment management

Units should have a machine that is fit for purpose. Optimal characteristics include portability, high-quality image processing, correct range of probes for examinations undertaken, relative ease of use, and rapid boot-up time, with battery backup. Machines that can be cleaned easily between patients are desirable, to limit the risks of transmission of infections (see Infection control, p. 280). There should be an adequate hard drive, with the ability to store both patient and operator details. Being able to add patient details at the end of an examination is desirable, in order that examinations undertaken in an emergency (e.g. during cardiac arrest) can be appropriately stored. There should be appropriate ports to enable upload to central digital storage systems and download of anonymized studies to external drives.

intensive care society
care when it matters

British Society of Echocardiography
Affiliated to the British Cardiac Society

Appendix 5 - FICE Logbook Reporting Form

Patient reference & clinical details	Date	Views
		(please tick)
	Operator	
		PLAX
(Do NOT use patient details. Any documents leaving clinical area must be anonymised)		PSAX
	Machine	A4C
Ventilation & haemodynamics		SC4
	Image quality	IVC
	Good	Lungs
	Average	Other
	Poor	

FICE assessment (please circle; *U/A = unable to assess*)

Q1. Is the LV dilated? YES NO U/A
Notes:

Q2. Is the LV significantly impaired? YES NO U/A
Notes:

Q3. Is the RV dilated? YES NO U/A
Notes:

Q4. Is the RV severely impaired? YES NO U/A
Notes:

Q5. Is there pericardial fluid? YES NO U/A
Notes:

Q6. Is there evidence of severe hypovolaemia? YES NO U/A
Notes:

Q7. Is there pleural fluid? YES NO U/A
Notes:

Other comments:

Conclusion, clinical significance & suggested actions:

Is expert referral required? (circle) **Yes** **No**

Signed: _____ Countersigned:_____
(Trainee) Mentor/Supervisor)
This is a training report only, and should not be used to influence clinical management without expert verification.

30

Figure 34.1 Focused Intensive Care Echo (FICE) reporting form.
Reproduced with kind permission from the Intensive Care Society.

Lung ultrasound reporting form

Date of study					
Patient details/cross reference	Any documents leaving clinical area must not include patient identifiable information.				
Name of sonographer					
Image quality		Good	Acceptable		Poor

		Lung sliding	B lines	Effusion	Collapse/consolidation	
					Minimal	Significant
Right	Upper ant Point					
Right	Lower ant point					
Right	Post-lateral Point					
Left	Upper ant point					
Left	Lower ant point					
Left	Post-lateral point					

Comments or further details:

Signature	
Mentor sign off confirming findings	

Figure 34.2 Core Ultrasound in Intensive Care (CUSIC) lung ultrasound reporting form.
Reproduced with kind permission from the Intensive Care Society.

Equipment needs to be maintained correctly. All equipment, including probes and leads, should be checked regularly and replaced immediately if damaged. All operators must be aware of correct handling of the equipment to prevent damage. All staff must have received training in correct operation of the US equipment. US equipment needs to be serviced regularly, according to the manufacturer's recommendation.

Infection control

Within the intensive care environment, the US machine represents a significant vector risk for transmitting infections between patients. It is essential that all staff follow good infection control practices. This should include ensuring that probes and cables are disinfected immediately after each patient examination and that this is undertaken before placing the probe back into the storage rack on the machine (Box 34.4). US probes can be damaged by the use of incorrect disinfectants; purpose-designed antimicrobial sprays are available for cleaning US probes. The machine should be wiped down at the end of each examination. Cases have been reported of reusable containers of US gel becoming colonized with pathogenic bacteria, and so

---

Box 34.4 Process for ultrasound cleaning between patients

- At end of the examination, remove the sterile sheath (if used), wipe off the gel from the probe, and place it on the patient's bed.
- Decontaminate the hands.
- Wipe the probe and cable with an antimicrobial agent, as per manufacturer's guidance.
- Return the probe to the storage rack on the machine.
- Wipe down the machine's keyboard and control panel with an appropriate surface cleaner.
- Return the machine to a dedicated storage area, and reconnect its mains electric supply.

---

single-use sterile sachets are preferred. If these are unavailable, it is important that reusable bottles are replaced regularly (e.g. weekly). To ensure that infection control practices are effective, microbiological surveillance of the US machine is recommended; swabs should be taken for culture on a routine basis.

Audit, peer review, and continuing professional development

Audit of US practice should include (but not be limited to) practitioners' scope of practice, reporting of examinations, and labelling and storage of images. Peer review should occur to provide assurance that examinations are being conducted and interpreted correctly. Regular multi-professional meetings, where US examinations are reviewed, provide an excellent forum for peer review and continuing education. All practitioners must ensure that they maintain and develop their skills by ensuring that they undertake regular examinations and include POCUS within their portfolio of continuing professional development. Practitioners should be encouraged to maintain a logbook of their examinations in order to demonstrate their ongoing commitment and experience. They should also have access to a fully trained supervisor, who can provide encouragement, guidance for further development, and discussion about difficult cases.

✅ Multiple choice questions

Interactive multiple choice questions to test your knowledge can be found in the Online appendix at www.oxfordmedicine.com/focusedicu. Please refer to your access card for further details.

Further reading

Intensive Care Society. FICE accreditation pack link. Available from: http://www.ics.ac.uk/ICS/fice.aspx [accessed 10 September 2018].

Intensive Care Society. CUSIC accreditation pack link. Available from: http://www.ics.ac.uk/ICS/cusic.aspx [accessed 10 September 2018].

Index

A

A-lines 28, 129, 145, 195
abdominal aorta 157–9
abdominal aortic aneurysm 159
abdominal scan 169–76
    bladder 174–5
    bowel 174
    FAST 205, 206t, 207
    gall bladder 172–3, 175
    kidneys 173
    liver 170–2, 175
    probe choice 169–70
    stomach 173–4
absorption 11
accreditation 5
acoustic enhancement 29
acoustic impedance 11
acoustic mismatch 11
acoustic shadowing 26
acute cor pulmonale 183, 227
acute coronary syndrome 58
acute heart failure 58, 65
acute kidney injury 217–25
    calculi 221
    hydronephrosis 219–21
    imaging technique 218–19
    pyelonephritis 221
    pyonephrosis 221
    resistive index 223
    role of ultrasound 217
acute respiratory distress syndrome
    (ARDS) 225–33
    acute cor pulmonale 227
    complications 227–8
    diagnosis 226–7
    differentiating from cardiogenic
        pulmonary oedema 148
    excessive fluids 230
    extracorporeal membrane
        oxygenation 232
    hypovolaemia 228, 230
    inhaled nitric oxide 230
    intravascular volume status 231–2
    left ventricular function 227
    lung ultrasound 225–6
    PEEP in lung-protective
        ventilation 230
    prone positioning 230
    pulmonary arterial pressure 231
    right atrial dilatation 227
    right ventricular dilatation 227–8
    right ventricular systolic
        function 228, 231
acute respiratory failure 6, 193–7
advanced life support 185
aliasing 16

alveolar conditions 142–4
alveolar–interstitial syndrome 144–8
amplitude 9
angle of interrogation 22, 23
aorta 151–9
    abdominal 157–9
    thoracic 152–7
aortic dissection 52, 101, 156
aortic regurgitation 100–1, 103, 104
aortic root 153
    dilatation 100
aortic sclerosis 99
aortic stenosis 99–100
    aortic root dilatation 100
    bicuspid 100
    calcific 99
    colour Doppler 103–4
    continuous wave Doppler 104–5
    dimensionless index 105
    leaflet mobility 102
    left ventricle 100
    peak velocity 105
    rheumatic 100
aortic valve 97–106
    anatomy 97–8
    annulus 98
    bicuspid 100
    colour Doppler 103–4
    commissures 98
    cusps 97, 98
    echo assessment 101–3
    leaflets 97, 102
    obstruction 98–101
    orifice observation 102
    physiology 98
    planimetry 102
    replacements 105–6
    spectral Doppler 104–6
    vegetations 101
apical four-chamber view 40
apical long-axis view 43
apical three-chamber view 43–4
apical two-chamber view 43–4
array 10
artefacts 25–31
    acoustic enhancement 29
    acoustic shadowing 26
    edge shadowing 26
    linear 30
    mirror image 30
    near-field clutter 29
    refraction 30
    resolution 25–6
    reverberations 27–9
    side lobe 29–30
    technical assumptions 25

    tumble 221
    twinkle 221
arterial cannulation 243
ascites 139–40, 261t, 265t
asystole 185–6
atelectasis 143–4
atria 81–7
    anatomy 81
    cardiac tumours 85
    colour Doppler 86
    contrast studies 87
    dilatation 83–4
    dimensions 83
    physiology 82
    spontaneous echo contrast 84
    thrombus 84–5
    two-dimensional appearances 82–3
    wires and catheters 86
atrial appendages 81
atrial septum 81, 82, 83
    defects 86–7
    lipomatous hypertrophy 85
attenuation 11, 19
attenuation coefficient 11
audit 278
auto-optimization 19
axillary artery 162
axillary vein 162
    infraclavicular cannulation 240–1

B

B-lines 28–9, 129–30, 135, 145–8, 195,
    226, 227, 230
barcode (stratosphere) sign 129, 133
BART mnemonic 21, 161
baseline 21, 22
basilic vein 162–3
    PICC placement 242
bat sign 128
Beck's triad 89
bicuspid aortic valve 100
biplane method 63
bladder scan 174–5, 221–2
BLUE Protocol 6, 193, 194–7
bowel scan 174
box size and position 21
brachial artery 163
brachial veins 162

C

cardiac arrest 185–91
    advanced life support 185
    asystole 185–6
    cardiac rhythm 185–6
    cardiac tamponade 187–8
    differential diagnosis 186

cardiac arrest (*Cont.*)
  hypovolaemia 186–7
  myocardial infarction 189
  pacing devices 186
  pericardial collections 188
  pneumothorax 190–1
  post-cardiac arrest syndrome 191
  post-resuscitation lung ultrasound 191
  pseudo-PEA 186
  pulmonary embolism 190
  pulseless electrical activity 186
  ventricular fibrillation 186
cardiac output 121
cardiac rhythm 185–6
cardiac tamponade 89, 91, 94
  cardiac arrest 187–8
  percutaneous
    pericardiocentesis 188, 257–60
cardiac tumours 85
cardiogenic pulmonary oedema 148,
    195, 227
cardiomyopathy
  dilated 63
  hypertrophic 57, 64
  Takotsubo 58, 65
carotid Doppler flow 123–4
central venous pressure 118
cephalic vein 162–3
chest drains 254–5
Chiari network 85
cholecystitis 172
chordae tendinae 108, 109
chronic heart failure 58
chronic kidney disease 218
chronic pulmonary hypertension 78
cirrhosis 171–2
Coanda effect 21, 114
coaptation line 107
coaptation zone 107
colour flow Doppler 16, 21
  aortic valve 103–4
  atria 86
  BART mnemonic 21, 161
  mitral valve 112–14
  venous thrombosis 166
comet tails 29
common bile duct 172, 173, 175
competence 5, 274
compression 19
concentric hypertrophy 57
continuing professional development 278
continuous wave (CW)
    Doppler 16, 21–3
  aortic stenosis 104–5
contrast studies 87, 225
control use 17–21
cor pulmonale 183, 227
cricoid cartilage 246
cricothyroid membrane 246
cricothyrotomy 248–9
CT scan, trauma 205, 206*t*
curtain sign 131
curvilinear probes 10, 14, 18

D
deep vein thrombosis 193–4
depth control 18
descending aorta 153
diaphragm
  anatomy 125
  paralysis/weakness 149–50
  ultrasound assessment 130–1, 148–50
  weaning failure 203
dilated cardiomyopathy 63
dimensionless index 105
dissection flap 156
documentation 275
Doppler imaging, principles 15–16
Doppler shift 16
duplex kidney 218
dynamic range 14–15, 19
dyspnoea 193–7

E
e' 65, 67, 123
E-point to septal separation 61–2
eccentric hypertrophy 57
edge enhancement 15
edge shadowing 26
E/e' 65, 67, 123
emergency medicine 3; *see also*
    FAST scan
empyema 252
endocardial cushion defect 87
endocarditis
  aortic regurgitation 100–1
  mitral regurgitation 109, 112
  sepsis 213–16
epicardial fat 91
equipment management 275, 278
extended FAST (E-FAST) 207, 209
extracorporeal membrane
    oxygenation 232
exudate 139, 140
eyeballing 59, 71

F
failure to wean, *see* weaning failure
false lumen 156
far field 12
FAST scan 205–10
  extended (E-FAST) 207, 209
  intra-abdominal free fluid 205,
    206*t*, 207
  liver trauma 207
  pitfalls/limitations 209
  pleural fluid 207
  probe choice and settings 205, 207
  technique 207–9
femoral vessels 163–4
  catheterization 241–2
FENICE study 118
field marker 36
fish-mouth view 39
fluid responsiveness 117, 118
  carotid Doppler flow 123
  determining 76–7, 182

fluid resuscitation
  ARDS 230
  starting 118–20
  stopping 120–1
fluid tolerance 118
focus 12–13, 19
focused cardiac ultrasound (FoCUS) 4
focused ultrasound
  definition 4
  development 3–4
  limitations 6
  risks 6
  terminology 4
Foley catheter 175
foreshortening 31, 59
fractional area change 62, 74–5
fractional shortening 61
frame 10
frame rate 17, 21
Frank–Starling relationship 117, 179
frequency 9, 18

G
gain 18, 21, 22
gall bladder 172–3, 175
gallstones 172
gel use 12
governance 273–8

H
haemodynamic instability 179–84
haemopericardium 90–1
haemothorax 139
harmonics 18
heart failure
  acute 58, 65
  chronic 58
  with preserved ejection fraction 58, 64
  with reduced ejection fraction 58, 64
hepatic arteries 170, 171
hepatic veins 170
hepatorenal angle (Morrison's
    pouch) 173, 207
horseshoe kidney 218
hydronephrosis 175, 219–21
hypertrophic cardiomyopathy 57, 64
hypotension 183
hypovolaemia 118, 119
  ARDS 228, 230
  cardiac arrest 186–7
  sepsis 211–12
hypoxaemia 193–7

I
image
  optimization 17–24
  pre-processing 14–15, 17
  storage 275
infection control 278
infective endocarditis, *see* endocarditis
inferior vena cava
  cardiac tamponade 94
  collapsibility 75–6, 120, 230

renal calculi 221
renal cell carcinoma 85, 221
renal cysts 175, 218
renal perfusion 222–4
renal transplant 218
reporting 275
resistive index 222–3
resolution 25
    lateral 13–14, 25–6
    temporal 10, 21
revalidation 274
reverberations 27–9
reverse doming 103
rheumatic valve disease 100, 109
Riedel lobe 175
right atrial appendage 81
right atrium
    anatomy 81
    ARDS 227
    cardiac tamponade 94
    dilatation 83, 227
    dimensions 83
    pressure 75–6
    thrombus 84
right ventricle 69–80
    anatomy 69–70
    apicalized (false apex) 31
    ARDS 227–8, 231
    blood supply 70
    cardiac tamponade 94
    dilatation 227–8
    eyeballing 71
    fractional area change 74–5
    haemodynamic instability 183
    loading 70
    mechanical ventilation 183
    overload 120–1
    physiology 70–1
    preload 119, 121
    pressure overload 70, 183
    pulmonary embolism 77–8
    pulmonary hypertension 78
    S-wave velocity 79
    sepsis 213
    size 71–2
    systolic function 70, 73–5, 79, 228, 231
    TOE 53
    tricuspid annular plane systolic
        excursion (TAPSE) 73
    ventricular interdependence 70–1, 183
    views 71, 78
    volume overload 70, 183
    wall thickness 73
right ventricular inflow view 43
right ventricular outflow view 43
ring-down 29

S

S-wave velocity (S') 65, 79
safe triangle 252
saline bubble contrast 87
sampling volume 23
saphenous vein 163

scale 21, 22
seashore sign 128–9, 133
sector width 20–1
secundum ASD 87
sepsis 211–16
    endocarditis 213–16
    hypovolaemia 211–12
    pulmonary hypertension 213
    tolerance to volume loading 212–13
    ventricular function 213
septic shock 63, 118
serum-ascites albumin gradient 264
shock 52, 181t
shred sign 142
side lobe artefact 29–30
signal attenuation 11, 19
signal intensity 11
signal reflection 11
Simpson's method 63
sinotubular junction 153
sinus of Valsalva 98, 153
sinus venosus ASD 87
small bowel obstruction 174
sound waves 9
    interaction with tissue 11–13
spatial pulse length 13
speckle-tracking 213
spectral Doppler 21–3
    aortic valve 104–6
    see also continuous wave Doppler;
        pulsed wave (PW) Doppler
spontaneous echo contrast 65, 84
staghorn calculus 221
stomach scan 173–4
stratosphere sign 129, 133
stroke volume 121
subclavian artery 162
subclavian vein 162
    catheterization 240–1
subcostal four-chamber view 40–1
subcostal inferior vena caval view 41–2
subcostal short-axis view 44
superficial femoral vein 164
superior vena cava collapsibility 53, 120
suprasternal view 44
sweep speed 22
systemic vascular resistance 213
systolic anterior motion (SAM) 57–8, 64

T

Takotsubo cardiomyopathy 58, 65
tamponade, see cardiac tamponade
temporal resolution 10, 21
thoracic aorta 152–7
    aneurysms 154–5
    dilatation 154–5
    dissection 156
thoracocentesis 254
thyroid cartilage 246
time gain compensation 15, 19
tissue Doppler imaging (TDI) 16, 23
    left ventricular diastolic function 65, 67
    right ventricular systolic function 79

tissue harmonic imaging 18
tissue valves 105–6
tracheal rings 246–7
tracheostomy, percutaneous 245–9
training 5, 273–4
transducers 9–11
transoesophageal echocardiography
        (TOE) 47–53
    complications 48–9
    contraindications 48
    focused 51
    indications 50
    probe frequency 18
    probe technology and use 47
    scan planes 49–50
    specific uses 52–3
transplant, renal 218–19
transthoracic echocardiography
        (TTE) 35–45
    anatomical factors 35
    apical four-chamber view 40
    apical long-axis view 43
    apical three-chamber view 43–4
    apical two-chamber view 43–4
    fish-mouth view 39
    image acquisition 37
    parasternal long-axis view 37–8
    parasternal short-axis view 38–40
    probe frequency 18
    probe kinematics 36–7
    probe orientation 35–6
    right ventricular inflow view 43
    right ventricular outflow view 43
    standard views 37–42
    subcostal four-chamber view 40–1
    subcostal inferior vena caval view 41–2
    subcostal short-axis view 44
    suprasternal view 44
transudate 139
trauma, see FAST scan
tricuspid annular plane systolic
        excursion (TAPSE) 73
tricuspid regurgitation velocity 67
tumble artefact 221
twinkle artefact 221

U

ultrasound pulse 13
ultrasound wave 9
ureters 173, 221–2
    jets 175, 222

V

vascular access 237–44
    advantages of ultrasound
        guidance 237–8
    arterial cannulation 243
    echogenic needle tips 243
    femoral vessels 241–2
    hands-free probe holder 243
    internal jugular vein 238–40
    needle guides 243
    peripheral venous access 243

vascular access (*Cont.*)
    peripherally inserted central catheters
        (PICCs) 242–3
    post-placement ultrasound 243–4
    probe choice 238
    scanning technique 238
    self-aspirating bulbs 243
    subclavian vein 240–1
vascular assessment 161–8
    axillary vessels 162
    differentiating arteries and veins 161
    femoral vessels 163–4
    image optimization 161
    internal jugular vein 162
    lower limb vessels 163–4
    probe selection 161
    subclavian vessels 162
    upper arm vessels 162–3

venous thrombosis 164–8
vegetations 100–1, 109, 112
veil sign 131
velocity–time integral (VTI) 22, 122–3
vena contracta 104, 113
veno-venous extracorporeal membrane
        oxygenation 232
venous thrombosis 164–8
ventilator-associated pneumonia 196–7
ventricular fibrillation 186
ventricular function
    sepsis 213
    weaning failure 204
ventricular interdependence 70–1, 183
ventricular septum
    motion 77
    rupture 189
volume loading 211–12

W
wall echo sign 175
wavelength 9
weaning failure 199–204
    cardiac dysfunction 203–4
    diaphragmatic function 203
    lung aeration 199–200
    pleural effusions 201–3
    respiratory causes 199–203
write zoom 21

X
X marks the spot 253–4

Z
Z-tract approach 263
zoom 21